The Future Loves You

ARIEL ZELEZNIKOW-JOHNSTON

The Future Loves You

How and Why We Should Abolish Death

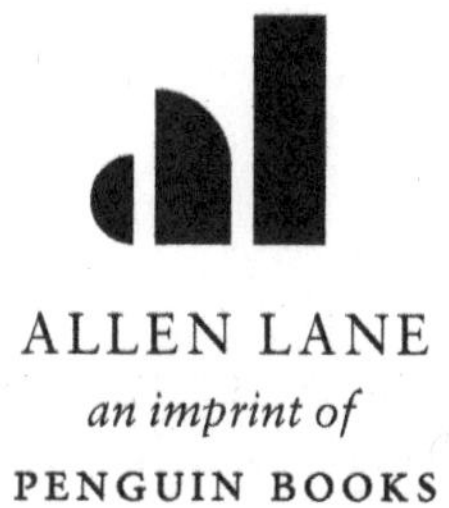

ALLEN LANE
an imprint of
PENGUIN BOOKS

ALLEN LANE

UK | USA | Canada | Ireland | Australia
India | New Zealand | South Africa

Penguin Books is part of the Penguin Random House group of companies whose addresses can be found at global.penguinrandomhouse.com.

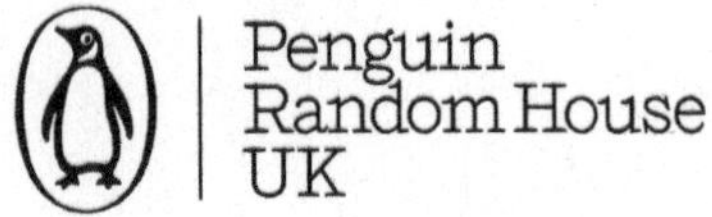

First published in Great Britain by Allen Lane 2024
001

Set in 10.5/14pt Sabon LT Std
Typeset by Jouve (UK), Milton Keynes
Printed and bound in Great Britain by Clays Ltd, Elcograf S.p.A.

The authorized representative in the EEA is Penguin Random House Ireland, Morrison Chambers, 32 Nassau Street, Dublin D02 YH68

A CIP catalogue record for this book is available from the British Library

ISBN: 978-0-241-65589-4

www.greenpenguin.co.uk

*To all those who nurtured, worked, and innovated in earlier times,
so that we may live now*

Contents

Introduction

If you'd been born before the twentieth century, you would probably have died before you reached your current age. A disturbing proportion of all humans who've ever lived never made it through their first month of life. Of those who survived the treacherous first few weeks, another considerable fraction succumbed to pneumonia, diarrhoea, or some other deadly disease before the age of five. In total, from the dawn of humanity up until the late 1800s, one in two people never made it to fifteen.[1]

Even during the twentieth century, there was still an unsettling chance you wouldn't have lived to your present age. Prior to the roll-out of antibiotics in the mid-1940s, many infections easily treatable by modern standards would have been a death sentence. Until blood pressure medications became prevalent in the 1960s, hypertension frequently led to fatal strokes or heart attacks. And before inhaled corticosteroids became widespread in the 1970s, it was not uncommon for asthmatics to die from a severe attack. Plenty of our grandparents and great-grandparents didn't make it to the twenty-first century because the treatment they needed came too late in the twentieth.

But out of the 120 billion humans who have ever lived, you're fortunate enough to live now. Whether it is a pill, an injection, or a life-saving surgery, today's medicine has a much greater chance of being there for you when you need it most.

Despite this, it's easy to take the marvels of modern medicine for granted and overlook our extraordinary fortune. Often, the importance of living late enough to live longer still only becomes apparent when the pace of medical progress becomes personally pressing. For

Elizabeth Hughes, whose life was suspended between the past's privation and modernity's salvation, nothing could have been clearer.

***

Up until she turned eleven, Elizabeth had been a bright and bouncy girl, sporting a cheeky smile under her dark, cropped hair and grazed knees from adventures in Central Park. But on the cusp of her adolescence, as her friends began to shoot up and outgrow their stockings, Elizabeth began to lose weight. Ravenous though she was, the food she ate seemed to simply vanish without explanation or effect. Then, one day, Elizabeth came down with diarrhoea so severe it almost killed her; in the aftermath, her doctor diagnosed her with diabetes. The condition was untreatable, and she would likely be dead within the year. In 1919, this was just the way it went.[2]

Or, at least, that was the way it had gone until very recently. In their desperate search for anything that would keep their daughter from death, Elizabeth's parents stumbled upon a new clinic, over the river in New Jersey, claiming it could keep diabetic children alive for years instead of months. Dr Allen, the clinic's director, explained to them that – since the disease was due to too much sugar in the blood – starving diabetic children could paradoxically extend their lives. Their daughter would be lingering on the threshold of death, but at least she would remain in this world a little longer.

Though, while the treatment could extend Elizabeth's life, it's unclear whether she would have actually counted the time it offered her as living. The regimen required restricting Elizabeth to no more than the most basic nutrients needed to survive: a few eggs for protein, some boiled vegetables for fibre, and a piece of fruit for essential vitamins. The diet left her perpetually emaciated and cold, unable to grow, barely able to move. She was to remain in this state, eking out whatever minimal existence she could, until death eventually took her.

Even so, the therapy 'worked', for a while at least. After three years of languishing in this limbo, Elizabeth was, quite incredibly, still alive. The dietary restriction had prevented her from succumbing to fatal dehydration, dangerously acidic blood, or any of the myriad ways untreated diabetes can kill a person. She had also avoided wasting away to nothingness, an ever-present concern for a therapy almost as fatal as the disease it treated. These were far from the joyous, carefree years that childhood is supposed to provide. But as long as Elizabeth endured, so did her parents' hope that a cure would one day be found.

That day arrived on 30 July 1921. Unlike the many other children who had faded away in Dr Allen's clinic, Elizabeth had got sick just a little bit later, and had held on just a little bit longer. And so she was alive when, through a series of experiments investigating the function of the pancreas, the scientists Frederick Banting and Charles Best became the first to isolate insulin. While diabetic children have lost the ability to make this hormone, which enables the body to regulate blood sugar, it still works if injected into them. Though the resulting twice-daily prescription is not exactly a cure, for someone on starvation therapy, its effects are just as miraculous.

When Elizabeth received her first dose, a few days shy of her fifteenth birthday, she weighed 20 kilograms, little more than skin and bones.* Three months into her treatment, she weighed 48 kilograms and had returned home. She went back to eating, to playing, to school. She went on to university, got married, and had three children of her own. Unlike the millions of diabetic children that had come before her, she got the chance to live.†

***

But in the end, of course, Elizabeth still died. Six decades and 42,000 injections after being given mere months to live, a fatal heart attack ended her story. Unlike type 1 diabetes, which kills almost no-one directly today, we still lose millions of people a year to cardiovascular disease. Even with pacemakers, bypasses, stents, and statins, there is frequently nothing we can do to help.

It would be comforting to believe that all those struck down by heart disease are very old, content with the time they've had and ready to pass on. But the truth is that many instead suffer Elizabeth's fate: dead at seventy-three, ten years younger than the average in many

* For reference, a typical girl her age would weigh about 52 kilograms, but even the smallest girl her age would likely weigh at least twice as much as Elizabeth did.

† I first heard of Elizabeth's story on Nate DiMeo's excellent podcast *The Memory Palace*.[3]

wealthy countries at present. The brutal reality is that, out of all those who die from the disease each day, a disquieting number felt they still had more life left to live.

This is no less true of people who perish from any other fatal disease. Cancer kills countless patients who were still desperately waiting for that new clinical trial, or that next therapy, which did not come soon enough. Multitudes die while stuck on organ donation waitlists, their kidneys or livers failing before a replacement can be found. So many people reach their end feeling robbed of time, knowing they might have survived if only they'd been able to hold on a little longer.

These innumerable personal tragedies unfold because, even though medicine has developed greatly between the 1920s and the 2020s, it is still far from maturity. Sure, we should be grateful for the many advances that have helped global life-expectancy to more than double from thirty-two in 1900 to seventy-two today.[4] But, even so, the breakthroughs are not coming fast enough to give everyone as much time as they might want. Our grandparents, our parents, our friends, and sometimes even our children are still dying all around us. Metastatic cancer, dementia, end-stage heart failure, and every other invariably fatal disease stand as testimony to the fact that one day we, and everyone we love, will die.

Perhaps we should just stop fighting and listen to those who urge us to accept death in whatever form it comes and at whatever age it finds us. After all, if desire for life only exacerbates our suffering, then maybe the wisest thing is to give it up. Yet while this may be a noble sentiment, it is hard to encourage those who still have so much left to live for to not see death as an opponent. And, as much as people may bravely face their fates, the hundreds of billions of dollars we spend globally on medical research every year suggests what many really want are cures rather than conciliation.

So scientists grapple instead with a seemingly unending task. Now that they've neutered threats like smallpox and typhus, their attention has turned to the new and emerging diseases lying in wait in the shadows of our elder years. But, try as researchers might, many of these maladies lack effective treatments, and for a disturbing number we do not even know their cause.

That is not to say there are no grounds for hope. Some scientists, through recognizing that age is the greatest risk factor for almost all diseases, envision a new line of attack. Perhaps, through the development of generic anti-aging drugs, there may be a way to prevent diseases before they even emerge. Hopefully this approach will one day yield fruit. Yet with all of these treatments still over the horizon, the bitter truth is that, for many of today's generation, these breakthroughs will come a moment too late.

Thus, as privileged as we are to live now, we experience a frustration our ancestors did not face. They died of pneumonia, without the knowledge that a simple antibiotic could have spared them. Instead, we die from cancer, knowing full well that treatments arriving in the years and decades to come would likely have saved us. While medicine's progress makes us optimistic for the future, it also makes the limits of current technology heartbreakingly salient. As with Elizabeth's story, these days we understand only too well that an entire lifetime can separate 'almost' and 'just in time'.

***

Facing the gravity of our circumstances, it's no wonder that a blend of desperation and optimism propels some of us over the edge of anticipating medical advances and into the expanse of science fiction. For example, take people who pursue *cryonics*, the practice of having one's body pumped full of antifreeze and suspended upside down in a flask of liquid nitrogen. Motivated by what they see as a clear historical trend of medical progress, its adherents believe that freezing the bodies of the clinically dead will allow for their eventual resurrection when more advanced technology one day becomes available.

In doing so, cryonicists are not putting their faith in a treatment that will keep them active, healthy, and happy, like Banting and Best's discovery of insulin. Instead, they are pursuing something more in the spirit of starvation therapy, a means to buy time through the dark days before a better treatment comes. They believe a person in this state, while not fully alive, is in a sort of stasis, akin to Elizabeth's three years in Dr Allen's clinic. But, cryonicists claim, they're also not truly dead, and so long as that's the case, there's hope for them yet.

Perhaps. The problem is, we've seen charlatans try to sell this kind of fantasy before. Ancient priests with magical talismans, medieval alchemists with rejuvenating elixirs, and now cryonicists promising future resurrection by means of medical miracles. Without acceptance by the medical establishment, little distinguishes cryonics from the snake-oil salesmen of earlier times. Unsurprisingly, few people buy it: despite much media attention over the years, fewer than 1,000 bodies have been preserved worldwide since its origins in the 1960s.

Indeed, cryonics as practised has many of the hallmarks of a pseudoscience or cult, including quasi-religious claims of an afterlife for those who perform arcane rituals, a lack of engagement with mainstream medicine or endorsement by esteemed scientists, and large upfront payments required for services that have no guarantee of success. None of these features inspire confidence that the frozen clients of cryonics will ever see another spring.

Many doctors and researchers are therefore understandably outraged that, even though cryonics has not been medically validated, some organizations are still happy to charge people small fortunes for the procedure. Sure, if you're already a billionaire with nothing left to buy, why not spend $200,000 on a chance at immortality? But for the rest of us, cryonics looks likely to be just another case of swindlers tricking people out of their money with impossible promises of longer, healthier lives.

***

Still, the fact that cryonics is unscientific and its claims are unsubstantiated doesn't make the core idea of preserving the dying to enable their future revival fundamentally unsound. Within this science fiction is a kernel of truth: with sufficient understanding of how the brain enables a person to be who they are, it might be possible to place a dying individual in a state from which they could one day be revived. For it to actually work, though, we would need answers to two critical questions:

1. How exactly does the human brain enable a person to be who they are?
2. How does the brain decay during death?

Armed with answers to both of these, it's possible that we really could devise a way to halt the decay of brain structures crucial to personhood, and keep someone in indefinite stasis until sufficient medical advances could one day restore them to health. Cryonicists likely fail here, as their methods harm the brain's structural integrity and do visible damage to its crucial circuitry. But perhaps neuroscientists could do better?

Certainly, in the past decade, it has become clear that neuroscience can offer sufficient answers to the two critical questions about personhood and death, even to the point of being able to directly manipulate the relevant brain structures. Neuroscientists now know how to erase, insert, and force the recall of specific memories. Doctors are increasingly providing prosthetic implants to functionally replace portions of the brain. The last few years have even seen the successful development of procedures arguably capable of perfectly preserving a human brain.

Perhaps, then, it is time to seriously evaluate the potential of a *brain preservation* procedure to buy more time for those we would otherwise consider beyond medical help. At the very least, the required starting assumption – that a person is to a large degree defined by the unique structure of their brain – is now entirely uncontroversial among neuroscientists and doctors.

That is not to say that it is clear whether or not any technique could actually be devised to preserve someone's brain and body in a manner compatible with their eventual revival. Evaluating the merits of any proposed protocol would require thorough examination. At the lowest level, we would need to know the technical details of how it supposedly stabilises the microscopic biological features that store someone's memories, personalities, desires, and other psychological traits. At the highest level, we would have to understand how the procedure fits into the philosophical frameworks through which we understand life, death, and personal identity. Only then would we have any idea of whether preserving the dying might someday be feasible.

This book is, in large part, a report of just such an investigation. Through a wide-ranging journey across normally disconnected topics in medicine, neuroscience, and philosophy, we will examine the viability of brain preservation. And surprisingly, should you read on, you may come to the same conclusion that I have: that there already exists at least one well-designed brain preservation procedure offering a credible possibility of indefinitely delaying death.

***

You should know from the outset that most of my neuroscientist colleagues have so far been reluctant to explore this space. This is quite understandable, as new medical techniques heralded with bold claims have a track record of being mostly useless, sometimes dangerous, and only very rarely valuable. Vitamin megadosing, abdominal decompression in pregnancy, and radionics are just three examples of complicated, scientific-sounding pseudotherapies originally proposed by scientists or doctors that turned out to be ineffective or harmful. As no researcher or clinician wants to be associated with such quackery, most have so far shied away from exploring brain preservation more seriously.

As a consequence, the majority of neuroscientists have either not heard of brain preservation or have summarily dismissed the notion without even looking up from their laboratory benches. This has kept the scientific community from providing a clear evaluation of the feasibility of brain preservation, meaning there is currently no expert consensus on the issue at all. The absence is understandable, as investigating every crackpot-sounding claim wastes time that researchers could otherwise spend curing diseases or solving fundamental mysteries. Unfortunately, though, history shows us that sometimes not paying attention to weird new ideas can go terribly wrong.

***

In the nineteenth century, a leading cause of death for new mothers was postpartum infection, known then as 'childbed fever'. In 1846, at Vienna General Hospital, obstetrician Ignaz Semmelweis became fixated by the observation that, of his two maternity clinics, the first had a death rate of one in ten, while in the second it was 'only' one in twenty-five. On examination, the sole difference he could find between the two was that the first clinic was used for teaching medical students, while the second was staffed exclusively by midwives. Semmelweis was unsure why this would make a difference, until the tragic but serendipitous death of a cherished colleague led to a breakthrough realization. Following an accidental scalpel injury while performing a post-mortem examination, his friend quickly died of a disease closely resembling childbed fever. Semmelweis reasoned it was contamination from cadavers that was causing the fevers, as medical students handled cadavers while midwives didn't. Following this hunch, Semmelweis instituted a policy of antiseptic handwashing for medical staff before entering the maternity clinics. The childbed fever mortality rate dropped from 10 per cent to 2 per cent almost immediately. Astounded by the success of his findings, he was sure the practice would be quickly and widely adopted.

Instead, Semmelweis was largely ignored or derided by his colleagues.[5] After speaking publicly about his discoveries, he lost his job in Vienna. He took an unpaid position at a hospital in Budapest, where he again managed to dramatically reduce childbed fever. Yet, after publishing the results, one journal remarked 'it would be well that our readers should not allow themselves to be misled by this theory at the present time'. He sent out copies of his findings across Europe, only to receive silence or criticism in return.

The problem was that he was going up against the conventional wisdom at the time that fevers were caused by miasmas: invisible, foul-smelling particles suspended in the air. So unsuccessful was his quest to change the consensus that in his frustration he wrote an open letter accusing obstetricians of mass murder. While you may be unsurprised to learn his colleagues did not find this approach persuasive, he had a point: hundreds of thousands more women would die of childbed fever before antiseptic techniques became widely adopted decades later.

In a particularly cruel twist of fate, Semmelweis himself became a victim of the medical establishment. In 1865, he was forcibly admitted to a mental asylum at the recommendation of his colleagues. Only two weeks later, he died from an infection after being severely beaten by the guards. He was forty-seven.

* * *

For fear of being seen as weird and suffering the same professional fate as Semmelweis, scientists, doctors, and the general public are sometimes agonizingly slow to accept paradigm-changing research. To ensure brain preservation does not go down the same path as antisepsis, this book is written to dispel its outlandishness for all three of these groups.

Rest assured, the text is truly written for everyone. There will be no jargon, nor assumed knowledge about any of the topics we will cover. Neuroscientists will see how the work they have been doing in their individual subfields, when taken together, all clearly points to the conclusion that a person can be preserved. Doctors will be provided with a showcase of the astounding progress made by neuroscience in the past decade, and the impact this could have for their practice were its implications more broadly understood. Everyone, including those with no scientific or medical training at all, will come away feeling we should be setting our expectations higher before giving up on the dying.

While I'll try my best to make the journey smooth, I admit it's still quite the wild ride. The key thing to hold onto as we press onwards is that millions of children died from diabetes until, one day, Elizabeth didn't. Billions of women died from infections following childbirth, but nowadays this is almost unheard of, at least in wealthy countries. So many causes of death now eradicated were once thought to be inevitable, natural, and immutable. Sometimes inspiringly quickly, other times tragically belatedly, science and society together wiped them from the Earth. Now, with the advent of brain preservation, I don't think that you, or anyone you love, has to die at all. Just let me explain how.

PART ONE

Why

You may have heard that longevity and anti-aging research are increasingly becoming big business. While that's not exactly true – research spending on preventing aging still pales in comparison to that on cancer or heart disease – there are indeed scientists and entrepreneurs seeking out ways to dull death's scythe. How far are they likely to get? And what would the consequences be if they succeeded? To assess these questions, we need to start with some context.

In the first chapter, through learning about different species with lifespans far longer or shorter than our own, we'll explore the biology that determines why people's lifespans are currently the length they are. And, as we do so, we'll come to understand that the seeming naturalness of our eighty-ish years is in actuality just an accidental outcome of conflicting evolutionary forces.

Now, there is a chance this new-found knowledge may unsettle your sense of how long a lifespan ought to be, and create tension with the common intuition that extending lifespans would have deleterious social, political, and environmental consequences. In acknowledgment of these reasonable worries, in the second chapter I will walk through the pros and cons of the case for abolishing death. Through touching on everything from climate change to psychological surveys of the dying, I will make clear that, even though the concerns are understandable, the case for empowering people to choose their own fates is still overwhelmingly strong.

I
Why Don't We Get More Time?

The light that burns twice as bright burns half as long.
Dr Eldon Tyrell *

Having turned 190 in 2022, Jonathan still lives as though his best years are ahead of him. Perhaps his optimism is a reaction to surviving a youth mired in hardship. Despite being born among the beautiful white beaches, coral reefs, and turquoise waters of the Seychelles, his childhood was grim and fraught with danger. Jonathan saw many of his siblings die, abandoned by their parents, and to this day he does not speak of his youth. In 1832, this was just to be expected.

He made a change at the age of 50 by moving to Saint Helena, a tropical island off the western coast of Africa. There he lived a safer and more comfortable life, socializing with the natives and ingratiating himself with the local elite. So successful was he in this regard that he ended up living at the governor's mansion, and even entertained the future King Edward VIII when the British monarch visited the island in 1925.

But with security comes boredom, and Jonathan's comfortable lifestyle led him to suffer a midlife crisis in his 130s. He found himself disrupting croquet matches by sitting on the ball, upending benches at the tennis courts, and generally making a nuisance of himself for lack of anything better to do. His frustration seemed interminable, until he found a younger girlfriend named Emma in 1962, herself a recent

* This quote is often attributed to the *Tao Te Ching* by Laozi but seems to have actually originated in the film *Blade Runner*.

immigrant to the island. They lived contentedly together for thirty years, but the arrival of the handsome Frederica in 1991 caused complications. Introductory tours around the island soon morphed into an illicit affair. It seemed that, even in his 160s, Jonathan was still capable of getting into scandals.

His age finally catching up with him in his 180s, Jonathan had a bit of a health scare in 2015. He lost weight, had trouble eating, and felt generally lethargic, as though his many years were at last weighing down on him. Yet luckily, after switching to a more varied diet of fruit and vegetables, he's started feeling much better and even looks younger. Though he's gone blind from cataracts and lost his sense of smell completely, he's grateful his hearing is still excellent and his energy has returned.

Today, at the age of 190, Jonathan is still going strong. He leads an active love life, feeling most alive and vocal when in the throes of passion with Emma or Fred. He walks every day, often wandering around the well-groomed gardens of the governor's mansion. He is no longer frustrated like he was when he was younger, instead appreciating the simple joys of sitting on the lawn and eating a banana. In his old age, all Jonathan wants is to enjoy his time in the sun in the presence of those he loves. Considering the fact that he's a 200-kilogram Seychelles giant tortoise, he just might do so for decades to come.[1]

***

While I don't begrudge him his years, it's hard not to feel it's a little unfair that Jonathan may well outlive me, despite him being 161 years my senior. My parents, grandparents, great-grandparents, and great-great-grandparents have all lived and died within the span of Jonathan's life. Are Seychelles giant tortoises really so much nobler than humans that they deserve to spend more than three of our lifetimes on island paradises?* When on holidays, sitting on the beach, I also feel like I could spend a couple of hundred years that way.

Much greater, though, than any sense of injustice is my feeling of confusion. Why do some tortoises like Jonathan live to 250, while a human is celebrated for reaching just a third of that?[2] It's easier to see

* I think a strong case can be made that they are, yes.

why we get the time we do by taking a step back from our usual human-centred perspective and thinking about life more broadly.

OF MICE AND MEN AND WHALES

The purpose of life is to stay alive, at least from an evolutionary perspective. Not because all living things consciously desire to continue living, or because life is inherently valuable to the universe. Rather, it's due to the straightforward rule that in our hostile environment creatures that do not actively try to keep existing tend to stop existing.

This law is enforced by a statistical process that is very simple, yet profound in its implications. *Natural selection* mandates that creatures better suited than others to their environment will become more common over time, no exceptions. Beyond this, though, there is no micromanagement of the particular strategy a creature may choose. In a cold environment, dogs grow fur, seals have layers of blubber, bears lower their body temperatures and hibernate, birds migrate to warmer areas, and many insects lay cold-resistant eggs and then freeze to death. If some crazy species wants to try the unusual method of surviving winter by stealing the skins of one species and burning the dead bodies of another, natural selection nods its approval. There is no such thing as cheating; any strategy that works wins gold, and any that falls behind is eliminated.

Considering the seasonal demise of insects gives us our first clue to why lifespans vary between species. Their deaths, come winter, highlight the fact that natural selection operates at the level of traits and genes, not at the level of individual animals. To illustrate the point, imagine two different species with two different strategies for surviving the winter. We'll call them Woollies and Eggies. Woollies grow a woollen coat each autumn that they use to keep warm throughout the winter. Each year a Woollie becomes a little bit larger and can grow a slightly warmer woollen coat, meaning that if they survive their first winter these animals will typically make it to thirty. In contrast, Eggies have no insulation of any kind and will freeze to death at the first cold snap of the season. No Eggie will ever live to see their first birthday. Despite this, the Eggie species survives because each autumn Eggies lay cold-resistant eggs that hatch come spring. The genes enabling the egg-laying trait survive from year to year, even though the individual Eggies themselves do not.

Genes have no sentimental attachment to the hosts obliged to carry them around. All they care about is their survival through any means necessary. This cruel truth alone goes a long way to explaining the suffering one can see everywhere in the natural world.

The case of the poor mouse provides a telling example of the indifference of genes. The house mouse species is an evolutionary success story, with a global population at least in the billions. Perpetually ravenous and undiscerning in their taste, they are able to survive on any food lying around in pantries, dumpsters, granaries, forests or fields. With a gestation period of three weeks and litters of about seven pups each, they put even rabbits to shame. Since any individual female can give birth to more than five litters a year, mice will increase in numbers rapidly when given the chance. If they happen across a new food source, such as the full granaries of a bumper harvest or the virgin vegetation of a previously undisturbed island, mouse plagues will quickly overrun the area. These traits of the house mouse are very successful, and thus the genes encoding them are extremely common in the world.

In stark contrast to the success of their species, the life of a typical house mouse is rather terrible. In the wild, they rarely survive a year, susceptible as they are to predation, starvation, and disease. They are highly anxious creatures, avoiding light and the scents of cats, rats, and other foreign mice. Male-on-male violence is a common cause of death. Even their infancy is fraught: when mothers become stressed while rearing their pups, cannibalism is a not infrequent result. The life of an individual mouse is nasty, brutish, and short. However, their genes are entirely unfazed by this suffering, as quick reproductive cycles mean any individual mouse is soon replaced. The collective behaviour of mice is sufficient to keep their genes around, and for natural selection that is all that matters.

To observe a very different evolutionary strategy, let's shift from a mouse's burrow to the frigid waters of the Arctic circle. Here live bowhead whales, 70-ton leviathans wielding 5-metre triangular skulls that they use to bash through the ice to make breathing holes.

When not smashing ice, they spend much of their time slowly cruising the depths at human walking pace while looking for food. They do this with their mouths wide open, filtering the water through sieve-like plates extending from their upper jaws to trap microscopic animals. This simple way of foraging food gives them plenty of time to serenade each other, which they do with great frequency and complexity during their breeding season. A female bowhead needs to be picky in her musical taste, as the breeding process will take about thirteen months and she can only perform it once every three to four years.

One of the negatives of this prolonged breeding cycle was ruthlessly demonstrated by nineteenth- and twentieth-century whaling. During this period the bowhead whale population was decimated, dropping from over 50,000 to around 3,000 individuals.[3] While the introduction of an international ban on commercial whaling has had them steadily increasing from that low point, their number today has only recently reached a fifth of their pre-whaling population.

Despite this devastating decline in numbers, an ironic result of whaling is that it provides unexpected insight into the lifespan of the bowhead whale. In May 2007, an Inuit whaling crew in Alaska, exempt from the commercial ban, found a harpoon fragment in the flesh of a fresh kill that had been manufactured in the late nineteenth century. This indicated the whale was probably at least 115 years old when it died, and possibly far older. The archaeological finding supported pre-existing evidence from chemical analyses of the eyes of bowhead whales suggesting that they may live up to about 250 years.* As a result, these whales are recognized as the longest-living mammals,

* Eye lenses are one of the few anatomical structures in mammals that do not have their constituent molecules continuously replaced as an animal ages. The constancy of these molecules provides a means by which to date the animals. Lenses contain a biomolecule called aspartate, which, just like gloves or shoes, can come in a left- or right-handed variant while still being made of exactly the same parts. Living things only create the left-handed aspartate. However, once made, this aspartate will start to spontaneously reform into the right-handed version. A baby bowhead whale starts with 100 per cent left-handed aspartate in their eyes, but over time this will tend to an equilibrium of 50:50 left : right molecules. In a process similar to radiocarbon dating, examining the exact ratio of left- to right-handed aspartate present in the lens can identify the age of an animal.

with two or three typical human lifespans passing for each one of theirs. That is to say, in the absence of predators before whaling began, bowheads had no need to rush into settling down and having kids.

Why do mice live fast and die young, while some whales alive today have been singing to each other since the first railways were being built? Why doesn't natural selection produce hardier mice or faster-breeding whales? The answer is the result of a cost–benefit analysis. As we'll see next, lifespan is determined by how costly creatures are to make and how long they are expected to last.

WHAT DETERMINES LIFESPAN?

Over time, everything starts to age, accumulate damage, and break down. No piece of machinery lasts forever, no matter how well crafted. Similarly, despite there being a wide range in lifespan between species, no individual creature lives forever. In this hostile world, full of countless dangers, something eventually goes wrong. An animal may break its leg and starve to death, or be hunted by a predator, or be thirsty and unable to find water, or suffer any one of innumerable fates. A whole other set of dangers exists at the microscopic level too. A creature may die from radiation-induced mutations, broken bits of biomolecules clogging up their cells, waste-product accumulation in their arteries causing blockages, or maybe parasites invading their body and stealing needed resources. While different animals can be better or worse at resisting these problems, all succumb to fate in the end.

Given this, the relevant evolutionary question for a species is, 'How many resources should I put into maintaining my individual members against danger and disease, as opposed to ignoring these problems and just increasing their breeding rate?' If there were no tradeoffs necessary, then all species would tend towards immortal members with short reproductive cycles, but this is not possible. Food an animal spends growing a larger and more resilient body is food it cannot spend growing new offspring. Cellular mechanisms to safeguard against mutations requisition energy away from other processes and slow down cell growth. There is no free lunch, and there is no free lifespan either.

This obligatory tradeoff results in some species putting more resources into longevity at the cost of reproductive speed, while others do the opposite. Which of these is the better choice depends on the environmental conditions the species lives in, as is clearly shown when what seem like very similar species have dramatically different lifespans.

The American robin is an orange-bellied songbird with an average lifespan of two years in the wild and ten years in captivity. In contrast, the Australian sulphur-crested cockatoo is a white parrot that lives about thirty years in the wild and can achieve upwards of seventy years in captivity. Why is the cockatoo's lifespan more than ten times that of a robin? Robins are, quite simply, much likelier to be killed at any given time. Only 25 per cent of robins survive their first year, in part due to predation from snakes, squirrels, and even other birds. In contrast, sulphur-crested cockatoos have far fewer predators and thus are less likely to be randomly killed at any moment.[4] You can see from their different lifespans in captivity, a circumstance under which the animals are removed from the threat of predation, that the tradeoff is built into the very bodies of the birds themselves.

Thinking about deaths in captivity prompts another question: what causes an animal to progressively sicken and die, even in the absence of external sources of danger? In other words, why do we have inbuilt expiration dates?

Aging is defined as the damage and dysfunction that a creature accumulates over time until it is unable to maintain itself any further.* At the cellular level, whether or not there is a primary underlying cause of aging, or instead many contributors, is still very much in dispute. Regardless, it's clear aging is not a result of just one or two bodily systems eventually malfunctioning. Instead, most parts of an organism are constantly accumulating damage, with the degradation just becoming more and more apparent over time. Much like our cars, washing machines, and laptops, our very cells are depreciating assets. Young animals seem healthy not because they aren't damaging

* Technically there are a few other processes that could also contribute to aging without constituting damage per se, such as the continuation of age-inappropriate developmental processes.

themselves, but because the damage hasn't yet had time to become obvious.

While everything in an animal is breaking down over time, the cycle of cell reproduction provides a particularly direct example of what can go wrong. All organs of an animal are constantly producing new cells while removing old ones, which helps repair damage and maintain optimal function. As an example, your skin cells completely replace themselves every month and a half, while your liver replaces itself about once a year. Unfortunately over time these cells become worse and worse at maintaining and replacing themselves, which is known as *cellular senescence*.

There are a few known mechanisms contributing to cellular senescence, and possibly others yet unidentified. One cause is the shortening of protective caps at the ends of DNA sequences. DNA inside cells is kept bundled up in coils called *chromosomes*. Chromosomes have protective caps at their ends called *telomeres*, much like those on shoelaces, which protect them from degradation or accidentally fusing with other chromosomes. Each time the cells replicate and replace themselves these caps shorten a little bit. If the caps become too short, the DNA itself starts to deteriorate and the cells become unable to do their jobs properly. This can lead them to become dysfunctional or unable to replicate, inducing senescence.

Another cause of cellular aging is the accumulation of *mutations* in older cells. Mutations are changes in the precise sequences of the genetic code that makes up the DNA carried by each cell. Each time a cell replicates there is a small chance of mutation, but it can also happen during repair processes after DNA has been damaged by exposure to radiation, oxidation, viral infection, or other factors. This mutation accumulation can render cells unable to perform their functions or can cause issues with their replication cycle. Once again, this can lead to the cessation of replication and induces cellular senescence. Worse still, particularly unfortunate mutations can produce inappropriately increased replication, the cause of cancer.

One more cause of cellular aging is the decreasing ability of our cells to control which genes are turned on and off, a separate issue from genetic mutations. Despite almost all cells in an animal containing the same genes, different cell types are able to perform very different roles by having different genes switched on or off. Liver cells have a particular combination of genes only active in liver cells, as do heart cells, as do skin cells. The process of activating and deactivating particular genes is called *epigenetics*, and (surprise, surprise) it too can go wrong with age. Epigenetic dysfunction is much like an identity crisis: cells stop knowing what kind of cell they are, and thus stop being able to do their jobs properly, leading to senescence or cell death.

Given that different animals live for markedly different lifespans even in the absence of external threats, it's clearly biologically possible for cellular aging to occur at vastly different rates. We also know our bodily expiration date comes from a tradeoff between earlier reproduction and a longer-lasting body. But why specifically is this exchange demanded at the cellular level?

The main problem is that the forces of biology rarely like keeping things neat and simple. It's usually not the case that one gene determines one trait, like having a single gene determine eye colour. Instead, individual genes tend to have effects on many traits, like how our gene for making melanin, called OCA2, also affects our eye colour, skin colour, and, bizarrely, our sleep. Unfortunately this means that genes can have beneficial effects on some traits while having detrimental effects on others. A gene may decrease the risk of developing cancer by 50 per cent in middle age while slightly increasing susceptibility to infection as a child. Another gene may decrease how much food a baby needs to eat to survive, but induce earlier menopause in that same child later in life. Essentially, genes affecting multiple traits may present tradeoffs between improving early reproductive success at the cost of accelerated aging and a shorter lifespan. This phenomenon is known as *antagonistic pleiotropy*, with *pleiotropy* meaning 'affecting multiple or unrelated traits'.

Antagonistic pleiotropy is the main factor determining the typical lifespan for a member of a species. In the carefree life of a whale, who had essentially no predators until humans invented boats and harpoons, it makes sense to have genes that slow down reproduction if they also dramatically reduce the rate of aging. The whale is going to be around for centuries, so delaying having kids for a year is more than made up for in the lengthier reproductive life the whale will enjoy. At a cellular level, this choice of slow aging over fast reproduction can be seen in the whale's risk of developing aging-related diseases such as cancer. A bowhead whale has roughly 1,000 times the number of cells a human has, which you think would increase their risk of mutation, and thus cancer, by 1,000 times. In reality, whales develop cancer at lower rates than humans. The principle also works the other way round. Natural selection may favour a mouse pup possessing a gene that helps them survive infancy better than their siblings, even if that same gene precipitates brain degeneration by their first birthday.

This proposal is not just compelling on theoretical grounds. There are experiments demonstrating how the genetic variation responsible for antagonistic pleiotropy, and consequently lifespan, adapts in relation to changing environmental conditions. One natural experiment started 4,000–5,000 years ago when a population of opossums became isolated on an island off the coast of Virginia, freeing them of their natural predators. Over this period, the newly liberated opossums have appreciated a 20 per cent increase in lifespan compared to their less fortunate mainland cousins, along with a delay in entering their reproductive age.[5]

This finding has been corroborated in the laboratory, with scientists performing the role of predators. One demonstrative experiment consisted of flies kept in vials with either high or low rates of predation over many generations, where predation consisted of the scientist randomly killing some proportion of the flies. Over successive generations, the heavily predated flies developed faster and became fertile sooner, while the insects free from harassment began to enjoy longer lives.[6]

Natural and experimental results agree that the equilibrium governing lifespan can and will change in response to the forces driving natural selection. Now, how does all this play out with humans?

SIXTY IS THE NEW FORTY, EIGHTY IS THE NEW SIXTY

Given human life expectancy has gone from about thirty years on average for our hunter-gatherer ancestors to about seventy years for the global average today, you'd be forgiven for assuming natural selection has recently given us a new lease on life. It may seem our emergent position on the top of the food chain has converted us from animals predetermined to die in our mid-thirties, to a species newly endowed with the superpower to push our years to a hundred and beyond. Yet, a sceptical reader might notice that this remarkable improvement seems to be undermined by texts from several thousand years ago, such as the Book of Psalms, declaring 'The days of our years are threescore years and ten; and if by reason of strength they be fourscore years [. . .]', meaning seventy to eighty.[7] Their scepticism would be made stronger still if they knew of teeth retrieved from ancient graveyards showing a degree of wear only achievable by people who had reached at least their sixties.[8] Something here just doesn't add up.

The average hunter-gatherer lifespan might have been thirty years, but there's a lot of confusion around what the term *average* actually means. It can have three related but distinct meanings (Fig. 1a). *Mean* lifespan is the sum of all the years lived by some population divided by the number of people who lived them. This is what is most commonly meant when people say 'average'. *Median* lifespan is the age by which half of the people have died, while *modal* lifespan is the most common age for people to die. These last two, median or mode, are commonly what people envisage when they think of a 'typical' lifespan. For humans, the mean lifespan has increased dramatically in the last few centuries. But this is not because our oldest die later, rather because our youngest die less. The modal lifespan, the one that definitionally most of us enjoy, has improved much more modestly, from around seventy in hunter-gatherer societies, to around eighty years globally today.[*,9] As long as you make it through childhood, you're likely to live only about a decade longer than your cave-dwelling ancestors.

To understand why the modal human lifespan doesn't match that of our friend the Seychelles giant tortoise, it's helpful to put these numbers in their evolutionary context. Humans diverged from our great ape cousins approximately 7 million years ago. The maximum

* I am still slightly unclear on whether the modal lifespan for hunter-gatherers applies in general, or only when excluding those who die in their first year(s) of life.

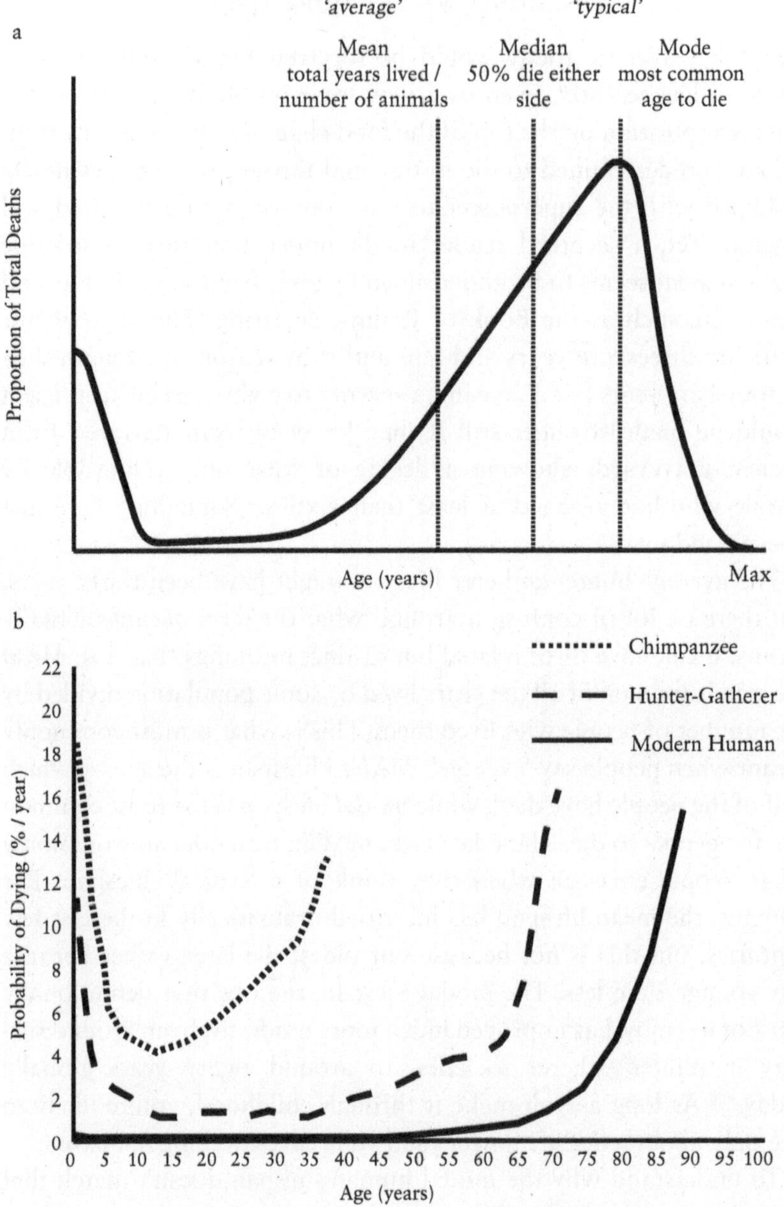

Figure 1. a) A stylistic plot of how the mean, median, and modal lifespan of a species can all be different. b) Modern humans have almost completely removed infancy-related mortality compared to hunter-gatherers and chimpanzees, but only somewhat delayed aging-related mortality compared to hunter-gatherers.[10,11,12]

reported lifespan of wild chimpanzees, gorillas, and orangutans is around forty to sixty years, suggesting this may have been the case for our last common ancestor too.[13] During the time that humans descended from the trees, started running, developed sophisticated tools, and learned to speak, our modal lifespans likely expanded to the roughly seventy years of hunter-gatherers. Presumably our increasing intelligence made us savvier at finding food, our weapons helped us fend off predators, and our language enabled us to better take care of each other. All these factors would have decreased external sources of mortality and thus shifted the pressure of natural selection towards lengthening our lifespans.

Despite this, remarkably, the two major killers threatening both us and our hairier great ape cousins remained the same. These are infectious disease and within-species violence. Infections kill around 70 per cent of wild chimpanzees and hunter-gatherers, while violence and accidents account for about another 20 per cent.[9,14] In fact, the annual mortality curves for contemporary hunter-gatherer populations and chimpanzees look remarkably similar, with the human curves just being shifted rightwards (Fig. 1b). While evolutionary improvements moved our lifespans beyond the forty-year maximum of our ape ancestors to around seventy, disease and violence likely kept them from being pushed even further. So many hunter-gatherer children died young that they only had a mean life expectancy of thirty at birth, rising to fifty if they made it past fifteen.[9] This meant that during their childhood, their remaining expected years to live actually increased as they got older!

The astounding rise in mean human lifespan since the Industrial Revolution has been driven largely by vastly diminished premature death from disease. The disarmament of infectious disease as our most dangerous enemy is one of the crowning achievements of human civilization. The data is very clear that many of us alive today owe our lives to sewers, vaccines, and antibiotics.

That being said, those of us who've already made it past our teenage years have less to be thankful for when looking forwards. A hunter-gatherer who survived the culling zone of childhood was probably going to die at around seventy, while the modal American dies at around eighty-five today.[9] Fifteen years is certainly nothing to be ungrateful for. But is it not reasonable to expect that, given we have what would appear to be god-like powers to our ancestors' eyes, like the ability to fly through the heavens and conjure light and music from metal tablets, we could also outlive them by more than a measly decade-and-a-half?

As special as we may feel, antagonistic pleiotropy is not just constrained to birds, opossums, and flies, but determines human lifespans too. Problematically for us, though, significant genetic changes to species can take thousands of years, and we've had proper hygiene and medicine for less than two centuries. For the most part, as far as our genes are aware, we might as well still be back on the ancestral African savannah. Public health and modern medicine have done wonders for mean life expectancy, but they've relied on the fact that in the absence of external killers human bodies were already designed to last considerably longer than thirty years. In contrast, pushing modal lifespans beyond seventy-ish years is going to require forcing human bodies past their design specifications.*

Evolution's ignorance of our altered environment is on display in what are undeniably tragic diseases for the modern world. For example, consider individuals with Huntington's disease, a progressive neurodegenerative disorder afflicting people with debilitating symptoms at around forty and killing them around sixty. Humans can still have dependent children at the age of symptom onset, so the disease may impact the ability of its sufferers to contribute to child rearing. As such, we would have expected natural selection to remove the disease-causing gene from the human population over time. That is, unless having a gene which causes Huntington's disease later in life confers some compensatory benefit earlier. It turns out there is evidence that this is the case, with people who develop Huntington's appearing to have both less cancer earlier in life and more children later.[16] This may well be happening with other genetic diseases too, and indeed with aging generally.

Perhaps Huntington's disease was not quite as tragic in an earlier

* There is some reason to be optimistic that we are at least partially achieving this, even though there is insufficient evidence to be confident that the trend will continue indefinitely. In developed countries, modal lifespan has been increasing at least linearly for the past 180 years, and possibly even at an increased rate since the 1960s.[15]

time, when a typical lifespan was ten years shorter and the chance of dying from disease was ever present. But the modest advances we have made so far in pushing for a longer typical lifespan have made it all the more heartbreaking to witness the suffering of those allocated even less time than the rest of us. The irony is that the very genes which may have helped you be fit and fertile when you were young may kill you as you get old.

Unfortunately, keeping the elderly healthy for longer is likely to be a lot harder than preventing young people from dying prematurely. Vaccines, the great saviour of humanity, merely involve a safe trigger for the immune system to practise responding as it would to a natural infection. Antibiotics are usually simple, single molecules that jam up the cellular processes of bacteria so as to provide aid to the natural immune response. In comparison, geriatric diseases such as cancer and dementia are much harder to deal with than the poxes and plagues of the past. This is because, instead of simply assisting natural cellular processes, curing these diseases involves trying to persuade cells to perform tasks they were not designed for. Evolutionary pressure deals with cost-benefit analyses in the same way as manufacturing. If the design requirements don't ask for something to be built sturdy enough to last past its expected use date, the easier and cheaper option is not to bother.

Researchers have made some impressive progress with fixing a few of these cellular processes, but not enough to make a huge difference to human lifespans as of yet. Immunological cures for some cancers can involve genetically re-engineering a patient's immune cells, a technically complex process which makes previously incurable cancer treatable. But even curing cancer entirely would only increase life expectancy by about three years, as many diseases of the aged remain untreatable.[17] An elderly patient cured of cancer is likely to soon develop heart disease, or dementia, or kidney failure, or ... the list goes on.* We still don't even know what causes most cases of dementia, let alone have viable treatments on the horizon. Most of our

* The majority of those who make it over 110 suffer from *amyloidosis*, a condition where misfolded proteins lodge in the blood vessels, which can contribute to subsequent organ failure.[18] If you're wondering which disease to worry about once we've solved Alzheimer's and cancer, this is probably it.

medical progress so far has worked with what evolution already left us, but significantly pushing modal lifespans upwards is likely to require going beyond our current genomes. If that's the case, what's the plan?

UNLEARNING HELPLESSNESS

Historically we've had seventy to eighty years if we were lucky, and that was it. Nothing we could do, nothing we could buy, nothing we could sacrifice would forestall the inevitable. Hunters, gatherers, kings, peasants, priests, alchemists, scholars, and farmers all died within seven to eight decades in almost every case. The same blessing of human intelligence that let us conquer the Earth also cursed us with awareness of our own mortality.

Helpless as we were, it is unsurprising we developed many coping strategies for normalizing and accepting death. We've done a remarkable job convincing ourselves that if there's nothing we can do about it, it must be because things are supposed to be that way. Yet, shockingly to modern sensibilities, this was also the outlook held about pain by some doctors and intellectuals prior to the advent of anaesthesia.[19]

Before the mid-nineteenth century, measures for reducing pain during traumatic medical procedures were ineffective, dangerous, or both. Mixtures of herbs, opium, and alcohol were used as analgesics if available, but these provided insufficient pain-relief for surgery. Methods of actually rendering patients unconscious were extremely dangerous. One consisted of compressing the arteries supplying blood to the brain – that is, strangulation to the point of unconsciousness. Another was to administer knock-out blows to the head, inevitably leading to at least concussion and possibly brain damage.

The anaesthetic options available to patients should have improved after 1799, when the potential medical use of nitrous oxide, also known as laughing gas, was first published in London by Humphrey Davy. Unfortunately, the clinical use of anaesthetic gases was not publicly trialled for another fifty years. In 1846 the dentist William Morton demonstrated their use through administration to a patient about to receive surgical removal of a neck tumour. Given the procedure was successful, one would have assumed the medical and general community would roll out this new technology as quickly as possible.* Disturbingly, one would be wrong.[20]

Though proponents and advocates did spring up quickly after the 1846 demonstration, a number of medical and religious authorities also rose up in opposition. In 1847, doctors at a meeting of the South London Medical Society made claims such as 'pain in surgical operations is in a majority of cases even desirable, and its prevention or annihilation is for the most part hazardous to the patient'.[21] The French physiologist François Magendie questioned whether there was any advantage in suppressing pain, arguing 'it was a trivial matter [for patients] to suffer'. The first president of the American Dental Association, Dr William Atkinson, even went as far as to say 'I think anesthesia is of the devil [. . .] I do not think men should be prevented from passing through what God intended them to endure.' Particularly horrific were the claims made that women should be denied anaesthesia during childbirth, as pain during labour was prescribed by God and subverting it would be 'unscriptural and irreligious [. . .] reprehensible and heretical in its character'.

Thankfully there were sufficient pioneers to continue to develop and promote anaesthesia despite the critics, while the turning point for its normalization likely came when Queen Victoria requested anaesthesia to aid her in the birth of her eighth child in 1853. Although anaesthesia did not cease to be dangerous then, and even today complications from anaesthesia still occasionally happen, no modern medical professional would claim it is a 'dangerous folly to try to abolish pain'.

When I see a modern philosopher claiming that 'death gives meaning to life' or read historical accounts of anaesthesia being against the will of God, I am reminded of the phenomenon of *learned helplessness*.[22] If an animal is placed in a stressful situation from which it cannot escape, it will eventually stop trying. Surprisingly, though, after giving up, they will often not even try to escape later if a route out does become available.

Psychologists in the 1960s first demonstrated the effect using dogs placed in harnesses which delivered mild electric shocks.[23] Normally,

* Following, of course, research into the potential medical complications of anaesthesia.

dogs placed in a harness that zapped them would readily press a button to terminate the shocks. However, something different happened with a separate group of dogs who were initially pre-trained with a harness where the shocks were inescapable. When subsequently placed into a different test harness, with access to a button that would terminate the shocks, these dogs would just whine when the experiment commenced rather than press the button to end their suffering. This second group of dogs had learned escape was impossible, and thus didn't even try to fix the problem when circumstances changed.

This is the situation I believe we are in today with respect to human lifespans. For all of human history until very recently, there was nothing we could do to forestall aging-related death. In response, we normalized it. Some medical literature even uses the oxymoronic term 'healthy aging' without irony, despite the fact that currently 100 per cent of people who age sicken and die. A more accurate term would be 'slowest possible age-associated disease progression', which acknowledges that individuals vary in how quickly they develop aging-related disorders without pretending that the minimal decline rate is not still a decline. Still, the phrase 'healthy aging' is reflective of our society's inability to attend to the harms of aging itself, instead misguidedly focusing on individual age-related diseases. Unfortunately, this narrow-sightedness leads us to pursue the wrong solution of playing whack-a-mole with each new aging-related illness while neglecting alternative approaches.

The most egregious examples of these wrong solutions are medical interventions that prolong lifespan without prolonging quality of life. Imagine Betty, an eighty-seven-year-old lady with advanced dementia who contracts pneumonia. She is sent to the hospital for intravenous antibiotic treatment, but the move exacerbates her confusion and she becomes delirious. As a result she is terrified her doctors and nurses are trying to harm her, and tries to escape by painfully pulling out her intravenous lines and rolling out of bed. In her fear and distress, all she achieves is a broken hip. Whether it's antibiotics, a hip cast, or any other hospital intervention, the treatment is doing nothing to address the aging that is the primary underlying cause of her suffering. Despite its futility, the effort to do 'everything we can to save Betty' presumably comes from a tacit understanding that most of us believe death really is something terrible to be fought. In this case, as in many, it is too little, too late. Tellingly, while doctors want to live long and healthy lives as much as anyone, they overwhelmingly decline treatment if faced with Betty's situation. Knowledgeable as they are about the counterproductiveness of the treatments available at this late stage, they are unwilling to suffer their side effects.[24]

Not as bad, but still misguided, is an excessive focus on research into individual aging-related diseases at the expense of elucidating the mechanisms of aging itself. In 2021 the National Institute of Health in the US aimed to spend less than 1 per cent of its budget on basic research into aging and senescence, in comparison to about 5 per cent on Alzheimer's disease alone.*[,25–27] This is akin to spending more money on designing treatments for burns and smoke inhalation than ensuring buildings are fire safe in the first place. As of 2022, the US Food and Drug Administration does not even classify aging as a disease-process and thus won't approve licensing for therapeutics seeking to forestall aging directly. This regulation reflects the mindset that because aging is normal it is unworthy of consideration. Much like the dogs, medical research is to a large degree not even trying to escape the root cause of the problem.

That said, I would still be pessimistic about our chances of living past our nineties, even with far greater investment in anti-aging research. In order to avoid death, the improvement in life expectancy for one's age cohort has to be increasing at more than one year per year.† Yet this level of progress is not currently occurring. If promising

* The National Institute for Health had an overall budget of $41.4 billion, of which the National Institute on Aging (NIA) received somewhere between $3.2–3.7 billion. Within the NIA, the neuroscience division, which primarily focuses on dementia, received around $1.8 billion, while the fundamental aging biology division received roughly $0.32 billion. It's not always easy to clearly classify whether any particular research should be classified as 'basic science' or 'disease-focused', but these numbers give a rough approximation.

† This situation is referred to as *longevity escape velocity* and was coined by the biogerontologist Aubrey de Grey. *Escape velocity* typically refers to how fast one has to be travelling to break free of the gravitational influence of an astronomical object, for example 11.2 kilometres per second for Earth. By analogy, *longevity escape velocity* is the rate at which one's life expectancy has to be increasing in order to break free of the inevitability of aging-related death.

therapeutics to reliably delay aging were obviously on the horizon this would be less worrying, but that is not the case. The most effective methods we have currently for slowing aging are the tried-and-true regular exercise and a good diet. These work not by improving upon our genetic potential, but by counteracting the ill effects of our sedentary and obesity-inducing modern lifestyles. Unfortunately, because of the multifactorial nature of aging due to antagonistic pleiotropy, any single new drug or therapy is unlikely to have a large impact on its own.

This isn't to say the cause is hopeless – far from it. The fact that whales live more than twice as long as we do demonstrates it should be possible, in principle, to change human bodies to live longer. The lack of sufficient research funding here is deplorable, especially considering that, because aging affects everyone, even small achievements can have a big societal impact. Maybe with a combination of therapies which can reverse cellular senescence, lengthen telomeres, repair DNA damage, reverse epigenetic dysregulation, as well as clean up accumulated plaque from arteries and remove accumulations of broken biomolecule aggregates in brain cells, we could improve modal lifespans. A pessimist would retort that even if we dealt with the current concerns, antagonistic pleiotropy implies currently unknown aging processes would likely then rear their heads. Even so, optimists could reply that our technology will continue to improve, and researchers have already identified a number of interventions that cumulatively may make some impact.[*,28] Either way, we should still be trying, as the research infrastructure exists these days to make attempting escape worthwhile.

But for those of us without many years left, we need another strategy to circumvent the genetically imposed limitations of human lifespans before our time runs out. Current medicine just isn't up to the task of keeping us as active, dynamic agents while preventing us from accumulating progressive, eventually terminal damage. And, in the end, even the optimists need to acknowledge that if aging itself were

* If you want a more comprehensive overview of the anti-aging field, I'd highly recommend reading *Ageless* by Andrew Steele, which provides a recent and thorough analysis that finds room for optimism without overhyping things.

cured, we'd still eventually die from virulent infections, traumatic accidents, violent assaults, or other life-limiting events.

As we'll see later in the book, there is a way around this using technology already existing today. The trick is to realize that, although we can't halt damage accumulation while remaining biologically active, we can pause aging indefinitely by taking someone out of biological time. How exactly we can achieve this is the subject of Chapter Seven.

But, before we arrive there, we should first think hard about the consequences for a world in which aging is abolished and everyone lives as long as they desire. In the next chapter, we'll ask whether this would even be a good outcome. Spoiler: I believe this would be a better world for Jonathan, chimpanzees, and humans alike.

2
Why Save Everyone?

Whoever saves a life, it is considered as if they saved an entire world.

The Talmud

On 2 November 2054, Professor Ai Tanaka pushed the button to send the mice one week into the future. It had taken a staggering 600 billion yen and five years of labour from her team at the Tokyo Institute for Advanced Physics to reach this pivotal moment. Earlier experiments with the prototype had demonstrated that items placed inside the device's chamber could be propelled forwards without themselves experiencing the passage of time. However, there was a big difference between observations of precise clocks or measurements of radioactive decay, and determining whether living, breathing animals could endure the journey. Despite having meticulously triple-checked the simulations, her hands still trembled with uncertainty.

—

Even as the mouse enclosure shimmered back into existence precisely one week later, Professor Tanaka's apprehension remained. The mice were alive and apparently unharmed, but she waited for her technicians to assess them. They confirmed the mice had lost no weight, experienced no changes in their menstrual cycle, and remembered their mazes too well for a week to have passed. Only then did she give in to her excitement. The physics was indisputable, the models impeccable, the experimental results in perfect harmony: they had built a genuine, functioning time machine.

Staff gathered in the institute's lunchroom, glass in hand, Professor Tanaka proposed a triumphant toast to their diminutive, furry pioneers.

'To the first ever chrononauts!'

Full of celebratory spirits, it wasn't long until the team had drained the bottles purchased in anticipation of the occasion and were making plans to continue the festivities at a whisky bar across the street. Tanaka urged them to secure a table, promising she'd join them after she'd shared the news of their success with her mother.

—

Keiko Tanaka had just swallowed an oxycodone tablet when she noticed her daughter's call. The potent painkiller hadn't taken effect yet, and a searing pain lanced through her right hip as she stretched across the table to retrieve her phone.

Until four years ago, Keiko had prided herself on being in excellent health. At the age of eighty-two, she could keep up with even the youngest women in her callisthenics class, and she had always been gratified by the surprise of her doctors when they learned that her only regular medication was a vitamin D supplement.

But then she found a lump in her right breast.

Now, four years down the gruelling road of surgery, radiotherapy, and chemotherapy, she found the exercise of getting from her bed into her wheelchair more painful and exhausting than any callisthenics class had ever been. That was to say nothing of the small pharmacy of medications that had made a home on her bedside table. Keiko was grateful for the time these treatments had bought her, but the road had been hard.

And it was only getting harder still. With new metastases in her bones and her liver, Keiko's doctors had finally broached the difficult discussion of whether they should cease active treatment.

'Hello Ai-chan. How did your mouse experiment go?'

'I have great news, but first I need to come talk to you about something important. I'll be there in thirty minutes.'

Keiko gently placed the phone down and began tidying the table of empty blister packs and adhesive wrappers, making room for tea. But on Ai's arrival, it was clear the usual routine wouldn't be happening tonight. Instead, an unusually energetic and possibly tipsy Ai insisted on taking Keiko to her laboratory.

'You look very excited, dear. I assume the mice survived then?'

'Yes Mama, but that's not all. Let me explain as we go . . .'

As they rode the subway beneath central Tokyo, the more Keiko listened to Ai's plan, the more she felt her medication was making her delirious. Yet, once they reached the institute, the sight of a mouse enclosure lying forgotten on a technician's desk sent a shock of alertness through Keiko, the likes of which she hadn't experienced since before she'd fallen ill.

When first diagnosed with cancer, it was anger, not sadness, that Keiko had felt most. Keiko wasn't finished with life. She reasoned she should have at least another decade or two of languid evenings filled with tea and conversation with friends; of busy weekends, strolling with Ai and her grandchildren through the local gardens; of long days to work fastidiously on her next novel. With life expectancy for Japanese women around ninety-one, she felt cheated that she would die before her peers.

Her illness, however, was entirely indifferent. And as her health deteriorated over the next four years, Keiko was bludgeoned into begrudging acceptance. Mostly, this was because the tumours growing inside her seemed to feed on what made her life worth living. Chemotherapy made her head too cloudy to write, nausea repelled her from her precious cups of sencha tea, and her crumbling bones made it impossible for her to play with her grandchildren. At the end of four years of suffering, exhaustion, and constant pain, Keiko had surrendered to the idea that death wouldn't be so terrible.

That was, until her daughter wheeled her up to the entrance of the small, steel-lined room that formed the heart of the prototype enclosure. In the physical presence of the device, Ai's suggestion that another life was possible suddenly felt real. Abruptly, Keiko's acceptance of death vanished. In its place stood a billowing storm of fear and hope that threatened to shatter her frail body.

She wanted to live. *Live*. She didn't want to wither and die, to feel nothing and become nothing. She desperately, more than anything, wanted to live!

But that didn't stop Keiko from being afraid of what awaited her on the other side.

'Ai-chan, are you sure there will be people on the other side to help me? Why would they care about an old, sick lady from the 2050s?'

Ai glanced away from the control panel she was manipulating to power up the machine. Wiping her tear-stained face, she met her mother's gaze with a smile.

'Mama, what do you think I would do if my great-grandmother suddenly appeared here, sick with tuberculosis or another treatable disease? Just leave her to die? Or rush her to a hospital for antibiotics?'

Keiko swallowed this thought as her daughter completed the setup. The plan was to send her far enough into the future that advancements in medicine would be able to treat her cancer. Just as medicine had improved tremendously over the past century, who knew what marvels awaited in the next?

While the plan made sense, a storm churned inside Keiko's belly. Confusion. Terror. Hope. Yet, as Ai dialled in the final settings and wheeled her into the chamber, what Keiko felt more than anything else was pride in her daughter.

'I love you, and I am so proud of you. If the future has people as brilliant and caring as you are, I'll be okay. I trust you, my darling. Do it.'

'I love you too Mama.' Ai replied through tears. She pushed a button, and Keiko vanished. 'I'll see you later.'

***

Now, I understand that this science-fiction story may seem needlessly far-fetched for a serious nonfiction book. Time machines belong in the realm of the imagination, and my limited knowledge of physics leads me to suspect they will remain there forever. Yet, fantastical as the framing may be, in chapters to come I'll show you how present-day technology is functionally equivalent to Ai's time machine.

Although you are very likely sceptical of the claim, I ask you to at least entertain it for now. Because, if you think there's any chance at all it could be true, it's best we have an important discussion before we go further. Would you, if you found yourself in Keiko's situation, use the device and send yourself into an ambiguous future? Pause, and take a moment to really consider it. Why would you? Why might you not? Contemplate how your friends or family members might choose, particularly if using the device had already become a widely accepted medical practice for the dying.* In the following passages, I'll share some information on how others have responded to this question. But, before you proceed, I encourage you to take a minute to genuinely reflect.

***

Okay, let's head to the data. While psychologists haven't specifically investigated this time-machine scenario, they have run surveys on related questions. An immediately notable finding is that if you ask people how long they would like to live, without providing any further context about the quality of life they will enjoy, respondents generally opt for an additional decade beyond the years they are statistically likely to get.[2,3] Intriguingly, though, while most people only choose around ninety years for themselves, 68 per cent of them believe others would prefer at least 120 years.†

As always, however, context matters. Perhaps unsurprisingly, it turns out that, no matter their actual age, the younger and healthier people feel, the longer they would like to continue living.[2,4,5] This holds for populations across the world, from Europe to Japan. Another key determinant of desired lifespan seems to be optimism toward the future. This finding becomes particularly evident when presenting various lifespan-extension scenarios.[6] When nothing is specified about what their future will entail, the majority of people state a preference for no longer than eighty-five years or so. However, when those same reticent people are guaranteed mental and physical vitality in their old age, 70 per cent of them switch their answer to at least 120 years. This data makes clear that most people, if they knew they would be safe and healthy, would like to live far beyond their current life expectancy. It is

* These kinds of 'reversal test' thought-experiments are very useful for recognizing situations we currently accept as normal, but which we would not countenance if the world were somehow different to begin with. As such, they give us a tool for eliminating status-quo bias.[1]

† Might this, perhaps, be a projection of their own desire for more life onto others, without wanting to seem greedy themselves?

not an excess of life that they wish to avoid, but rather the infirmity, isolation, and insecurity that can accompany old age.

As such, whether or not you would choose to employ the time machine may well depend on your beliefs about what awaits you on the other side. Should you remain in the present, oblivion beckons, threatening to snuff out your consciousness forevermore. Venture through the device and you pass into an alien era, never to return. Either option is terrifying, and both deserve consideration. Yet only the device will let you live. Let's explore whether it would give you a life worth living.

THE FUTURE IS A FOREIGN COUNTRY

Imagine you, like Keiko, elect to take your chances at a longer life. Confined to your wheelchair, dying of some fatal illness, you find yourself wheeled into the time machine's enclosure. The attendant departs, closing the door behind them, and for a fleeting moment you are suspended between fear and hope, experiencing your last second of the twenty-first century. Then, as the time machine is activated, an alarm sounds, and the faint light peeking through the door's window begins to shimmer and pulse. Another second yields a brilliant flash of light, and all of a sudden you've arrived. You find yourself in the future, a temporal refugee entering a foreign land, in desperate need of aid. What awaits you next? There are at least three distinct possibilities.

The first and darkest to consider is that there is no-one there to meet you. Peering through the window of the time machine's door reveals a decaying, moss-draped structure showing no signs of human presence. It seems there has been some calamity in the years since your departure: perhaps a global nuclear war has left the Earth an apocalyptic wasteland, or some terrible pandemic has eradicated enough of the world's population to destroy civilization. These and other *global catastrophic risks* are genuine concerns; the philosopher Toby Ord assigns some variant of this calamity a one-in-six chance of occurrence in the next one hundred years.[7] If such a fate has come to pass, you will soon meet the same end as the rest of humanity. This is a distressing conclusion. Still, you are no more dead than you would have been had you remained in your own time.

In the second scenario, while an intact building materializes behind the door's window, the door itself remains stubbornly closed. Instead, an apologetic voice emanates from a speaker, informing you they cannot receive you at this time. They explain that their current medical technology is insufficient to cure the disease that afflicts you. Perhaps that is true, or perhaps they simply lack the capacity or inclination to take in temporal refugees. Either way, moments after the voice ceases, you hear the alarm sound and see the light through the door's window shimmer once again. Your odyssey is not yet complete.

In the third and final case, the machine's door opens once the shimmering subsides. Awaiting you is a medical professional, standing a few metres away beneath a sign suspended from the ceiling proclaiming 'WELCOME TO THE FUTURE!' Approaching you, the medical worker confirms your name and asks whether you consent to treatment. Slightly dazed, it takes you a moment to say yes. With your assent, the worker rolls up your left sleeve and presses a patch onto your upper arm, then manoeuvres around you to grasp your wheelchair and guide you out of the time machine enclosure. They mention they are taking you to an 'Integration 101' session, but their words barely register, as your attention is captivated by the holographic displays and robotic attendants you are rolling past. Gradually, as the initial shock of time-travelling wears off, you notice you feel considerably less sick than earlier that day. By the time you reach the induction room you feel healthier than you have in years. Scared as you still are, a sense of relief is mounting. Perhaps everything will turn out all right.

This is obviously not an exhaustive list of all the possible outcomes that could await you if you were to use the time machine. Instead, these three imaginary scenarios capture the essence of what one could expect to happen when making use of the real brain preservation technology we will explore later in this book. But before delving into the mechanics of how brain preservation operates, we should first decide if we would use the device were its success guaranteed.

Would you prefer to be a temporal refugee, to brave the uncertainty and dislocation of an undiscovered future, or to accept the totality of death and be yourself no more? That is the question we must grapple with when deciding whether time-travel is a venture worth embarking on.

Let's examine the third scenario, where an individual like Keiko arrives in the future, frail and at the brink of death, only to be restored to youthful vigour by the medicine of this later age. Blindly leaping towards this world demands a considerable amount of trust that the future offers better outcomes than the present. In our contemporary milieu, shaken by catastrophic pandemics, climate nihilism, political rupture, and growing inequalities, trust in the future may seem fraught. However outside of this subjective vantage point, from which the future *feels* bleak, statistical and historical trends offer more optimistic evidence. On reflection, a more objective view suggests that if we take a leap of faith towards the future, we'll likely fall safe on soft and springy ground.

For example, straightforward extrapolation from historical trends of the past 200 years implies that people of 2154 may well be vastly healthier and wealthier than us today. In the 1850s, global mean life expectancy was thirty years, compared to about seventy in 2011. The total output of the entire world's economy was worth around $1.5 trillion (in 2011 dollars), the same as the output of just Australia alone in 2011.[8] If these trends in health and wealth persist, it seems reasonable to anticipate a marked improvement in living standards by 2154.

However, grants of health and wealth alone will not guarantee happiness for Keiko. Moving to a foreign land under duress is inherently traumatic, especially so if one is forced to travel alone. Keiko will be feeling lonely, cut off from her daughter and her grandchildren. She's likely feeling isolated, too, from the unfamiliar society of the future, with no friends or social connections in this foreign time. Deprived of family and friends, she may have lost her sense of purpose – once derived from caring for her grandchildren and making tea for her friends – now all of them are gone. Consumed by nostalgia, Keiko may struggle to embrace this future, even with all her physical and material needs met.*

If she does make attempts to integrate into her new home, she may

* *Nostalgia* literally means 'homesickness', from the Greek *nostos* ('homecoming') and *algos* ('pain/grief/distress'). In Keiko's circumstance the term provides a very appropriate combination of its original meaning with the more modern sense of 'sentimental longing for a past time'.

well be quickly overwhelmed. Contemporary language has evolved enough that, while still intelligible, it demands significant concentration to understand. Social norms are very different; to her horror, some people stroll through the streets nude but for their virtual reality goggles, while others have replaced their appendages with shiny cyborg modifications. Keiko learns in her first induction class that most people of this era live, not as nuclear families, but in long-term, multi-family houses. Topping it all off is her complete incomprehension of the prevailing technology – the mobile phone she brought with her is now as archaic as a stone tablet, yet she lacks any understanding of how to interact with whatever it is people are using in 2154.

Rather than giving into despair, though, we can look to comparisons with the stories of present-day refugees and migrants for demonstrations of how these potential problems, though serious, can be surmounted. Certainly, their experiences suffice to show how travel can be a worthwhile alternative to death. In particular, there are cases where elderly individuals have moved from developing countries to cities in technologically developed nations – such as from refugee camps to the United States, or twentieth-century migrants travelling from east Asia to Australia – that give us a possible approximation of how time travel may go.[9,10]

Analysis of the experiences of elderly migrants finds that their life satisfaction correlates with their ability to access social support and preserve their heritage identity.[11] Language classes and instruction on the use of transport and technology are among the most crucial forms of support, empowering people to freely navigate their new environments and form new habits and relationships. Invitations to community gatherings such as religious groups, sports teams, and art groups, where people are invited to participate in the cultural practices and festivities of their new land, provide the seeds for new friendships and purpose. But beyond mere assimilation, the most successful outcomes for migrants and refugees occurs when integration into their new society is fused with maintenance of social and cultural connections with their old community. An elderly Vietnamese migrant to Australia who celebrates the 'New Year' twice – once on 31 December with her friends from church and again with her family for Lunar New Year – is likely to be much happier than a migrant who celebrates only once, being either unable to participate in the social fabric of their new home or else severed from the culture and practices of their old place.

What insights can we glean from the experience of modern geographical migrants and refugees to inform the hypothetical scenario of temporal refugees? Primarily, that efforts made at either end of the time machine journey would be helpful for improving their wellbeing.

Aside from merely addressing their physical ailments, future societies willing to take in temporal refugees could foster their wellbeing by providing avenues for cultural and social integration. Regardless of the era's technological landscape – self-driving cars, routine spaceflight, or interacting with artificial intelligences – equipping new arrivals with the knowledge to navigate these systems will make a big difference. Whatever future societies may look like, those willing to accept their ancestors into their communities would likely also go to the effort of making them feel welcome.

These efforts would be bolstered considerably if time travel usage among dying individuals became widespread enough to ensure there would be a large community of temporal refugees to support each other. Each additional person saved by the journey benefits the lives of all others who have travelled before them by improving connections to their ancestral home-time. Living in the future with perfect physical health and your material needs taken care of is probably worth the leap, but sometimes you might want to hang out with people who remember the good old days when food was grown instead of printed and humans could still beat robots at football. Saving *everyone* ensures that no-one who chooses to brave the future is necessarily permanently isolated from their friends and family.* Widespread usage enables the best of both worlds – bring your old culture and community along while enjoying the technological fruits of a more advanced age.

Obviously, all these hopes are contingent on the assumption that future generations would be willing and able to share the future with us. This is no small assumption, as it depends on two uncertain requirements. Firstly, that our descendants possess spare resources to provide and care for their ancestors. Secondly, that they have the

* In principle, family and friends dying at different times could synchronize their arrival times into the future, and could adjust together.

motivation to do so even if it were technically possible. In a world that is already overpopulated and struggling to support its pre-existing population, neither of these conditions would be met. Nor are our dying likely to find a warm welcome should they arrive in a world polluted and depleted of resources, particularly if this was a consequence of the actions of our earlier time. There is even the risk that our 'primitive' moral values and dispositions may spoil our eligibility for refuge and aid in the eyes of our future descendants. The indifference of future generations is enough to doom us – if they feel no gratitude and love towards their ancestors, why bother to prepare for their arrival?

So, even if the time machines function seamlessly, they are still useless if either we or our descendants believe their universal usage by the dying would be detrimental to the world. Collectively, we may conclude that dying is a necessary sacrifice to guard against the dangers of overpopulation and ecological collapse, social stagnation, or wealth inequality. In this case, individuals like Keiko may be intentionally prevented from arriving at the other end of the machine, even if the alternative is their certain and irrevocable death.

For now, let's examine these first few concerns one at a time and assess whether they justify destruction of the time machines. The issue of wealth distribution and equitable access to life-saving technology, such as time machines or their equivalents, is so important it will be the focus of the final chapter of this book.

OVERPOPULATION

When considering life-extension technologies, the first worry for most people is overpopulation. At present, with a global population of around 8 billion in the early 2020s, we struggle with excessive fossil-fuel usage, insufficient food and clean water, urban sprawl, and unaffordable housing. This already leads to social unrest, inequality, and the mass extinction of non-human species, let alone what could result if our excesses lead to ecological collapse. Given that climate change, an effect of pollution carried out by humans in the present and recent past, is likely to lead to significant suffering for our grandchildren, it may seem absurd to propose increasing the future population size by saddling our descendants with our dying. Surely universal use of the time machines would lead to an unsustainable future?

This is a reasonable concern at first glance, yet it warrants further investigation before we panic and ban the time machines. For a comparable earlier example of premature hysteria, we can look to those who were already concerned about overpopulation when the world had fewer than 1 billion people. In 1798, the English scholar Thomas Malthus posited that human populations would always grow to exhaust all available resources, leading to food shortages, disease, or stagnation of living standards.[12] As one of seven siblings himself, at a time when Europe still suffered famines, it was presumably not difficult for him to conceptualize what has become known as a *Malthusian catastrophe*.

Overpopulation concerns have persisted since Malthus's time, with the most notable recent example being the book *The Population Bomb* by Paul and Anne Ehrlich. Published in 1968, when the world population was 3.5 billion, the Ehrlichs predicted hundreds of millions of people would starve to death in the 1970s, causing a dramatic rise in the global death rate. Even though this did not happen, many continue to share the Malthusian concern that the Earth cannot sustain the food production necessary to feed an ever-growing population.

Yet, contrary to historical and contemporary Malthusian expectations, the human population growth-rate has actually been declining since the 1960s, even as agricultural production advances at an accelerating rate. Current projections estimate the world's population will peak at around 11 billion in 2100, after which it will steadily shrink.[13] Thankfully this decrease in population growth is not due to food scarcity and mass starvation. Instead, as countries become healthier, wealthier, and more educated, families are choosing to have fewer children.

Ignoring migration, for a developed country to maintain its population size it needs to maintain a fertility rate of 2.1 births per female. As of 2021, the US and UK had a rate of around 1.6, Japan of 1.3, and China of 1.16.[14] The lowest in the world is South Korea at 0.88, a number so far below replacement that the country's population is expected to shrink 40 per cent from its current size by 2100. This demographic trend is sufficiently pronounced that in many developed countries the number of births has already dipped below the number of deaths, leading some demographers to have concerns that *under*-population is the more serious issue in the long run.

As the global population approaches its peak, the world is now feeding close to ten times more people than when Malthus began forecasting the ills of overpopulation. This suggests that the real issue is perhaps not so much the absolute number of people on our planet, but instead how wisely and efficiently our available resources are managed. Be it with respect to food, energy, water, land, or any other goods that people need to live, there is evidence that it is resource mismanagement, rather than absolute population size, that results in the environmental and/or institutional damage that can ultimately shrink a population.

Just such a circumstance may have occurred a few centuries ago on the island of Rapa Nui, also known as Easter Island, over a thousand of kilometres from any other landmass in the remote eastern Pacific Ocean.* Rapa Nui is famous for its numerous, awe-inspiring stone statues called Moai, some of which tower up to 21 metres (70 feet) tall. These statues may have been crafted by powerful chiefs seeking to immortalize themselves or their ancestors, their grandeur and expense memorializing the leader's status for eternity.

When Europeans first reached the island in 1722, they were mystified as to how the Rapa Nui people, the indigenous Polynesian population, could have constructed such monuments given the lack of resources available. While a colonial European mentality that dismissed the technological capabilities of indigenous peoples is a key ingredient in the historical 'mystery' of how the Moai came to be, the question of how the statues were resourced remains. With a population of only a few thousand there was limited human labour, and a complete absence of large trees meant assembling the ladders and tools needed for construction would have been impossible. How could these awe-inspiring statues have been created, given these constraints?

* The island lends its name to the immunosuppressant and potential anti-aging drug *rapamycin*, which was originally isolated from bacteria in soil samples taken from Rapa Nui. The first Europeans to sail to the island sighted it on Easter Sunday in 1722, and named it Easter Island.

One interpretation of the archaeological data on Rapa Nui suggests that the island used to have a much larger population until it destroyed itself through ecological collapse. Analysis of pollen left behind in ancient mud samples indicate that the island was once home to a variety of large trees. Assessing the number of pollen particles present in mud samples from different time periods, researchers suspect the number of trees started to decline with the arrival of the Polynesian population around 900 to 1200 CE, and had disappeared entirely by 1600.[15] This evidence complements archaeological analysis of the number of buildings and farms on the island, which imply a population peak of around 15,000 – much higher than when Europeans arrived. The collapse theory hypothesizes that this larger population depleted the island's tree supply, with total deforestation leading to soil erosion, diminished agricultural production, and ultimately starvation.

As always with science, the real story may be more complex. Alternative interpretations of the archaeological data challenge the collapse theory. Some suggest that the deforestation was a result of climatic changes in rain patterns, others that the pre-contact population was never large and thus there was no peak to collapse from.[16] Despite all this, the possibility that Rapa Nui's population underwent ecocide-induced collapse serves as a cautionary tale of resource mismanagement precipitating ecological and social catastrophe.

On the other hand, there are instances where ingenious resource-management has saved millions from starvation while simultaneously preventing environmental damage. When the Ehrlichs claimed that millions would perish from hunger in *The Population Bomb*, they focused on developing countries like India that 'couldn't possibly feed two hundred million more people by 1980'. Not only did this catastrophe fail to materialize, but India has since often been a net wheat exporter.

The reason for this comes from a series of improvements to agricultural practices beginning in the 1960s known as the *Green Revolution*.[17] Rather than bloodshed and anarchy, this revolution led to such improvements in agricultural productivity that, for a given unit of land, farmers produce roughly double the amount of food today as they did in the 1960s.[18] Notably, this was achieved not simply via flagrant use of fertilizer and pesticides, but in great part through clever selective breeding of crops to fundamentally improve their vigour and productivity.

The Green Revolution was the result of hard work by many, but two particular agricultural scientists stand out as emblematic heroes: Yuan Longping and Norman Borlaug.

In his youth, Yuan Longping survived the terrible famine caused by agricultural malpractice during China's Great Leap Forward, in which tens of millions starved.[19] The memory of the hunger stayed with him, and over his career he worked tirelessly to improve agricultural productivity.* In his research, he conducted a series of investigations to develop hybrid rice varieties that could combine the positive attributes of multiple independent strains, such as fast plant growth and disease resistance. By 1999, the widespread adoption of hybrid rice was estimated to be feeding an additional 100 million Chinese than would otherwise have been possible. China's population had been 650 million in 1960, when Yuan survived the Great Famine. By his death in 2021, he had personally helped ensure improved agricultural practices could deliver a population over twice its earlier size an abundance of nutritious food.

Norman Borlaug, who won the Nobel Peace Prize in 1970 for his contributions to feeding humanity, is a much better-known figure of the Green Revolution. Similarly to Yuan, Borlaug strived to selectively breed wheat varieties of higher yield and disease resistance than their ancestral strains. His and his colleagues' work has been credited with feeding over a billion people, an incredible achievement. However, an underrated aspect of his legacy is his contribution to reduced deforestation. By enhancing agricultural productivity on existing farmland, there is less need to convert untouched forests into new farmland. Globally, the Green Revolution is estimated to have saved an area of land equivalent to the United Kingdom from being transformed for agricultural production.[18]

In 2019, the world produced at least 30 per cent more food per

* During the Cultural Revolution in 1966, Yuan was denounced as a counter-revolutionary and almost imprisoned before he was rescued by national leaders who saw the value of his research.

person than was actually required to feed everyone.* The Malthusian population bomb has been thoroughly defused. As with so many problems, ongoing instances of food insecurity are not due to exceeding nature's bounds, but because of humanity's own poor governance.

***

Yet modern Malthusian concerns tend to be centred more around climate change than food and famine. It may seem that sending our dying into the future, and thus increasing the future's population size, would make averting emissions-induced climatic catastrophe even harder than it already is. Although plausible, I think this argument is wrong for two reasons. Firstly, because climate change is a problem that needs to be solved in the coming decades, long before our dying could make it through the other end of the time machine. Secondly, because I suspect sending people through the time machine would actually make climate change easier to solve.

If humanity maintains the same rate of greenhouse gas emissions as seen in the early 2020s, then the Earth's average surface temperature is likely to warm around 3.2°C by 2100.[21] As you're likely aware, even though three degrees might not sound like much, it is enough to cause serious damage to both humans and the environment. For example, due to rising sea levels and other factors, areas vulnerable to floods will see somewhere between 2.5 and 3.9 times more damage than if warming were restricted to 1.5°C. Inland communities will not be spared either, suffering increased intensity and frequency of droughts, heatwaves, hurricanes and other extreme weather events.†

As bad as that sounds, humans are likely to have it fairly easy compared to the fate of our furry, feathery, and fishy cousins. Up to 29 per cent of all land species, along with an untold number of marine creatures, would be expected to go extinct. As a result, failing to address climate change may add humans to the list of causes of mass

* In 2019, global per-capita calorie production was around 2,920, whereas an adult needs about 2,250 calories per day.[20]

† The risks also extend beyond direct weather events. Rising temperatures will allow mosquitos and other horrible tropical parasites to extend their geographic range, spreading diseases like dengue fever and malaria over broader swathes of Eurasia, the Americas and sub-Saharan Africa.

extinction events, whose other infamous members include the meteor that killed the dinosaurs and continent-sized volcanic eruptions.

To mitigate these consequences, the ambitious goal of the global community is to limit warming to 1.5°C. Hitting this target requires deep reductions in emissions by 2040, reaching net zero by 2050, and then achieving negative emissions by actively removing carbon dioxide from the atmosphere for the rest of the century. While challenging, this goal is by no means theoretically impossible. Instead, the problem is that many countries have been lacklustre in their efforts to implement the long-term plans and changes required for net zero to happen.

This is especially disappointing because, with proper planning, tackling climate change doesn't demand drastic sacrifice or a return to Stone Age living standards. For instance, take Australia and France. Both are rich, developed countries, yet they lie at opposite ends of the emissions spectrum. In 2021, Australians emitted 15 tonnes of carbon dioxide per person, with the French polluting only a third of that.[22] This meant that Australia emitted more greenhouse gases in total than France, despite there being 40 million more French than Australians.

This is particularly embarrassing for Australia given its natural abundance of sunshine hours, windy days, uranium ore, and other sources of low-carbon energy. The only absence has been long-term investment in the infrastructure required to transition away from fossil fuels. All this is to say, the problem is not that the world is due to reach a maximum population beyond which climate change prevention becomes impossible. Instead, just as with food supply, far greater populations could be sustained if only resource coordination could be better handled.

Beyond the issue of resource management, I also mentioned that the practice of sending our dying through time machines would actually make climate change easier to solve. My logic is simple: if people expect to be alive in the future, they have greater incentive to ensure that the future turns out well. For instance, younger Americans are reportedly more concerned about climate change and supportive of measures to phase out fossil fuels.[23] A charitable view might attribute this to young people being more sensitive to the suffering of other human and non-human beings than previous generations. Those of a more pragmatic mindset may instead focus on how children aged ten or younger in 2020 are likely to experience a fivefold increase in extreme weather events during their lifetimes under the current trend of 3°C of warming, while those already over fifty-five share no such risks.[24]

Although many older individuals care about climate change, and some young people are indifferent, a massive contributor to the discrepancy in concern between these age groups undoubtedly stems from young people having more at stake. Frustratingly for them, then, the actions needed to avoid climate change cannot be made by the young alone. The limiting factor for reducing carbon emissions is in large part political inaction, and very few politicians are young. Looking at the data available, the average member of the US Congress was about sixty in 2021, for the Chinese Politburo it was sixty-two in 2017, while for the UK Parliament it was fifty-one in 2019. These politicians are roughly 60–70 per cent through their expected lifespan, so it would be unsurprising if their vision reaches a little less far ahead than the youngest generations. They may fear the political repercussions of inaction on climate change, or worry about their grandchildren, but few of them are likely to live long enough to suffer the worst of its consequences under the status quo.

Yet in a world where both politicians and private individuals could expect to personally live to see the consequences of climate change inaction, their behaviour might be quite different. They would understand that when they emerge from the time machine, they would inhabit a world shaped by their younger selves. If they had succeeded in limiting warming to 1.5°C and heralding an era of abundant, pollution-free energy, then the old codgers could expect a warm welcome. However, should they fail in this task and arrive in the future on the wrong side of history, an icy reception would be the least of their concerns.*

* * *

So that's why, in the short run of the next century or so, overpopulation due to time machines would not be such a concern. During this period, population size will be determined more by the birth rate than the death rate. We already produce enough food to feed our current

* Sorry, I couldn't resist the puns.

population, and there's no reason to expect improvements in agricultural productivity will stop. Climate change is a critical concern, but it's more a problem of short-term thinking than population size. If anything, sending our dying through time machines would likely improve conditions for future societies by encouraging long-term planning and counteracting the demographic decline expected after 2100.

It's true that, in the long run, abolishing death's inevitability while maintaining a positive fertility rate will result in an ever-growing population size. However, if we're considering that long a run, note that we are nowhere near the theoretical limits of the population our civilization could sustain given advancing technology. The Earth receives enough sunlight every hour to power global energy consumption for a year. If that's not enough, scientists are making progress in replicating the Sun down here on the ground through fusion plants, which could provide nearly limitless clean energy within the next century. There is still plenty of room for human habitation too: not only are many cities largely comprised of sprawl that could be densified, but only 1 per cent of global land is currently built up at all. And that's only considering the territory available on Earth using existing infrastructure strategies. The cost of launching objects into space is getting lower and lower: in the 1980s it cost $65,000 to put a kilogram into orbit via the Space Shuttle; nowadays it costs $2,600 on a Falcon 9 rocket, and SpaceX's upcoming Starship aims to do it for just $10.[*,25,26] Space colonization may seem like ridiculous science fiction, but so too would hormonal contraception and high-yield disease-resistant crops have seemed to Thomas Malthus back in 1798. If properly managed, there is enough to go around on Earth and in the heavens.

Lastly, before moving on, it's worth reflecting on just how disturbing the argument is that we should reduce our environmental impact through aging- and death-mediated population control. The same logic can be used to argue against any medical research that lengthens lifespans. Should we cease research on cancer and heart disease cures because survivors will go on to produce carbon-dioxide emissions?

* When converting to inflation-adjusted 2021 US dollars.

These diseases primarily affect the elderly, and they've already had time to lead a full, long life. Should we go further and mandate euthanasia at seventy to eliminate the carbon footprint of the elderly? After all, anyone who's lived that long has already achieved a typical lifespan by the standards of their ancestors. If these proposals seem absurd, so should the notion of denying access to time machines for dying individuals. If a suggested solution involves the involuntary deaths of billions of people, it's wise to keep searching for alternatives.

SOCIAL STAGNATION

After overpopulation, out of all the potential ills of life-extending technology like time machines, a fear that they will impede social progress is typically the next objection raised. The concern might be phrased along these lines:

> In the past, people committed countless acts of inhumane behaviour, from the support of slavery and oppression of women to acts of cruelty for mere amusement. Although these practices are not as widespread today, some of the same prejudices and narrow-mindedness still exist, especially among the elderly who often hold more conservative views. Their resistance to change hinders the adoption of positive progressive policies such as paid parental leave, while their lack of concern for the environment is destroying the planet. Not only that, but their selfishness has led to wealth concentration, exacerbating economic inequality.
>
> The natural process of generational turnover is thus necessary for the gradual improvement of society, as outdated beliefs and traditions give way to more enlightened practices. If time machines prevented the deaths of the elderly, politics would stagnate, institutions would crust over, and wealth would accumulate even further into the hands of a gerontocracy.
>
> Also, even if future generations were able to mitigate the negative impacts of their time-travelling ancestors, they may still view the new arrivals with the same disgust and contempt that we would hold for our own slave-owning, witch-burning, heretic-torturing forebears. Our

descendants would probably make the time-travellers feel unwelcome and unloved, possibly even leaving them to die upon arrival.

Although the concern is understandable, this argument is flawed. The main issue is that it ascribes supposedly immutable social attitudes to both previous and current elderly generations, while overlooking the role of cultural context in shaping people's actions.

It might be tempting to believe that people today are naturally more moral and upstanding than their predecessors, but the assumption is doubtful. While it's impossible to test directly, there exist situations that provide suggestive evidence to the contrary. Take Yusuf Abdi Ali, a war criminal turned Uber driver.[27] In the 1980s, Ali was a commander in the Somali national army where he allegedly tortured, maimed, and killed hundreds of people in the service of a dictator. Yet two decades later, in 2019, Ali was working quietly and peacefully as an Uber driver in the United States.* The banal evil wrought by Ali and others is often directed by circumstances and structures, not the twisted mind of an individual in a vacuum. Put a criminal in a different context and give them different options, and you'll find people often make very different choices. This is not to excuse the crimes of our ancestors, nor to exonerate individuals of all responsibility for their unjust actions, but simply to note that the character of our ethics is always refracted through our circumstances.†

Perhaps paradoxically, though, while our behaviour is more shaped by our external environment than we may care to admit, our internal proclivities are substantially more static. To a large degree, once people become adults, they stay essentially the same. To provide some

* He even had a rating of 4.89 stars out of 5.

† The worst-case fears of a dictator attempting to use the time machine to resume their totalitarian rule in the future are not particularly worrisome either, unless the time machine somehow makes them immune to imprisonment or assassination. Being a dictator is such a dangerous job that it is one of the few circumstances where profession may displace age as the greatest risk factor to one's ongoing survival. A typical dictator holds power for about twelve years before dying, and informal analysis shows that if dictators did not age at all they would only survive another four years on average before dying by the bullet of an assassin or by the hands of a rebellious citizenry.[28]

quantified evidence, psychological tests show core personality traits are set early on in life and become extremely stable by the time one reaches thirty.[29]

Don't take that to mean people don't change at all across their lives. In general, people do tend to become a little less open to new experiences over time, as well as becoming more agreeable and less neurotic as they mature. Rather, what this means is that while external circumstances may change dramatically, the internal nature of human personality is far more boring and stable than our culture gives us credit for, mired as it is in notions of heroic redemption and sinful corruption that spring from popular narrative and religion. When contrasting the shifts in a particular person's personality over their lifetime with the kinds of differences apparent between distinct individuals, the intrapersonal changes in personality and perspective are comparatively miniscule. In other words, we have a great deal more in common with our past selves than with other people.

You might read this as proof that the elderly are unfit to assimilate into the new world beyond the time machine, but this stability of human personality does not mean the elderly are incapable of changing their minds. Older scientists seem to adopt paradigmatic changes in their field at the same rate as their younger colleagues, such as the publication of evolutionary theory by Darwin in 1859, to take a historical example.[*,30] Or, to provide a more recent case, as the winds of

* You may have heard the saying 'science progresses one funeral at a time', meaning that geriatric professors refuse to accept new theories and use their eminent positions to stifle developments. This is a common paraphrasing of an excerpt from the autobiography of the theoretical physicist Max Planck. The original text reads 'A new scientific truth does not triumph by convincing its opponents and making them see the light, but rather because its opponents eventually die and a new generation grows up that is familiar with it.'

Given scientific discoveries are amongst the greatest ways in which a society's living standards can be improved, this is not a charge we should dismiss lightly. It turns out the evidence for senior scientists blocking scientific revolutions is mixed. On the one hand, older scientists seem to adapt to paradigmatic changes as quickly as new ones, as given by the example of Darwinian evolution in the main text. On the other hand, there are some data to suggest that, for more incremental scientific progress, elderly and eminent scientists may indeed inhibit new entrants and ideas into their field.[31] What is clearer is that the productivity of scientists tends to decline once they reach their forties, which may well be related to the cognitive decline that all people suffer as they age.[32,33,34] social opinion shifted in favour of legalizing same-sex marriage in the US, support increased faster than can be explained by generational turnover alone.[35] As we'll increasingly see, it's not so much that the old cannot change their minds as that without social pressure they often do not want to.

For example, a huge factor behind varying levels of enthusiasm for change among different age groups is that older segments of society wield remarkably disproportionate amounts of power compared to their demographic size. Whether this constitutes appropriate deference to the accumulated wisdom of our elders, or an egregious abuse of misappropriated power, depends on your point of view.*

To illustrate the point with specific details, let's take Australia as a representative example of a Western country.[36] The most egregious disparity is that the approximately 20 per cent of the population under eighteen, whose outcomes will be lifelong affected by the political decisions of the present, have infinitely less voting power than the 16 per cent aged over sixty-five. Simultaneously, these seniors control 30 per cent of private wealth, despite them being net recipients of government aid after the age of around fifty-eight. Much of these benefits comes in the form of subsidized healthcare and pensions, paid for by the income taxes of younger working people. Given fewer than 50 per cent of those in their mid-twenties to thirties own homes, while more than 80 per cent over sixty-five do, this may seem unjust. Indeed, these hard numbers are emblematic of a more general fact: in everything from governance and institutions to businesses and asset ownership, seniors have outsized influence relative to their demographic size.

It's not surprising then that, like any other influential group, seniors are more resistant to changes in the status quo than those with less

---

On that note, Thomas Huxley, one of the early proponents of evolutionary theory, went even further by saying 'men of science should be strangled on their 60th birthday, 'lest age should harden them against the reception of new truths, and make them into clogs upon progress . . .' I am unsure whether Huxley continued to endorse that statement once he himself turned sixty, but given he lived until seventy I assume not.

* And probably your current age.

power. Policies that sound progressive and equitable to young ears may sound dispossessive and destabilizing to older listeners.*

Unfortunately for these seniors, perennially critical of those darn 'kids these days', eventual changes to the status quo are inevitable. In our current world, with its absence of hypothetical time machines, the forces of aging and death do indeed make space on the stage of power for younger generations of leaders, while our forebears trample behind the curtain and into the history books.

So how would society evolve if the aged never exit the stage? While the elderly might sustain their lives, were time machines to exist, the devices would be unlikely to similarly preserve their influence. The reason being, should seniors travel a hundred years or more into the future, the prevailing conditions they once exploited would have vanished.

In terms of wealth, their extended absence would likely have led to their fortunes being distributed to inheritors or appropriated by others. Even if their assets were held passively in trust for their return, technological and societal changes in the intervening years – such as artificial intelligences and universal basic incomes – would likely significantly diminish or eliminate their value.

As for social structures, seniors would surely arrive into a transformed world. The specific political, business, and institutional networks that they once navigated would have transformed or been replaced by entirely new entities. Fresh faces in politics, industry, academia, entertainment, and religious institutions would have emerged, bringing with them different relationships and interaction norms. Understanding and exploiting the loopholes of the past would likely be of little use in this drastically different future.†

* Similarly, the greater fluid-intelligence and cognitive flexibility of youth is better suited to a world in flux than the crystallized knowledge of those with accumulated wisdom. A cute demonstration of these differences: raw intelligence peaks in one's late twenties, but performance on the *New York Times* crossword puzzle does not peak until people reach their sixties.[33,34]

† Even if time travel alone was somehow insufficient to neutralize the theoretical threats posed by seniors to future societies, there are ways to mitigate their potential abuses of power. Attempts to squirrel away wealth could be defeated through redistributive taxation policies. Efforts to reassert outdated political positions by

Indeed, rather than retaining power, it is more likely that seniors who step through the time machine would find themselves in a youthful state with respect to more than just their physical health. Like teenagers, they would possess little wealth and only weak social networks, being reliant on caregivers for some degree of support while learning to navigate their new lives.*

Reception of the elderly and terminally ill into the future is thus only possible with the consent of our descendants. This gives future generations existential control over how temporal refugees integrate into the world, and even if they should arrive at all. Consider the parallel situation of potential parents weighing the conditions in which they would want to raise a child, what values they would want to teach them, and whether or not they are willing to bring a life into this world at all. Parents, much like the leaders of this possible future world, have all the say.

Accordingly, the only reliable source of power remaining to seniors passing through the time machine would be the same force that otherwise helpless children regularly wield over adults – love.† Every traveller is someone's grandmother or grandfather, their uncle or aunt, their mentor or kindly neighbour. A person sent forward fifty years to when their heart disease could be cured might be greeted by adults with fond memories of their grandparent picking them up from kindergarten to go eat ice-cream. At the other end of the time machine,

---

time-travelling politicians could be prevented by laws outlining term limits. Just because the elderly control disproportionate power in the present, it does not follow that they are intrinsically bad people who should be left to die without their consent to nullify their potential negative impact.

* The science-fiction novel *Rainbows End* by Vernor Vinge explores this idea. It follows a protagonist who is cured of Alzheimer's disease but must return to high school to learn how to navigate a now futuristic world.

† In another respect, though, seniors would arguably have some unique gifts that children do not: knowledge and wisdom from the old world. The reason humans can live in luxury in dense cities while chimpanzees have only sparse communities dotted in parasite-infested forests is that we are highly capable of passing on complex information from one generation to the next. As good as we are at capturing this knowledge in oral traditions, writing, video, and other formats, all these media are imperfect. With living, breathing, talking contemporaries of historical wisdom, society may do considerably better at remembering the lessons of history.

with the roles reversed, it may be the grandchildren's turn to spoil and lavish their grannies and grandpas.*

***

Still, the primary problem for hopeful time-travellers may not be that future generations look upon them with fear, but rather with disgust. In today's world, many of us gaze back in horror upon the actions and beliefs of our ancestors, with no shortage of barbarity around the globe. People with European ancestry had forebears who either directly participated in or indirectly benefited from the Atlantic slave trade. Those with a Japanese background know many great-grandparents committed atrocities while colonizing Korea, China, and much of Southeast Asia. Central Americans can look to the ubiquitous human sacrifices of the Aztec and Maya, North Africans the cruelty of the Barbary pirates. Even looking back before agricultural civilization, all humans can trace their lineage to hunter-gatherer societies who perpetrated shocking levels of violence by modern standards. Should we not be afraid that future generations will judge us as harshly as we may judge our own ancestors?

There is no shortage of contemporary failings for which we might be critiqued. Systemic racism and social inequality persist in even the wealthiest and most developed nations. Many countries continue to commit environmental vandalism through carbon-dioxide emissions despite the scientific consensus on the harm this will do to future generations. Few change their dietary practices in response to concerns about the suffering perpetuated by factory farming, let alone worry about its potential to cause catastrophic future pandemics. It is not hard to imagine our descendants looking back at us with horror and disgust at our primitive and selfish practices.

Despite this, to see all our ancestors as monsters and victims would be to paint with too broad a brush. For example, consider the philosopher and reformer Jeremy Bentham, who in 1759, at the tender age of eleven, was aghast to learn of the limited rights of women to

* As each grandparent is in turn someone's grandchild, this chain of love could, in principle, be extended indefinitely to those who need to make a journey of any length of time.

vote, divorce, or hold political office.[37] These feelings spurred him into a career spent pushing for women's rights, slavery abolition, anti-colonial endeavours, corporal punishment abolition, homosexuality decriminalization, and animal-welfare improvements. This is a progressive agenda even by the standards of the 2020s, let alone in 1759. This demonstrates that sometimes, through thoughtful reflection, people have anticipated moral reforms centuries in advance.*

But even when considering those who were less explicitly progressive than Bentham, for many of us in wealthy nations, it's hard to avoid hypocrisy in criticizing our ancestors while enjoying the fruits of their contributions to technological and social progress. From those who first cultivated wild grains in the Middle East to Fritz Haber's invention of industrial fertilizer production, it is not just Borlaug and Yuan we have to thank for our daily bread. Similarly, many modern social-justice movements can trace their roots all the way back to early democratic reformists in ancient Athens and medieval England. It's impossible to say if those who worked to breed aurochs into modern cattle, or enshrine civil rights in the Magna Carta, knew their actions would have effects centuries and millennia later, yet their efforts laid the groundwork for our modern world.

Most people throughout history have just been trying to get by day-to-day and provide for their families. It is difficult to judge these masses as monsters without similarly condemning ourselves, and, critically, the same will likely be true for our descendants. As *Homo sapiens*, with our biology largely unchanged for the past 100,000 years, we all still share the same human imperfections and desires. This is not to argue that all morality is relative, and that the atrocities committed by our ancestors were acceptable because times were different then. Instead, it is to say that when we tally our ancestors' sins, we should also consider their efforts to improve the world, if not their

* That's not to say that Bentham was a complete paragon of virtue who held no objectionable opinions. He invented the concept of the *panopticon*, a prison where inmates never know whether they are being watched or not, in an effort to compel convicts into self-regulation. His reformist philosophy was also used to justify social welfare practices where impoverished individuals were coerced into living under harsh conditions, in the name of providing a disincentive to unemployment.

fundamental humanity, just as we hope our own descendants will do for us.

That being said, there are some very good reasons to worry about how future generations will perceive our legacy. In parallel to the claim that politicians would act with more haste on climate change were they to anticipate living to suffer its costs, there are historical examples of when people may have acted better had they known they would personally bear the consequences of their actions. For example, while the horrors of slavery are blatantly apparent to modern eyes, even Thomas Jefferson, the third US president, knew that slavery was problematic.[38] As a junior lawyer he had represented enslaved people seeking emancipation. Later in his career he signed a law attempting to ban their importation into America. He even wrote in his autobiography that 'Nothing is more certainly written in the book of fate than that these people are to be free.' However, he owned hundreds of enslaved people and did little to push for abolition during his time in office. Had Jefferson believed he would be alive to endure the judgement of those freed in 1865, or the civil rights movement in the 1960s, perhaps he would have acted better.

In contrast, in circumstances where historical figures acted with explicit concern for their descendants, it is nearly impossible to look back upon them with anything but gratitude and love. In 1866, the British parliamentarian John Stuart Mill, a follower of Bentham's philosophy, gave an address to parliament on the troubles that contemporary coal mining might cause for future generations.[39] Now, Mill was not quite so forward-thinking as to have anticipated climate change. Instead, he worried that exhausting limited coal reserves would leave future Britons in economic hardship. Remarking on the negligence of such a decision, and considering what opportunities in posterity had been already sacrificed for modernity, he stated:

> it is our duty to pass it on, not merely undiminished, but with interest, to those who are in the same relation to us as we are to those who preceded us. So shall we too deserve, and may in our turn hope to receive, a share of the same gratitude.

John Stuart Mill died of a bacterial infection in 1873 at the age of sixty-six. I am sure that if a dying Mill could have instead been transported to a modern emergency department, no doctor would hesitate to administer him antibiotics. I am less confident that the same could be said for Jefferson, were he to arrive today into the care of a doctor who'd experienced a lifetime of grievous racism. I think about these two often when I imagine myself, sick and dying, passing through the time machine. If my life were to pass into the hands of a medical worker in a future era, I would feel much more comfortable if I expected they would feel my past actions had positively affected the world in which they live.

DISCARDING PALLIATIVE PHILOSOPHY

At this stage, I suspect some readers will feel I'm wilfully ignoring one huge and obvious objection to 'time machines'. Sure, it's possible the hypothetical social and environmental consequences of mass temporal migration could be avoided with decent preparation, and maybe our descendants would be willing and able to welcome us into their time. Truthfully, though, these probably aren't many people's biggest concerns. The really juicy issue with the death-deferral proposal is that it ignores a fundamental predicate of thousands of years of philosophical, spiritual, and cultural practices that teaches us that death is a natural and necessary part of life.

As far back as we have records, philosophers have been claiming that life's ending should be accepted, if not actively embraced. The ancient Greek Socrates proclaimed that death, like dreamless sleep, is a deliverance from the pains of life.[40] The Roman emperor and Stoic philosopher Marcus Aurelius claimed that 'Death is a cessation [. . .] of the service to the flesh.'*[,41] Nor is this constrained only to the Western canon: in different forms and in different texts, a philosophy of death acceptance can be found across diverse cultures, geographies, and times.

* This is entirely unrelated, but my favourite Marcus Aurelius quote is 'At dawn, when you have trouble getting out of bed, tell yourself: "I have to go to work – as a human being."' Even emperors struggle to get out of bed to go to work! Imagining Aurelius finding it hard to rise two millennia ago is one of the strongest reminders I have that humans throughout history are all pretty similar.

Just as ubiquitous are the warnings from poets that attempting to escape death constitutes the gravest kind of arrogance, hubris, and selfishness. A tale holds that the first emperor of a unified China, Qin Shi Huang, died horribly from drinking an elixir he believed would grant him immortality, but that actually contained poisonous mercury. In the Hindu story of the 'Churning of the Ocean of Milk', which appears in the *Vishnu Purana*, the search for the nectar of immortality threatens to release a poison that could destroy creation. In ancient Greek myth, Sisyphus is forced to roll an immense boulder up a hill for eternity as punishment for attempting to escape his mortality by wrapping Death in chains. Throughout history, these tales have prescribed that people should accept their mortality, lest they face consequences worse than death.

Throughout millennia and across disparate cultures, the philosophy of death acceptance has stayed remarkably consistent. Today, eminent thinkers such as the bioethicist Leon Kass continue to claim that a desire to live beyond one's eighties is 'an expression of a childish and narcissistic wish' and that 'the finitude of human life is a blessing for every human individual'.[42] The prestigious medical journal *The Lancet* convened a commission that even went so far as to say 'it is healthy to die' and 'without death every birth would be a tragedy'.[43]

Our modern myths and legends continue to echo the themes of the ancients. Voldemort, the villain of the popular *Harry Potter* books, commits his heinous acts in an attempt to seek immortality.* There are plenty of similar examples too. The powerful One Ring from *The Lord of the Rings* grants its bearer an extended life, but at the cost of steadily progressing corruption. In multiple instances in the *Star Wars* movies, the desire of a character to avert the death of themselves or their loved ones results in corruption by the dark side of the Force. The message is the same as it's always been – if humans don't know their limits and die when they're supposed to, they will suffer fates worse than death.

Correspondingly, the formal arguments given for why individuals

* In case the evil of pursuing a longer life wasn't clear enough, the author explicitly names Voldemort's henchmen 'Death Eaters'.

should accept their impending deaths have remained the same across history. In a section of text titled 'Folly of the Fear of Death', the Roman philosopher Lucretius justified death-acceptance by listing essentially the same arguments given today: that the finality of death provides an ending without which our lives would have no meaning; that if we lived longer, we'd become bored and lazy; that we can't be harmed by death because once we're dead we're not around to be harmed; and that life is suffering.[44] Having put all these points forward, Lucretius claims that through reflection and examination of these arguments we will come to realize that death is not to be feared but instead embraced.

The most popular contemporary argument, just as it was in Roman times, is that death provides a deadline without which our pursuits would feel senseless and boring. If not for the tick of a countdown clock, we would forever procrastinate. Why bother taking up Spanish classes or having children today if you could do it in a few decades? Consider how we assign value to activities by spending parcels of our precious limited time. As such, our culture awards merit to those who sacrifice time for expertise and effort. If everyone has endless time to learn how to draw life-like portraits, solve Rubik's cubes, or climb Mount Everest, the achievements become meaningless. Eventually, after years and years of this low-pressure lifestyle, we would run out of things to do. In the end, we would feel as though we were stuck watching the same dull television series over and over, trudging around in purgatory long past the point when our lives had meaning or purpose.

That is the commonly espoused claim, but is it accurate?

A generous critique might be that, even if you accept the claim, it's not clear where the deadline should be set. It certainly seems hard to imagine there are many objections to the previous extensions we have received. Our last common ancestor with our fellow apes lived around forty to sixty years, which seems far too short by today's standards. How is one supposed to make friends, raise a family, and fulfil one's passions in such a short space of time? With only sixty years you may not even live to see your grandchildren be born, let alone have the experience and maturity to run for public office.

Even the extension of fifteen years granted to our hunter-gatherer forebears over their pre-human ancestors seems brief to modern sensibilities. While not as bad as dying young, only making it to one's seventies is still less than many of us would wish for in this day and age. Importantly, people do not typically feel that suffering from a disease that removes decades from one's life is sufficiently compensated for by an increase in the meaningfulness of one's shortened existence. We cannot accept the death of a child because children represent opportunity; after all, they have 'so much more life to live'. But as medicine affords us the opportunity to live well for longer, the age of 'acceptable' death necessarily gets higher. If we're sure that forty or sixty years is lamentable today, and seventy still feels short, then how can we be sure a deadline of eighty-five is appropriate?* Maybe 120 would be better – more time, but close enough to still feel some pressure? Or maybe longer still?

On further thought, though: is it really the impending deadline that ensures we feel meaning when we go about our lives? This is not obvious when examining the main things that give people a sense of meaning and joy.

First and foremost among these are the connections people have with their family and friends. Let's admit that temporal boundaries can certainly make relationships feel more special and pertinent. A mother savours the charming nonsense stories of her rapidly maturing three-year-old. A summer fling feels all the more emotional because the days of passion are numbered. But, while limited timing may lead us to be more reflective about our relationships, that doesn't mean that those relationships are meaningful fundamentally because they change or end. The same mother loves with fervent passion even after her child leaves home. Most integral to the summer fling was the solid romantic chemistry, not the fact that it lasted a month. Those blessed with the good fortune to spend time with those they love do not derive additional pleasure from knowing these times will one day end. Instead, with every additional achievement celebrated together, failure softened with a shoulder to cry on, or lazy afternoon spent in each other's

* While the philosopher Francesca Minerva offers few definitive positions of her own in the book *The Ethics of Cryonics*, she does commit to the statement 'A trip of 80, 90, or even 100 years is not long enough; living takes a lot of practice, and death can wait.'[45]

company, healthy relationships are strengthened with unending growth. Ask almost any proud and caring grandparent if they are feeling sick and tired of spending regular time with their grandchildren and you'll learn an excess of hours is no object to love. This social source of love and joy is enough alone to dismiss the need for a deadline.

Next most important after love is the meaning provided by being impactful with one's time and energy. Whether it be an engineer taking pride in constructing a bridge that will be used by many, a nurse who knows their efforts will bring relief to a suffering patient, or an educator whose guidance and mentorship will empower the young to find their own sources of purpose, many take inexhaustible pride in their efforts to make the world a better place.

For others, the joy of leisure is reason enough to want to keep living indefinitely. Last year's football competition does not make this year's contest any less enjoyable. There are more good books written than can be read in a human lifetime, and yet talented authors just keep writing. In so many domains, there are an inexhaustible number of ongoing pursuits to be had, as long as one is still healthy enough to pursue them.

***

Despite my claims to the contrary, you may still believe that a typical ninety-year-old would be too tired and bored with life to set off on a time-travelling adventure. Surely the prospect of being young again would be totally unappealing to those who've already lived a full and meaningful life? To set things straight, let's set aside armchair philosophy and examine how people actually feel as they approach their deadlines.

Ask people of any age how long they'd like to live, and you'll see the stated age perpetually increases as they get older. A thirty-year-old may say eighty, but ask that same person when they're actually approaching eighty and, as long as they're still relatively healthy, they're likely to say one hundred or beyond. Survey the opinions of people specifically in their elder years and you will be quickly disabused of the notion that old people are finished with life. Generally, people always want at least a bit more time, and the healthier they are the more they want.[3,4,46]

If you go beyond general population surveys and instead explicitly

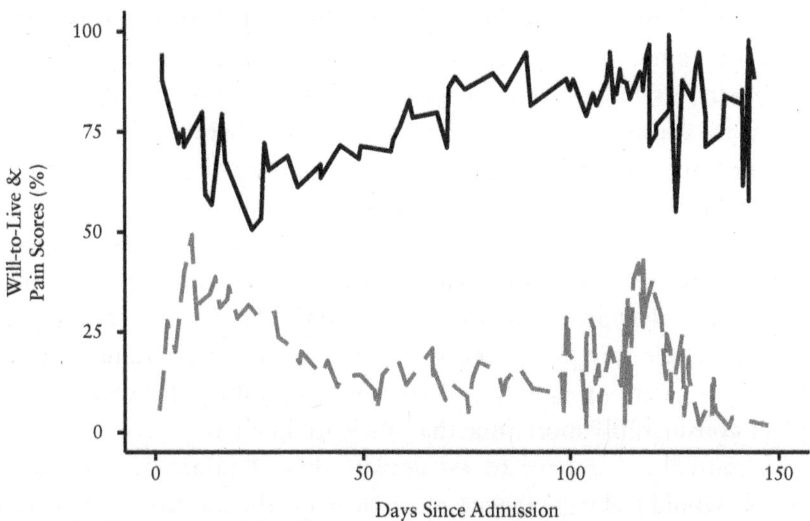

Figure 2. An 82-year-old woman dying from terminal bowel cancer was admitted for palliative care. Although her will to live weakened when her pain scores increased, she maintained a consistently high will to live even as death approached.[48] This is typical of most people in her position.[49]

ask the terminally ill how they feel as they approach their deadlines, you will find that most of them still have a strong desire to live. A representative quote from a medical worker supporting these patients is provided by the nurse Sarah Creed, saying 'Ninety-nine per cent understand they're dying, but one hundred per cent hope they're not [. . .] They still want to beat their disease.'[47] This anecdotal claim is backed by formal studies where elderly patients with terminal cancer were surveyed on their 'will to live', along with their pain, anxiety, and other physical and mental symptoms.[48,49] In one study that included individuals in their eighties, 69 per cent of patients expressed a moderate or high will to live despite facing imminent death (Fig. 2).

Notably, many of those who expressed a low will to live were suffering from severe nausea or other acutely painful symptoms, and regained their will to live once these symptoms were treated. This accords with other studies showing that will to live is associated with an absence of pain, anxiety, and disability.[50] Of those who reported a low will to live, all surveyed had no spouse and probable poor social support. Reminiscent of the correlation between poor social ties and poor outcomes in the reports of elderly migrant wellbeing mentioned earlier in this chapter, the only group who spoke about being ready to die were those who felt isolated and socially bereft.[10] It's not that people typically reach a point where they want to die, so much as they sometimes lose the things that make life worth living.

What these surveys suggest is that, so long as people are spared feeling severely ill or socially isolated, there is no obvious age at which they decide they are bored and finished with life. Whether it's surveys asking people how long they would like to live if guaranteed good health or querying elderly people who are imminently dying, most want considerably more time than they are likely to get.

Admittedly, it is hard to extrapolate these findings to guess how people would feel were they to reach their 150th, 200th, or 500th year, given we don't yet have anyone in this position to ask. Maybe people really would get bored one day. But even if such a time were to come eventually, most people do not want the end date they are currently set.

It would be unfair to disempower people by denying them the ability to choose to die one day if they so desire, just as the current inescapability of death is unfair for stripping people of control over their lives. But the use of the time machine, or any other life-extension technology, would not grant people inescapable immortality. Instead, it would grant them that most valuable of liberties – the power to make decisions about their life on their own terms.

***

Apart from the argument that life needs a deadline to be meaningful, there are other arguments made to convince people of the acceptability of death. One favourite among philosophers is that a person cannot be harmed by death because once a person is dead they are no longer around to be harmed. The reasoning is that one can't be harmed by deprivation of experience, as if you're not alive then your absence is no loss to you.

I am not sure anyone except a philosopher could find this

comforting.* By this logic, the death of a ten-year-old and a centenarian are equally non-harmful to both, as neither will subsequently feel deprived of whatever years they otherwise would have had remaining. This does not match up with the near-universal feeling that a child's untimely death results in them suffering greater harm, through deprivation of a full life, than that of a ninety-year-old. It is a simple step to extrapolate this reasoning to a person of any age who misses out on years they could potentially have enjoyed living.

One last claim sometimes made to justify death is that it provides a final relief for our pained and weary souls after a lifetime overwhelmingly filled with suffering. While that is sadly true for some unfortunate individuals, it is a flat-out wrong description of the lived experience of the majority of people. When asked to respond using a ten-point scale, where zero is 'not at all satisfied with their lives' and ten is 'completely satisfied', most people from most developed countries rate themselves as somewhere around seven.[52–54] These responses of overall satisfaction do not discount the fact that everyone experiences pain and suffering in their lives, but merely reflect that, in the minds of most, the good outweighs the bad.†

All that said, to give full justice to this argument, I must sadly inform you that in the last few years before death most people's life satisfaction does start to drop precipitously.[56,57] However, this does not mean that the dying come to embrace the relief of death. Even as their drop in wellbeing is ongoing, most people's will to live only

* To forestall the retort that this is an *ad hominem* attack instead of a real argument against the point, I should register that I am philosophically inclined, and I do take the notion seriously. However, to properly run through the argument's merits and criticisms requires a tedious formal philosophical analysis as well as digressions into related topics of population ethics and metaphysics. I believe this analysis ultimately leads one to dismiss the argument, so I am neglecting to do it thoroughly here for the sake of brevity. If you'd like to read a longer discussion of the issue, see Chapter Three of Ingemar Patrick Linden's book *The Case against Death*.[51]

† For a much lengthier discussion of the methodologies and data used to address this question, see the section 'How many people have positive wellbeing' in Chapter Nine of *What We Owe The Future* by William MacAskill. He concludes that the typical person's life contains more good than bad, and that 'If I were given the option, on my deathbed, to be reincarnated as a randomly selected person alive today, I would choose to do so.'[55]

negligibly diminishes with proximity to death. The reality is that the typical dying person is not glad to be finished with a life full of suffering, but aggrieved and saddened by the looming loss of what was previously a mostly satisfying life.[58]

***

I am reluctant to cast aspersions on the works of so many of history's great thinkers, but the arguments listed above – that death is acceptable because it is natural, because it offers protection from suffering, or because it creates meaning by circumscribing time – strike me as unusually weak when compared to the typical rigour of philosophical debate. This is not just my opinion: some contemporary philosophers have also noted the same issue.[51] This raises the question of why so many philosophers throughout history have put forth such unconvincing arguments on this particular subject?

The obvious suspicion is that philosophers have desperately wanted the inevitability of death to be acceptable, to assuage their own mortal fears.* Historically, death has always been an inescapable reality whether or not one considers it tolerable. That such a harrowing inevitability could occur without good reason is deeply unsettling. To acknowledge this perspective is to view the moral character of the universe as at best indifferent and at worst cruel. It would be so much more comforting if death's inevitability had some redeeming purpose to justify its otherwise conspicuous horrors.

Whenever there is a situation where we would prefer one possible state of the world to be true over another, we have to be very mindful of *motivated reasoning*. This is the kind of thinking where a person holds a belief not because there is strong evidence for its veracity, but because it is comfortable to believe. If someone who believes themselves to be a good driver is involved in an accident, they may blame the other driver, the weather, the road conditions, a mechanical problem with their car, or anything else, before considering the possibility that their own driving could be at fault. Or, as we saw last chapter, think of the priests who found it more palatable to believe women's

* To be slightly fairer to this group, a survey of analytical Western philosophers found that 45 per cent of them would take immortality if offered.[59]

suffering during childbirth was justifiable punishment for Eve's sins, rather than pain women had to endure due to the indifference of evolution. Ideally, philosophical instruction in rational thought is supposed to train people out of this fallacious mode of thinking. Yet philosophers are still human, and thus fallible. If Socrates is a man, and therefore mortal, he is disposed to believe that he is mortal for a reason.

On occasion philosophers have all but come out and explicitly said they have motivated reasoning with regards to accepting death. The Greek philosopher Epicurus stated 'Empty is that philosopher's argument by which no human suffering is therapeutically treated. For just as there is no use in a medical art that does not cast out the sicknesses of bodies, so too there is no use in philosophy, unless it casts out the suffering of the soul.'[60] Relieving suffering is certainly a worthy goal. But alleviating the suffering of the soul and mind is much more the role of clinical psychology than the cold logic of philosophy.

Philosophy literally means 'love of knowledge', an apt name for a discipline dedicated to the pursuit of truth. But, as is so often the case, the sweet highs of love come braided with the risks of real pain. In the quest for knowledge, one is sometimes forced to decide between clinging to a comforting false belief or begrudgingly accepting a hard truth. In such a circumstance, it is a perversion of philosophy to shy away from reality, no matter how harsh it may be. Although often painful, only by seeing the world for how it truly is can we hope to address the root causes of our problems and change the character of our world.

In medicine, a treatment that provides symptomatic relief without addressing the underlying problem is termed *palliative*.* These methods are often employed at times when, although a patient's disease cannot be cured, there is still much that can be done to ease their discomfort. A tumour causing pain by pressing up against a nerve may not be able to be surgically removed without killing the patient, but radiation therapy to shrink it may still relieve the patient's distress. Giving oxygen to someone whose lungs are failing from emphysema won't save them, but it will reduce their breathlessness. These are the

* Originally from the Latin *palliare*, meaning 'to cover with a cloak', i.e. to conceal.

jobs of palliative medicine, to minimize symptoms and maximize wellbeing for as long possible.*

I believe that, without acknowledging it, philosophers promoting death acceptance have been practising *palliative philosophy*. For all the earlier time in human history when nothing could be done about the inevitability of death, philosophy provided comfort when there was no cure that could be offered.

In the days before anaesthesia, belief in the purifying effects of enduring pain was similarly palliative. Yet nowadays, with better treatments, that old mindset has been so thoroughly unendorsed by the medical and general community that few know any ever held it. Just as the therapy for surgical pain changed with the advent of anaesthesia, so too should our treatment of the dying if we gain access to time machines. The costs and benefits have shifted: where before denial was the best of a bad deal, improvements in medical technology should now prompt us to acknowledge the pain we've been covering up.

For involuntary death, at any age, is a profound injustice, robbing us of everything that matters most. What if you didn't have to count the hours you spend in your lover's arms like a finite, depleting resource? What if illness could not permanently rob you of the opportunity to watch your children grow into the strong, kind, and successful adults you nurtured them to be? What if you could sit on soft, green earth beneath the setting sun, with new friends and old, with good meals and good music and other delights you've yet to name or know, all without cursing the coming night for stealing one more day from you that can never be returned?

Even worse, involuntary death does not just strip us of ourselves, it also cuts us away from those who need us. Our family, our friends, anyone who loves us and whose lives we are a part of are diminished by our absence. We mourn and grieve the dead not just for the life they have been unjustly deprived of, but because without their presence our own lives are diminished. Every grandparent, every friend,

* It may seem throughout this section that I am implicitly criticizing palliative medicine, but that couldn't be further from the case. Palliative care is an important and extremely undervalued medical field, often neglected because it is less sexy than curing diseases.

every child is a portion of ourselves torn away and lost. It is true that, even in the face of this loss, their presence and actions continue to live on in our memories. But there is no legacy, however mighty, that can wholly diminish the despair of knowing we can no longer be there for those who need and miss us.

Accordingly, even if it is taboo to say it explicitly, we already act implicitly as though death at any age is unacceptable. One need only observe society's spending patterns on medical treatments and research for ailments affecting the elderly. We spend huge sums of money to treat cancer, even though the typical patient is over sixty-eight.[61] Less than 2 per cent of people under sixty-five suffer from dementia, and most sufferers don't develop it until they're in their eighties.[62] If we really thought death was acceptable for people in their old age, why try so hard to find a treatment for Alzheimer's? Shouldn't we tell medical researchers that they're no longer needed once they can guarantee everyone makes it to eighty-five in reasonable health? That there is no need for non-palliative treatments after that age, as from then on patients should be allowed to die to serve a greater purpose? Would it not be hubris for doctors and researchers to try to treat diseases of advanced age, and utter selfishness of patients to expect any more life than they are naturally allocated?

Not at all. The sheer ambitiousness of the goal is too embarrassing for scientists to usually come right out and say it, but the ultimate objective of medical research is the elimination of all disease. Whether they acknowledge it or not, every researcher who contributes to tools to cure cancer, repair heart disease, and otherwise prevent specific causes of death, is chipping away at this overarching problem. There will be no downing of stethoscopes, scalpels, and microscopes until every last person is free to live as long and healthy a life as they choose.

I hope, dear reader, that for you the concerns of death remain an abstract, distant notion. From afar, you may presume the elderly version of you will at least accept, if not willingly embrace, your eventual fate. A courageous mentality to hold, but perhaps one that you are unlikely to maintain. For, when the end draws near, it is by no means certain that you will feel content and complete, as if you have finished everything you set out to accomplish and are ready to die. It is much more likely that you will be angry and upset with a body that is failing you. You will know how much your children will miss you, how much you could help them if you were only still able. You may well still want to play with your grandchildren, to see how their lives turn out and the people they become. You will likely still have books to read, places to travel to, new skills to learn. You might still have so much love to give, so many things to do. You might still be too young to die.

In this position, much like Keiko, you should be able to choose the time machine if you so wish. The case for saving everyone is clear: no one should be forced into oblivion against their will.

Unfortunately, time machines aren't real, and likely never will be. But that does not mean other forms of time travel are not possible, if only we think a little more creatively about how to achieve them. The problem is not that we aren't moving forwards in time; we do that every day. The issue instead is how to keep a dying person alive, in some way, shape, or form, long enough to be cured of what is killing them.

In the chapters that follow, we will walk through recent scientific findings that mean for the first time, unlike all the generations who came before us, this may actually be achievable. We'll first need to explore what exactly a person is and what precisely it means for them to die, after which we'll be in a position to see how it is that brain preservation provides the functional equivalent of a time machine.

The difference between stoically accepting fate and tragically succumbing to learned helplessness is only a matter of whether something can be done. I do not ask you to suspend your disbelief or scepticism, and I encourage you to deliberate the potential complications. But, insofar as universal access to brain preservation would grant people autonomy over their own lives, I beg you to take seriously the case for abolishing involuntary death.

PART TWO

What

If I've succeeded in convincing you that death is an evil to be fought, you may now be wanting to leap straight into action. But in order to defeat an enemy, it helps to take the time to understand them. Before we discuss procedures that might be able to halt death, we first need to talk about what it is.

We'll begin by developing a clear definition of precisely what it takes for a person to die, and how earlier ideas evolved as medical technology advanced from bloodletting to brain implants. This exploration will trigger questions pertaining to the neuroscience and philosophy of personal identity, consciousness, and memory, and we'll subsequently spend a chapter on each topic in turn.

By the time we've finished with medical cases of brain injuries leading to dramatic personality changes, theorizing on the internal experiences of artificial intelligences and octopuses, and experimental accounts of editing memories using viruses and lasers, we'll have a much better understanding of what a person fundamentally is. With that knowledge gained, we can finally turn to how to build the armour that can save someone from death.

3
What Is Death?

In the past few decades, medical science has rendered obsolete centuries of experience, tradition, and language about our mortality and created a new difficulty for mankind: how to die.

Atul Gawande, *Being Mortal*

Even if Trent's skull didn't break when he initially hit the concrete, it certainly did once the trailer fell on top of him. One second he was relishing the thrill of being pulled along behind a dune buggy, the next he was unconscious with his skull fractured in seven places. Following the injury he was rushed to hospital, where doctors began desperately trying to put his head back together. Half the task was just keeping him alive while they did so. Over several days of surgery his heart stopped four times, with more and more damage accumulating to Trent's body with each pause. Disappointingly, at the end of all this, though his skull was patched, he was yet to show any signs of consciousness.

The medical team decided continuing treatment at this stage would simply be forestalling closure for his family, as he had vanishingly little hope of recovery. His mother wearily agreed that her son shouldn't be left like this. She knew her son was generous, and that he would have wanted to donate his organs to help others with lives that could still be saved. However, with his heart still beating, Trent wasn't officially dead yet. Even though it had been several days and four cardiac arrests since he hit the concrete, there was one additional test the medical team needed to do before Trent could be declared dead: a final brain scan.[1,2]

***

Trent's story is a lot more complicated than it would have been a century ago. Back then, Trent would have been considered dead the first time his heart stopped, at the latest. In general, before the middle of the twentieth century diagnosing death was clear cut – alive if lungs breathing and heart beating, dead otherwise.* These days, determining when exactly someone dies is a lot murkier.

The first major complication came with the invention of mechanical ventilators, which blurred the link between breathing and life.† These devices could artificially inflate a patient's lungs if they stopped breathing on their own, and were initially invented to assist with respiratory failure during surgery.‡ Next came *cardiopulmonary bypass machines*, unseating the heart as the determinant of life by artificially circulating a person's blood. Using a series of pumps and tubes, someone could now have their heart stopped, operated upon, potentially even replaced with a transplant from another person, all without being considered dead. These days a person can be kept alive for weeks with neither functioning heart nor lungs using a technique called *extracorporeal membrane oxygenation*. This method involves draining a patient's blood into tubes, passing it through an artificial lung that introduces oxygen and removes carbon dioxide, then pumping the blood back into their body. Through these processes, death and the cardiorespiratory organs have been completely decoupled.

These once unimaginably futuristic technologies have severed the

* Actually, even back then this wasn't always quite true, as people would occasionally be pronounced dead only to regain signs of life later. Fears of being erroneously pronounced dead were great enough that in 1896 the London Association for the Prevention of Premature Burial was founded to try and improve procedures for doctors checking for signs of life prior to burial, and to ensure warning devices were placed in coffins that could be used in case these checks failed.

† Now unfortunately well-known due to the COVID-19 pandemic.

‡ I'm fairly certain that was the original intent behind their design, but note that they would have been inspired by the earlier 'iron lungs', which were used to help polio patients during recovery from paralysis.

definition of death from its origins and set it adrift. Where it will finally settle is not obvious, as there's no reason to think the end of these advancements is in sight. If we want to know what the final definition will be, the question to ask is 'How badly decayed does a human body have to be before a person could not, even in principle, no matter the technology, be restored to health?' This chapter is going to answer that question and provide a definition of death that applies at that limit. Let's start by considering what it currently takes for someone to be formally considered dead.

(MIS)PRONOUNCING DEATH

First of all, it's worth acknowledging that, when considering one's own life in isolation, a rigid definition of death isn't necessarily all that useful. While most people are concerned about their own survival, they're generally very unconcerned about the possibility that their survival may be ambiguous to them. Thought experiments and science fiction aside, knowing you haven't died because you're still alive is a perfectly workable definition.

As is so often the case, things become more complicated when other people are involved. People are not just isolated individuals, we come with tangles of responsibilities, obligations, debts, and other relationships. For example, meet Alex. She works as an engineer, has a spouse named Blake, and owns a house. It's not something we often like to consider, but what would happen were Alex to die? As a society of government agencies, unions, and mortgage brokers, we want to be very clear on the conditions under which Blake's aspirations for their joint life should end, the mutual obligations between Alex and her employer cease, and when her claims to property can be disregarded. As well as being legally significant, defining these conditions is of considerable emotional and practical importance. It marks when Alex's friends and family should mourn her just as much as when her property should be distributed to inheritors. While an individual themself has no need to know when they are dead, the others in their community certainly do.

Certain social statuses of individuals, like marriage and employment, are so consequential they are formalized by law. As such, let's consider the legal definition of death. There is a reasonable level of consistency in this across different jurisdictions.[3–5] Most commonly, a person is defined as dead if either or both of the following applies to their body:

1. Irreversible cessation of blood circulation.
2. Irreversible cessation of all functions of the brain, including the brainstem.

Considering we live in the age of cardiopulmonary bypass and extracorporeal membrane oxygenation machines, which can keep your blood circulating with the ease of a pool pump keeping a jacuzzi's bubbles flowing, it's immediately apparent that it will not always be straightforward to apply this definition.* For this reason, laws typically include a statement such as 'a determination of death must be made in accordance with accepted medical standards'. While pragmatic, this combination of underdefined law and deference to doctors is the foothill to a towering mountain of definitional problems.

There are at least two issues with the legal definition of death. The first is that what counts as 'irreversible cessation' is as much dependent on medical technology as it is on the damage to a person's body. Declaring an injured person dead or alive based on what medical equipment is available is a bit like saying perfectly edible food is already off because there's no refrigerator nearby. In other words, if we're defining death by properties other than those intrinsic to a person, we're on shaky philosophical ground. The second concern is the requirement that 'all' functions of the brain are irreversibly lost before a patient is declared dead. It turns out that this requirement is out of touch with both the beliefs and actions of doctors. While these issues can be safely ignored in the vast majority of deaths, we'll soon see exceptions illustrating how our current definitions of death are problematic.

In response to the decreasing emphasis placed on blood circulation with the advent of artificial cardiorespiratory technology, modern medicine became more concerned with defining death based on the loss of brain functions, commonly termed *brain death*. Later, we'll see how current and developing technology is increasingly rendering brain death as

* In practice the process of keeping someone's blood flowing is probably trickier than that of a pool pump, but the principle is the same. You understand the point.

obsolete a concept as cardiopulmonary bypass did for heart death. But, before even coming to how the functions of natural brain tissue could be replaced with prosthetics, it's worth focusing on how doctors already ignore the legal requirement that death requires the loss of *all* brain functions.

For example, consider the *hypothalamus*. A small, nugget-shaped region at the base of the brain, it is involved in regulating instincts, hormones, and many other basic bodily functions (Fig. 3). Contrary to the requirements of the second legal definition of death, the hypothalamus is often still mostly working in patients otherwise declared brain dead.[*,6]. While not at all compatible with the legal notion of 'whole-brain' death, this is quietly but consistently ignored by the medical community. Even stranger, there is other evidence suggesting there are often isolated 'islands' of preserved neural tissue in brain-dead patients, even though most of the rest of the brain has ceased functioning.[7]

While it doesn't affect day-to-day practice, the medical profession is well aware of the gap between the written letter of the law and actual implementation. Calls to resolve this have been made in prestigious journals, though this has had little impact.[8] Despite the tension, doctors issue tens of thousands of death certificates per day without worrying they are falsely pronouncing patients dead. Why are they so unconcerned? Because routine examinations can uncover sufficiently extensive brain damage indicating that patients have no hope of functional recovery, even if strictly speaking they do not meet the criteria for whole-brain death.

The following tests for brain function are generally applied, though with some variation between jurisdictions.[9] No proper examination is necessary if it is obvious that there is no possible brain function remaining, such as when a person's body has been incinerated, pulverised, or is clearly rotting. Otherwise, a combination of tests for residual cardiorespiratory and neurological function are performed. A doctor will check for signs of breathing or cardiac activity.[†] In addition, they will check for responsiveness to pain by pushing down on the patient's

* When they're left on cardiorespiratory support.

† As noted previously, this is more because if cardiorespiratory functions have ceased then brain functions will stop shortly thereafter, not because blood circulation alone is

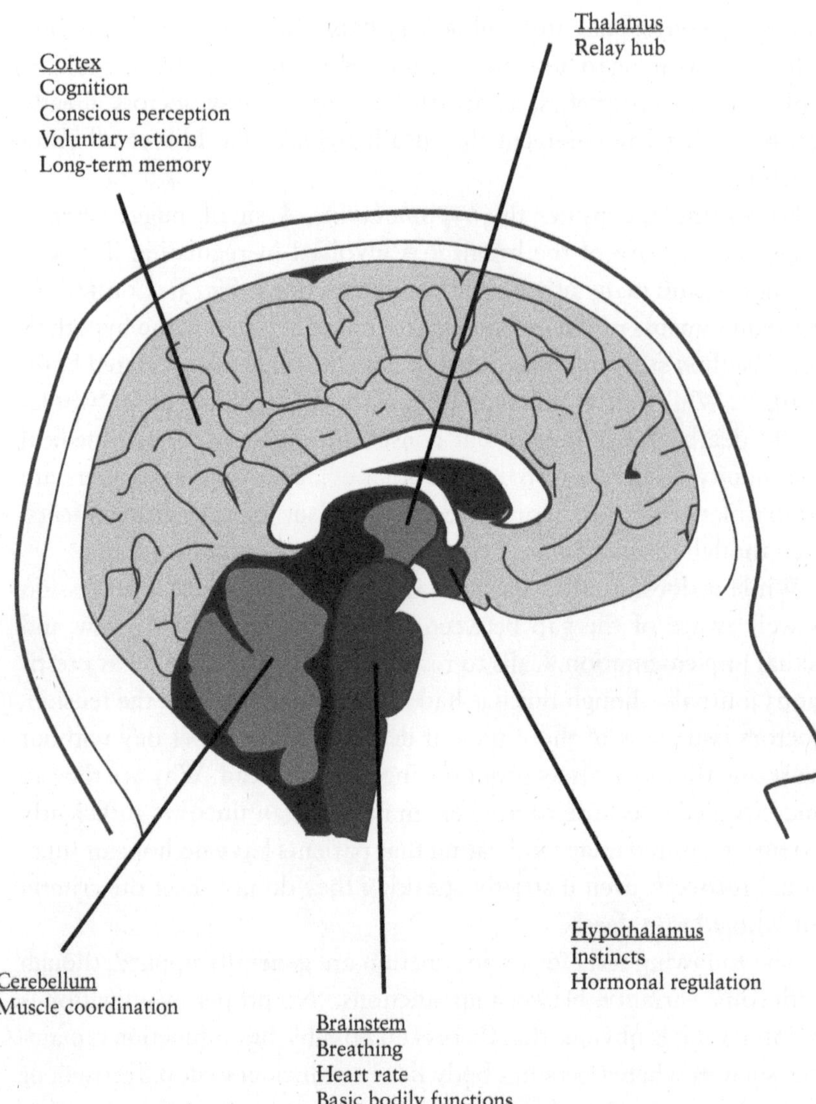

Figure 3. A side-on view of the middle of the brain.

forehead, and for a pupillary response by shining a light into their eyes. If none of these signs are present, the patient can be declared dead.

These simple tests are taken to be accurate indicators of death because they assess the function of the *brainstem*, a brain region critical for normal functioning. The brainstem is an evolutionarily primitive anatomical structure resembling the stem of a plant, connecting the spinal cord at its roots to the rest of the brain at its branches. It regulates certain basic functions such as breathing, heart rate, and the overall wakefulness of the rest of the brain. Damage to the entire brainstem necessarily entails permanent loss of consciousness and breathing, so checking for brainstem death is a convenient shortcut for assessing whole-brain death. The pupil shrinkage that doctors are looking for is useful because the clusters of neurons that control constriction are present in the brainstem, so a persistent absence of shrinking pupils is a pretty clear indication the patient won't ever be coming to again. The everyday bedside examinations described above are normally sufficient to declare a patient dead because brainstem death suggests widespread, irreversible cessation of important brain functions.

Yet, in the same way that doctors dismiss ongoing hypothalamic functions as signs of life in patients with brainstem damage, there are calls by some philosophers to recognize certain patients as dead even if some brainstem function is maintained. Sometimes much of the brain can be destroyed while sparing the brainstem, meaning the corresponding body may continue spontaneously breathing while doing little else. The *higher-brain* view of death, in contrast to *whole-brain*, claims that, in circumstances such as these, whether a person's body has a gag reflex is as irrelevant to whether they're alive as whether their fingernails are growing.[10] Advocates argue that if a person's reasoning functions are gone, their memories destroyed, with no self-awareness remaining, and in fact no capacity to experience anything at all, then the person is dead. Because evidence suggests that higher-brain structures such as the *cortex* support these functions, the argument goes, cortical destruction alone is enough to entail death.

So far, no jurisdiction nor medical association has endorsed the

---

taken to be important. If that were the case, every brain-dead patient could be 'revived' by hooking them up to a cardiopulmonary bypass machine.

higher-brain concept of death, even if actual medical practice suggests implicit support for the idea. There are several reasons why this is the case. The largest is that many people are disturbed by the idea that a spontaneously breathing human could be dead.* Another is that it is much more difficult to design useful diagnostic tools for higher-brain death than brainstem death.† A further issue is that there are no generally agreed-upon criteria for determining the degree of higher-brain damage required for irreversible loss of personhood. Without a widely accepted theory of consciousness it is difficult to tell the difference between a patient whom brain damage has left irreversibly unconscious and a patient possessing severely degraded consciousness.

Additionally, in the absence of similarly clear markers as in brainstem death, there are fears that criteria based on higher-brain death may erroneously mark patients as dead who may one day recover consciousness. Unless a better understanding of the exact brain mechanisms that underlie consciousness is found, or disregard for spontaneous breathing becomes widespread, the higher-brain concept is unlikely to become broadly adopted.

This decision to require destruction of the brainstem, rather than just the cortex, is thus more of a pragmatic choice than a rigorously defensible philosophical position. Doctors have been tasked with fulfilling the social need to identify when individuals die, and have chosen uncontroversial and conservative criteria to mark the boundary. Their aim is to declare dead only those with absolutely no hope of regaining consciousness, while being sensitive to differing cultural and religious views. They are also acutely aware that people are much more disturbed by falsely declaring living patients as dead than vice

* The American medico-legal case of Karen Ann Quinlan is a paradigmatic example. In 1975, she entered a persistent vegetative state at the age of twenty-one, after she stopped breathing for twenty minutes due to consuming alcohol and benzodiazepines. Imaging showed signs of irreversible higher-brain damage, and she was eventually taken off a ventilator after some legal controversy. Though her body continued breathing due to an intact brainstem and 'lived' for another nine years, she never regained signs of consciousness.

† In particular, doctors are worried about missing cases of *locked-in syndrome*, where a patient is completely paralysed but still conscious. Sophisticated behavioural tasks and brain scans are able to show evidence of this in a small number of brain-injury patients.

versa. As a result, doctors err closer to the whole- than higher-brain concept of death. In doing so, they take the safer route of declaring dead only those with such extensive brain damage that their irreversible loss of consciousness is uncontroversial.

This conservative choice is still controversial, though, as it may be killing more patients than it saves. Failure to declare patients with higher-brain death dead can mean that other, definitively conscious patients die who would otherwise live. Current organ transplantation practice follows the *dead donor rule*, which states that a person must be dead before life-prolonging organs can be procured from them. Some think it is deeply unethical that a patient with higher-brain death, who will never regain consciousness, is kept in care while their organs could be used to extend the life of one or more active, conscious, hopeful patients. Others think that taking donations from such patients would be an unconscionable act of murder, regardless of the positive consequences it may have. Another take is that even if doctors broadly agreed that higher-brain death should be considered death proper, this shouldn't be acted upon without clear public support. This comes from a worry that more organs would be lost from people withdrawing consent to be potential organ donors, due to fear of being wrongfully pronounced dead, than would be gained from the small number of cases of higher-brain death without brainstem death. The debate on this is not settled, though there are no signs any jurisdictions are considering shifting from the whole-brain definition anytime soon.

Regardless, all these definitions of death are unsatisfying if we want to know when a person is dead in principle, even in the face of considerably better medicine than we have today. None of the current definitions really try to address what it is for brain damage to be truly irreversible. To know where this point-of-no-return is, we need to examine how brain damage occurs in a dying brain at a deeper level than just loss of whole brain regions. I'm sorry, this is going to be even less pleasant to think about than the chapter has already been thus far. But if we want to know where the limit is, we need to look at exactly what would be happening in your brain if you were imminently dying.

FROM CARDIAC ARREST TO BRAIN DEATH: A TIMELINE OF DYING

Imagine Alex is at home sitting on the couch when she suffers an untimely cardiac arrest. Her heart is no longer pumping blood around her body, so her organs are suddenly starved of life-sustaining nutrients and oxygen. Poor Alex is now rapidly dying, her cells screaming for food and choking on their own waste products. Prompt medical attention could potentially save her. The question is, how long does Alex have before she is irreversibly dead (Fig. 4)?

About fifteen seconds after her heart stops beating, Alex's subjective experience will dissolve into unconsciousness.[*,11] This is so quick because the brain is disproportionately energy hungry, consuming 20 per cent of the body's energy, yet has essentially no reserves. Specifically, Alex's neurons are no longer able to regulate the release of *neurotransmitters*, the chemicals neurons use to send signals to each other, as this process is particularly energy intensive.[12,13] Without precise neurotransmitter release there can be no coordination of activity between neurons, a prerequisite of consciousness according to any scientific theory. Scalp recordings of her brain waves would correspondingly show a complete loss of cortical activity. If Alex does not receive medical attention soon her unconsciousness will become permanent. Things may seem dire, but at this stage there is still hope.

At about the ninety-second mark, Alex's neurons will run out of energy and become unable to send electrical signals along the branching dendrites and axons of their cell bodies.[14] In essence, this is similar to a phone line losing power – the line is still there, but it no longer functions.[†] At this point her neurons are no longer capable of information

* Probably at this stage, and definitely within one minute, Alex will also stop breathing. This doesn't really matter, as without blood circulation breathing is pointless.

† Neurons are unable to conduct electrical signals from this point onwards because of the loss of power to their ion pumps. Under normal conditions these pumps ensure unequal concentrations of sodium, potassium, and calcium ions are maintained inside and outside the neurons, which is necessary for electrical signalling. When cellular energy sources are depleted, these pumps cease working and ion concentrations equalize between the inside and outside of the neurons. The loss of the ion-concentration gradient results in the loss

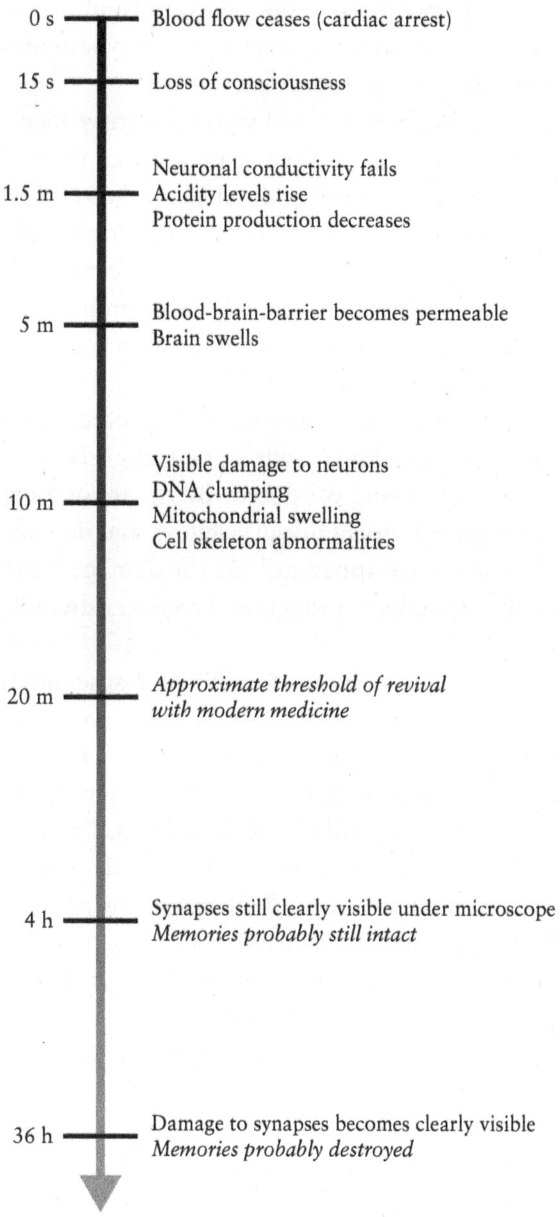

Figure 4. The timeline of changes to the brain following cardiac arrest.

processing even if they were receiving coherent neurotransmitter signals. Neuronal conductivity failure due to depleted energy supplies marks the beginning of the danger zone for Alex.

From here on out, her starving neurons will start to destroy themselves in their panic and desperation.[15] Molecular pumps that control the flow of ions like sodium, potassium, and calcium start to fail, flooding some areas of the neurons with ion levels they cannot handle. A particularly bad result of this is that abnormally high internal concentrations of calcium lead to dysregulation of mitochondria, the energy-producing organelles of the cell. The carbon dioxide they generate as a waste product cannot be removed by the blood and instead accumulates as acid.* Increasing acidity damages the proteins that make up the existing molecular machinery, while the lack of cellular energy means new proteins stop being produced. By the ten-minute mark, abnormal DNA clumping, mitochondrial swelling, and damage to the neuron's internal skeleton are apparent.[16] As the damage accumulates, Alex's chances of ever making a functional recovery dwindle smaller and smaller.

Without medical attention, Alex's chances of successful resuscitation are dropping at roughly 5 per cent per minute.[17] As time goes on, Alex's brain becomes so vulnerable that ironically even restarting her blood flow will invite damage. In part, this is because by the five-minute mark, the protective blood–brain barrier has partially broken down. This barrier normally exists to shield the brain from infection or dangerous chemicals that might be carried by the blood. Breaches in this cerebral sea-wall not only let fluid in, resulting in dangerous swelling, but also mean that the return of blood flow will allow inflammatory and toxic materials to enter her brain.[18] At this point, Alex's life is not so much hanging in the balance as rolling rapidly towards the edge of the abyss.

Probably within five to twenty minutes following cardiac arrest, Alex passes the threshold at which current medicine is able to restore her to consciousness.[19] If nobody finds and attempts to resuscitate her,

---

of a voltage difference across the surface of the cell, and with it the ability to conduct electrical signals.

* It's actually more complicated than this and includes steps involving bicarbonate buffers, lactic acid, and other enzymes, but this will do for now. Sorry.

she will reach the whole-brain definition of death once her brainstem is sufficiently damaged. But even if she is found and cardiopulmonary resuscitation (CPR) started early enough to prevent irreversible loss of spontaneous breathing, she may never regain consciousness.[20]

If she is resuscitated just before the transition to whole-brain death, her body may survive in a *coma*. In this state, enough brainstem neurons survive to command spontaneous breathing, but that's about all the behaviour her nervous system can muster.

Were Alex to be resuscitated a little earlier, she may instead end up in a *persistent vegetative state*.[21] In this case, a little bit more of the brainstem has survived, and Alex displays signs of a sleep-wake cycle as well as spontaneous breathing. This means that she may open and close her eyes for periods of the day, and even perform eye movements, but without showing any responsiveness or environmental awareness.[22] Unintuitively, perhaps, this is no clear indicator that Alex is somehow conscious. Sleep is such a primitive neurological function that it can even be found in animals without brains, such as jellyfish and worms.[23] Sadly, all Alex's sleep-wake cycle indicates is the survival of a simple brainstem circuit akin to an alarm clock, nothing more.

Resuscitated a bit earlier still and it becomes hard to tell whether Alex returns to consciousness or not. A *minimally conscious state* can occur if some of her cortex is spared in addition to her brainstem. In this case Alex would still show heavily impaired behaviour, but may be able to provide very basic responses, such as occasional eye movements in response to a yes/no question. Brain scans would show greatly reduced activity relative to a neurotypical person, but still significantly more than if she were in a comatose or vegetative state.

From here on, earlier resuscitation means increasingly better clinical outcomes. Patients may suffer 'only' from memory loss and other cognitive impairments, while a lucky few may not show detectable impairments.[24,25] If CPR and resuscitation is commenced early enough, Alex may even make a full recovery.

But even if no-one finds her, it's worth noting that the moment Alex slips past modern medicine's point of no return and suffers 'irreversible' damage is not indicated by a definitive change in the structure of her brain. On the one hand, her neurons would have stopped communicating long before this time, having been silent for many minutes now. On the other hand, much of the important structure of her brain will continue to exist for some time. In particular, the synaptic connections between neurons that store Alex's memories may well still be intact. Some mild swelling of the neurons is apparent five minutes after cardiac arrest, but not enough to destroy the synapses.[*,26] In fact, Alex's synapses are still clearly identifiable at least four hours after her blood flow has ceased, and often don't become difficult to make out until almost a full day has passed.[27,28] Not enough research has yet been done to determine the exact rate of synaptic degradation, and it's possible that molecular-level damage occurs to the synapses earlier than they become visibly damaged under a microscope.[†] But it certainly seems plausible that Alex's memories still exist for hours after she draws her final breath. While modern medical science is unable to repair the damage incurred from twenty minutes of neural asphyxiation, it's not at all inconceivable that better technology could push this window further out.

If future medicine could push the point of irreversibility from twenty to forty minutes, or further still, how are we to decide when Alex has died? Does it matter if we push this limit back through keeping the current neurons intact longer, or is replacing them fine? As one of the best-known defenders of the whole-brain view of death claimed in 1998, 'the idea of a mechanical, electrical, or synthetic brain [. . .] would force us to alter completely our concepts of death and personhood'.[29] As we will soon observe, this crisis in definition entailed by biotechnological progress is already at our doorstep. Once we take a look at the facts, we'll see why a philosophically rigorous replacement for current death definitions is needed before this technological trend develops any further.

* The review cited here by Krassner and colleagues is the most comprehensive review of this literature that I'm aware of.

† It's equally possible that the information in them actually lasts even longer, and that the visible damage can easily be compensated for through sophisticated analysis techniques.

NEAR-TERM TRENDS IN REVERSING BRAIN DAMAGE

Less than a century ago, the idea that someone could be alive without a functioning heart or lungs was so unbelievable that no real effort was made to define death with any more precision than 'the person stopped breathing'. Yet with ventilators, cardiopulmonary bypass machines, and extracorporeal membrane oxygenation there is now an arsenal of methods to revitalize your body at its untimely brink. So, after releasing a sigh of relief over our better chances of surviving heart attacks these days, we should take a deep breath and dive into exploring the equivalent methods scientists are developing to replace damaged brain tissue.

The most straightforward approach is replacement: exchanging dead brain cells with new ones that take on the functions of the old.[30] Cells in many other organs are capable of doing this, so this is a tried-and-true method elsewhere in the body. Skin can grow back if damaged, and replaces itself every month even if it isn't. The liver can regenerate to full size even if large chunks of it are destroyed. Both organs do this by using *stem cells*, immature cells that have two jobs. Individual stem cells may be kept in reserve, merely replacing themselves and ensuring a steady supply of new stem cells. Otherwise, they can fulfil their destiny by maturing and specializing into a non-replicating cell that performs a particular role. For example, a stem cell in your bone marrow may continue to reproduce itself for a while, before possibly maturing into an immune cell, or maybe a red blood cell. From a brain-repair perspective, the hope is that it may be possible to transplant stem cells into damaged brain regions, coax them to mature into neurons, and have those neurons support or replace the broken neural circuitry.

Unfortunately, if this was going to work easily it would probably have already evolved naturally, so it's unsurprising that developing stem-cell therapies for brain damage has been difficult. Unlike other organs, the adult human brain has either no or extremely limited capacity for natively making new neurons. This is probably because under healthy conditions, making new neurons would do more harm than good. One issue is that new neurons can destabilize existing neural circuitry, resulting in memory loss.*[31] Another is that the distances between brain regions are much greater in an adult than a developing brain, and there are no signposts for any newly growing neurons to find their way. In the same way it is much more difficult to retrofit cables into a pre-existing building than to install them initially while it's under construction, it is challenging for these new neurons to form appropriate connections. These problems mean that from an evolutionary perspective the costs of repair outweigh the benefits. Sadly for us, evolution finds it cheaper for a brain-damaged human to just die and be replaced than to spend the effort designing a brain that can repair itself.

Thankfully, medicine exists to counteract the cruelties of nature, and scientists have been undeterred from attempting to develop stem cell therapies to alleviate brain damage. The clearest successes so far have been seen in Parkinson's disease, a neurodegenerative disorder with relatively well-defined pathology. Part of the problem with the disease is that a specific population of dopamine-producing neurons in the brainstem start to die, and the subsequent loss of dopamine causes symptoms such as muscle control difficulties. Implantation of stem cells into this region can produce some degree of functional integration and recovery in certain patients, though the treatments have by no means cured the disease.[32] This work is inspiring, and attempts are being made to try similar therapies for trauma- or stroke-induced damage.

Unfortunately, these other cases are much harder to treat, due to the damage being less well-defined and the neural circuitry much more complicated. A recent study did show some promise in using stem cells to improve muscle control recovery in patients with traumatic brain injuries.[33] However, it's not clear whether the improvement was due to functional replacement of the dead neurons by new ones, or through some other mechanism such as an increase in non-neuronal support cells. This is a challenging area of research, and, despite a couple of promising results, there are many clinical trials that have failed to show benefits of stem cell therapy. Still, the work that does

* Most new neuron production is done in fetal development and early childhood, with neuron population size declining thereafter. Forgetting early childhood memories may be caused by the insertion of new neurons disrupting the circuitry that stores memories, an issue that goes away as neuron production decreases.

exist may provide a proof-of-principle that some brain damage is reversible through growing new neurons to replace the dead ones.

A different approach is to dispense with the difficulties of biology and to try and reverse brain damage through wholly artificial means. After all, the current definition of death is concerned only with 'irreversible cessation of all *functions* of the brain'. Only the continuity of the process is required, not the retention of the original equipment. If those with false teeth can chew, those with artificial lenses can see, and those with cochlear implants can hear, then presumably we should be unconcerned by replacing neural tissue with machines, so long as function is maintained.* This is the motivation behind *neural prostheses*, electronics implanted into the nervous system to replace dead neurons or augment the function of those that remain. This is not just the realm of science fiction – real world examples have already been deployed, with varying degrees of sophistication.

One of the newest and most impressive neural prostheses is a device that partially compensates for a loss of brainstem regulation of blood pressure. A careful balance of blood pressure is required for the brain and other organs to function – too low and you'll faint, too high and you run the risk of a stroke. Maintaining the correct pressure is a complicated balancing act for the cardiovascular system. It needs to keep blood flow to important organs like the brain constant, working harder or gentler depending on whether someone is running around or lying down. In a healthy person, sensors in the brainstem rapidly detect any changes in blood pressure and order the heart and blood vessels to compensate. If these sensors are destroyed, or their connection to the cardiovascular system severed by spinal cord damage, a person can develop debilitating dizziness, fainting, and other symptoms.

A thirty-eight-year-old man who suffered a broken neck provides a concrete example of how this circuitry can be manipulated. In 2021, in an effort to alleviate the patient's symptoms, a team of scientists

* Depending on your preferred theory of consciousness (for example, if you subscribe to integrated information theory), you may have concerns that the architecture of the machine needs to be structured in a particular way, as well as having the same input/output relationships as the original brain tissue. In that case, my point still holds for the subset of neural prostheses with neuromorphic designs. We'll discuss this in much greater detail later.

and doctors implanted a neural prosthesis onto his spinal cord.[34] To check whether his blood pressure is within the healthy range, the device uses input sensors that directly monitor blood pressure. If it detects a reading which is out-of-bounds, the device sends output signals to his heart and blood vessels that alter their activity and bring blood pressure back into the appropriate range. When activated after surgery, this neural prosthesis led to an almost complete resolution of his symptoms. In implanting the device to treat his illness, the surgeons had effectively replaced part of his brain and spinal cord.

Some success has also been seen in replacing loss of muscle control due to brain damage. As with the stem cell examples before, some of the earliest-developed neural prostheses have been used to treat Parkinson's disease. Again, because the damage in this disease is relatively well understood, the treatment is more straightforward. Brain regions that control muscle functions are regulated by dopamine-producing neurons in the brainstem, and in a patient with Parkinson's disease these neurons are dying. If the activity of those neurons can be replaced, then muscle control should be correspondingly restored. This is exactly the goal of *deep brain stimulation*, where electrodes are implanted directly into brain regions controlling muscle function. These implanted electrodes provide stimulation that compensates for the loss of brainstem dopamine neurons, partially replacing this section of the brainstem. Patients who receive these implants typically see about a 50 per cent amelioration in function, and this will hopefully keep improving over time. Older and cruder versions of these prostheses provided constant stimulation while turned on, while newer models are becoming better at mimicking natural brainstem activity.[35]

Going beyond the basics, neural prostheses are not just limited to restoring basic functions like blood pressure and motor control. Memory improvements have been demonstrated in a series of studies on a neural prosthesis in rodent and monkey models.[37,38] When researchers implanted the device into the hippocampus, a brain region important for memory formation, the device appeared to improve the retention of at least short-term memories. In doing so, the implant demonstrates the possibility of replacing not just the brainstem but also parts of higher-brain structures like the hippocampus.

Lastly, there is a particularly poignant example of a neural prosthesis reversing brain damage associated with disorders of consciousness.[39] Another unfortunate thirty-eight-year-old man, different from the previous example, had suffered a severe brain injury after being assaulted, leaving him non-verbal, unable to communicate, and probably unconscious. After six years of being cared for in a nursing home, the patient was re-evaluated with a variety of brain imaging techniques. These showed two relevant factors. Firstly, the damage he had suffered had been to non-cortical brain areas that controlled the activity of other brain regions, such as the thalamus. Secondly, despite the reduction in global brain activity and probable unconsciousness, there was some evidence for intact cortical structures. On this basis, the patient was implanted with a deep brain stimulator into his thalamus, the brain region between the brainstem and the cortex that acts as a relay hub for all cortical activity. The hope was that the patient's cortex could be 'woken up' by increasing activity in the thalamus, and therefore increasing activity in the cortical areas to which it connects. An immediate sign of success was seen about two days after the surgery, when the stimulator was first tested. Seemingly miraculously, though very much the product of hard scientific labour, the patient started opening his eyes and turning his head towards a voice. Over the coming months the patient's behaviour continued to improve as he became able to bring a cup to his mouth, chew food, and even communicate to a limited degree. Unfortunately, he could by no means be considered to have recovered completely, and he still required significant nursing care. Nonetheless this was clearly a success story, with his prosthesis able to somewhat reverse the loss of critical brain functions. If this patient could be restored to consciousness after six years of oblivion, there is hope that other cases of 'irreversible loss' may also turn out to be much more reversible than they currently seem.

Neither stem cells nor neural prostheses are mature technologies as of yet, and their limitations are still considerable. So far, they are only able to help certain patients with certain kinds of brain damage. Stem cell therapy struggles with issues of sourcing the cells, immune rejection, inducing the cells to grow into appropriate neuron types, encouraging the neurons to connect properly, and trying to make sure the stem cells don't accidentally give the patient cancer. Neural prostheses are also limited by immune rejection, as well as electrode size and stiffness, power consumption, targeting the right brain regions, appropriate stimulation patterns, and a list of other issues. Yet these issues are likely to be surmountable, and a lot of companies such as Elon Musk's Neuralink are throwing considerable resources at these problems. With time and money these stumbling blocks will be overcome through technological improvement, extending and expanding the scope of recovery for today's 'irreversible' brain damage.

It is clear that the current 'irreversible heart and/or brain cessation' definition of death is being rendered increasingly obsolete. Indeed, as doctors and bioethicists themselves admit, this definition has only ever been accepted on pragmatic grounds.[40] This uneasy status quo cannot hold, as advancing neuroscience is only going to make the inadequacies of the current definition more and more stark. As discussed in the beginning of the chapter, a definition of death is essential for any society. But as we've been seeing, once a society develops sufficiently advanced medical technology, a specific need arises for philosophically and neuroscientifically rigorous definitions of irreversibility and death. Now that we have an understanding of what happens in a dying brain, and how the damage might be reversed, we can provide exactly that.

DEATH IS THE LOSS OF PERSONAL IDENTITY

Let's jump back to Alex, who we last saw dying on the couch. It turns out she was found about thirty minutes after her cardiac arrest and has been taken to a hospital. Her distraught spouse Blake arrives shortly thereafter, inconsolable to find Alex frail and unresponsive, punctured by reams of cords, and breathing mechanically through a ventilator. Medical examination shows she has suffered brain death, and typically she would be pronounced legally dead at this point. But imagine instead that the doctors inform the distraught Blake that there is a new treatment they could try. Recent advances have enabled a brain from a recently deceased donor to be implanted into Alex's skull, taking the place of the damaged original brain. They reassure Blake by saying the procedure has been done many times with other organs such as kidneys, livers, and hearts, and, while doing it with a brain is more complicated, they've now got the procedure working with a decent survival rate. Unfortunately, they make clear that there will be some side effects. Alex will lose all of her memories, and will also have considerable personality change. She won't recognize Blake, and may well not even be attracted to them. 'Still,' the doctors say, 'performing the procedure means that Alex would survive, and that's what's important, right?'

I doubt anyone believes Alex would survive this procedure, despite the fact that a brain donation would ensure Alex's body did not suffer cessation of brain functions. In contrast, replacement of any other of her organs would be fine. No-one questions whether a liver- or lung-donation recipient has survived, so long as they emerge from anaesthesia after the operation. For some reason, though, transplanting a donor brain into Alex's body isn't the same. Almost everyone would agree that Alex died along with her damaged brain, and if anyone survives in Alex's body it would in fact be the brain donor.

Why is total brain replacement unacceptable? After all, replacing its subcomponents is no problem. A healthy brain, just like any other organ, is constantly replacing parts of itself: all of the ion channels, structural proteins, mitochondria, and other cellular components in Alex's neurons are constantly being removed and recreated. Given this is happening in everyone all of the time, it would be rather odd to say this level of replacement constitutes death. Furthermore, this natural process is similar to a thought experiment we'll consider formally in the next chapter, in which a person's neurons are gradually replaced with synthetic counterparts over time. Though importantly, in that case, the synthetic neurons maintain the same synaptic connections as their previous biological equivalents, meaning no information would be lost during the replacement process. If Alex had undergone that procedure, instead of a cardiac arrest and subsequent brain death, we'd have significantly less doubt about whether she had survived. What makes these natural or synthetic replacement cases different from brain donation?

Let's consider one final example before formalizing our intuitions. This time, imagine a case where, instead of global brain damage, Alex instead suffered only from a brainstem stroke. It destroyed the neural circuitry that regulated her breathing and heart rate, as well as that required to maintain wakefulness. But if her other brain areas are kept supplied with oxygenated blood, they should be able to survive and resume their functions if the damaged brainstem is replaced. As long as she receives a prosthetic or donor brainstem, Alex will once again have the same memories, personality, and behaviour as before her stroke. In light of this, it seems to me that so long as the procedure is successful, it is likely that both Alex herself and her family would be comfortable with the replacement of her brainstem. Why would this be okay, but not a whole-brain donation?

The key difference is that Alex's personal identity is lost in the case of whole-brain transplantation, a process that discards her memories, desires, intellect, and other aspects of her identity, but survives in cases of natural or synthetic replacement that retains them. Existing treatments like deep-brain stimulation can replace some of the functions of one's brainstem, and nobody is arguing that their usage kills the patient. It's not a large step to extend this to a neural prosthesis that replaces the breathing, cardiovascular, and wakefulness regulation of the brainstem entirely, in much the same way we don't feel someone dies when they receive a heart transplant. Pushing this even further, a future technology that could replace all neurons with functional artificial equivalents does not concern me, so long as this could be done without change of personality or loss of memory. In this case, the person with artificial neurons wouldn't feel any different, and no-one around them would notice a change in their behaviour.

Formally, this is the philosophical position of defining *death* as 'the irreversible loss of personal identity'.[41] By this definition, a person does not die once their heart stops or their brainstem fails to tell their lungs to breathe. Nor do they still exist if a sole surviving neuron is still sending signals, despite its 86 billion fellows having ceased. Instead, a specific person survives so long as the personality, memories, desires, and other core aspects that make up their identity still exist. To put it another way, it is when these core aspects of a person's self are irreversibly lost that the person has died.

This definition is similar to, but not quite the same as, the higher-brain concept of death. Under the higher-brain definition, a person dies once they irreversibly lose functions critical for personhood, such as consciousness. But it says nothing about whether a person needs to retain the psychological properties core to their identity in order to survive. By the higher-brain definition, a brain transplant or prosthetic implant that erases all aspects of a person's identity could still be said to keep the person alive. As per the hypothetical case of Alex above, this doesn't accord well with many people's intuitions of what it means to survive.

The personal-identity definition of death separates 'brain death' from the actual death of a person in the same way that cardiopulmonary bypass machines have separated 'heart death' from actual death.[42] Nowadays, we recognize that someone can still be alive even if their heart has stopped. In the same way, neural prostheses will increasingly allow people to live even when parts of their brain have died. We also understand that someone may have died even if their heart is still beating, such as when a brain-dead patient is left on a ventilator. Equivalently, it's possible to imagine a case where someone has died even though all their brain functions remain, not just the basics of the brainstem. Imagine a hypothetical procedure that wiped a person's autobiographical memories and personality while leaving their language, motor, and reasoning skills intact. This could maybe be done by randomly reconnecting a proportion of someone's cortical synapses while leaving the neurons alive.* This procedure would kill the original user of the brain by wiping out their personal identity, just as surely as in the brain transplant case. Afterwards, it is a new person who would inherit the brain, even while making use of the same neurons that existed before the procedure. The point being, while both heart death and brain death normally result in actual death, it's not obligatory for this to be the case. Rather, your survival depends on the maintenance of intricate neuronal connections in your brain that provide you your identity.

Death as the irreversible loss of personal identity is also known as *information-theoretic death*, which means much the same thing but with a different focus.[43] Information-theoretic death emphasizes that a person dies when the information that comprises their personal identity is irretrievably lost. Notably, this doesn't define someone who is asleep or anaesthetized as dead, where personal identity information is still present in the brain but not currently being accessed. It

* Perhaps through the selective transplantation of stem cells, or the use of targeted drugs to dramatically increase neuroplasticity in certain regions.

also doesn't include a person who has recently suffered cardiac arrest, as modern medical technology is often successful at restoring these patients to a point where they can regain consciousness and assert their identity again. Critically, it also doesn't include someone whose brain cannot be restored to function with current medicine, but who theoretically could be with better technology. In contrast, a person whose brain has been cremated is dead by information-theoretic standards, as no future technology could recreate their synapses from their ashes. 'Irreversible loss' is now finally defined in a physically absolute sense, meaning lost to medical technology unimaginably more advanced than that currently available.

To summarize, as long as personal-identity information survives, a person survives. It doesn't matter if the information is unused for a few hours, as in the case of sleep, a few days, as in the case of a medically induced coma, or longer still. As an analogy, consider the case of whether a specific text is said to still exist or not, such as *The Epic of Gilgamesh*. Under what circumstances can this tale of Gilgamesh's search for immortality still potentially enthral a reader? If *The Epic of Gilgamesh* exists as a book in a library, the text has definitely survived, even if no-one is currently reading it. If the book is shredded, it may become impossible to read for a time, but because the shreds could be put back together the text cannot be considered lost yet.* Perhaps the text is written on broken tablets that have lain buried for thousands of years, to be later found by people who cannot read the language in which it is written. Even then, if the pieces can be put back together, and the language decoded and translated, the text cannot be considered irreversibly lost. In the same way, so long as the synaptic connections and other neural information that record personal identity exist in some form, a person has not truly died.

Lastly, there is one significant concern with the personal-identity definition of death that is worth acknowledging. The problem is that information is not necessarily lost in an all-or-nothing fashion, but can instead degrade to a greater or lesser degree. A novel with a few

* For example, just after the American–Vietnamese war, the North Vietnamese reassembled shredded American intelligence documents and used the information to track down former US employees.

words missing is basically unchanged. With a few pages missing the story may become occasionally confusing, but is usually still interpretable. At a certain level of damage the book becomes incomprehensible. But how can the point at which the book is damaged to the point of destruction be defined? In the same way, what degree of loss of personal identity information can a person survive, and what level of loss constitutes death?

As was the case earlier, I cannot give a definitive answer as to where the line is, as I suspect in fact there is none. In reality, there is a blurry continuum, and where exactly the line is drawn is a matter of personal and societal choice. That is not to say that the choice is completely arbitrary; there are clear cases that can guide our intuitions and provide some boundaries. If someone drinks themself blackout drunk and loses a night's worth of memories, I think it's still clear the person has survived. On the other hand, if someone has suffered so much brain damage that all their memories are gone and the remaining personality is completely altered, I would consider the person dead. The exact degree of loss a person can survive is still a serious open research question for philosophers and neuroscientists, with such profound ethical implications that all of society should weigh in.

But we don't need to know exactly where the line is for the definition to still be useful. All we need is a conservative bound on how much information can be lost before a person dies, such that if they haven't lost that much, they definitely haven't died. As long as there is a way to stop that amount of information from being lost, then there is a way to save someone.

DELIMITING DEATH

This chapter covered a lot of neuroscientific and philosophical ground, so let's summarize. Recent advances in medical science have made traditional cardio-respiratory views of death obsolete. Current laws also include a whole-brain destruction view of death, but this definition is philosophically unsound and doctors routinely ignore it in actual clinical practice. Problematically, both these definitions define death based on irreversible loss of function, seemingly unconcerned that irreversibility is determined by the technology of the day. This results in the absurd position of a person being defined dead based on what medical equipment is in their vicinity rather than because of intrinsic properties of their body.

In response to these problems, I've shown how a definition of death based on irreversible loss of personal identity provides an intuitive and philosophically consistent view. Whether a person can move their legs, grow their nails, or beat their heart is ultimately irrelevant to their survival. Instead, a person survives so long as the potential remains for them to take joy in their successes, mourn what they have lost, remember how they have helped those they love, and otherwise express their identity.* A person dies when the neural information that comprises their personal identity is permanently lost in a physically absolute sense. It is this information-theoretic death that should be considered actual death, and it is ultimately this we must avoid if one seeks to survive.

I should acknowledge that this chapter has concerned itself with death as it relates specifically to people, rather than the alternate concept of 'biological death'. Although I think I've provided sufficient examples to show how these two can be distinguished, some people will still object that a distinction can be drawn between 'the death of a person' and 'biological death'. One position they may hold is that death should be commonly defined across biological creatures as 'the loss of an organism as an integrated whole'.[44] According to this view, a creature lives so long as its body, considered holistically, has properties that are greater than the sum of its parts. Examples of these properties may be maintaining an energy balance, excreting waste products, coordinating movement, or defending against infection. While loss of these properties is a useful indicator of death when considering biological systems, I think there are two major reasons why the definition is unhelpful for assessing when a person has died.

Firstly, there are many kinds of biological disintegration that can occur with seemingly no bearing on whether a person has lived or

* The idea that someone has partially died when they suffer severe brain trauma or other extreme changes to their identity is not, on this view, merely a metaphor, but a claim worthy of serious consideration.

died.* I don't feel that a person made quadriplegic due to a spinal cord injury has partially died. The same holds for a person with diabetes unable to regulate their blood sugar, with their intestines removed due to bowel cancer, or with immunodeficiency due to HIV infection. All of these are examples of significant degrees of loss in an organism acting as an integrated and coordinated whole, yet none of them even raise the question of whether or not a person has died.

Secondly, and more importantly, I and others do not think conceptualizing people as 'organisms with integrated wholes' captures what we care about when contemplating death.[45] Consider how individual cells within a human can also be examined through the integrated whole approach. They need to maintain an energy balance, excrete waste products, coordinate their cell skeleton in order to move, and have subcellular organelles to help them do all these things. These same cells die in their trillions every day and we shed no tears for them. Using the same term 'death' to describe the permanent cessation of both these cells and an organism of which they might be a part provides a convenient descriptive tool for a group of common behaviours. But its very breadth is also suggestive of its irrelevance when applied to the creatures we are actually concerned about. A decapitated human's body may be able to be kept alive indefinitely using extracorporeal membrane oxygenation and other medical equipment, yet it still seems as though the person has been lost. It is clear that we have a very different kind of reverence for the deaths of people compared to the deaths of amoebae, plants, sponges, or other organisms without personhood or personal identity.

At this stage you may still be filled with scepticism and caution around the conclusions of this chapter. 'If the personal-identity definition of death is so much better, why hasn't it already been broadly adopted?' As you may guess, the issue has less to do with the personal-identity view being philosophically unsound and more to do with a legacy of pragmatic medical choices. As with the higher-brain definition of death, the personal-identity view does not provide clear neurological diagnostic criteria for doctors to use on patients. The

* In fact, the problems are very similar to the case of the whole-brain definition of death.

view also implies the possibility of a person having died from severe cortical damage while their body continues to breathe due to residual brainstem function. No doctor wants to explain to distraught relatives that the still-breathing body of their family member is actually dead, particularly if they don't have a philosophical consensus and clear-cut diagnostics they can point at to defend their position. This is despite the fact that at least 50 per cent of doctors privately admit these patients should be considered dead.[46]

Until now, the benefits of shifting to a personal-identity definition over the current (pseudo)-whole-brain death view have not outweighed the costs. In the absence of strong motivating reasons for doctors and laypeople alike to adopt a philosophically rigorous definition of death, doctors have quite reasonably defaulted to relatively simple markers that are clinically well defined, as well as socially and emotionally palatable.

But what the medical community has not yet realized is that this calculus changes when we take improving medical technology seriously. At the point of no return, it is always harrowing to leave distraught relatives with a simple 'I'm sorry, there's nothing more we can do . . .' Yet in a society that made use of the procedures we'll discuss in a few chapters' time, a doctor holding the personal identity view would be empowered to add the much more hopeful '. . . for now.' Over time, we have been able to save more and more patients we would previously have considered dead. If this trend holds, it suggests that there may be ways to save people who would be considered dead by today's standards. In response, doctors could shift from the difficult task of determining when exactly death occurs to instead focusing on when current medicine is no longer able to help a patient function. From this viewpoint, the burden on doctors shifts considerably and accepting the personal-identity view becomes much more attractive.

This shift would bring official doctrine into line with what doctors actually do and resolve the ongoing tension in the medical community. It could also be done with very minor adjustments to the legal system. The law already considers a person dead when a doctor says so, and equating legal death with 'no longer treatable with current technology' would require minimal changes. There would remain difficult discussions around euthanasia, but these would be similar to those we already have to deal with, and, if anything, would be easier with a better definition of death. The only major changes to both medicine and law would be in how we handle people's bodies when they reach the point where modern medicine can help them function no further.

***

Returning to where we began, it turns out the true story of Trent's trailer trauma has a happier ending than unfortunate Alex's imaginary tale. In the end, pronouncement of Trent's death was cancelled when the doctors realized their prognosis was incorrect. The day before his final scan was scheduled, Trent started showing signs of awareness. Surprisingly, given his accident, it seemed that enough of his brainstem remained intact to command his heart and lungs, and enough of his thalamus for information to flow through the brain loops that enable his consciousness.

Do not be quick to judge the doctors for prematurely deciding further care was futile, as this outcome is by no means an indictment of their skills. It is instead their triumph, as Trent would surely have been irreversibly dead without the assistance of modern medicine. By repairing his skull and restarting his heart, they bought Trent the time needed for his identity to reassert itself.

But imagine other scenarios, where the pattern of damage had been ever-so-slightly different. What if Trent's brainstem or thalamus had not been spared, and he remained unconscious indefinitely? That which makes Trent Trent would still have been there, just inaccessible through natural or modern technological means. Or, alternatively, imagine he had suffered extensive but non-lethal damage to his cortex, leaving him conscious but with his memories erased and personality altered. Would it be correct for the doctors to question Trent's survival in either or both of these scenarios? As we'll see in the next chapter, to answer this question we will need to rigorously assess the exact conditions under which one's personal identity can survive.

4
What Is Personal Identity?

Know thyself.

Ancient Greek maxim

Before the accident, ordinary Phineas Gage had no reason to believe he would become one of the most famous medical case studies of all time.[1–3] Up until about 4:30pm on 13 September 1848, he was a fit and healthy twenty-five-year-old, working as a foreman for a railroad construction team in Cavendish, Vermont. As part of his team's preparations to clear a rock obstruction with explosives, Gage had just finished pouring blasting powder and inserting a fuse into a pre-prepared borehole. More specifically, in the final moments prior to the accident, Gage was in the midst of using a thirteen-pound, three-and-a-half-foot iron tamping bar to compress the powder, ensuring that on subsequent ignition its explosive force would be maximally directed into the surrounding stone.

There is no record of what exactly the fateful commotion was, but at some point during the tamping process Gage was surprised by a noise originating from the men working behind him. Startled, he turned his head sharply to the right and jerked his tamping iron into the wall of the borehole. As the iron scraped along the rock, sparks flew, igniting the powder. To Gage's misfortune, the subsequent explosion rocketed the tamping iron out of the borehole and directly into the left side of his face. The improvised projectile entered just above his jaw, exited out the top of his head, and ultimately landed fifty feet away, smeared with blood and brains.

In a seemingly impossible stroke of fortune, Gage was somehow still alive in the aftermath. Not only that, but within minutes he was lucid and even able to walk with some assistance. When he was first seen by a doctor around half an hour later, Gage exclaimed to his rather astonished physician, 'Doctor, here is business enough for you,' and said that he hoped 'he was not much hurt'. Given Gage's brain was clearly visible through two open wounds in his skull, the doctor's shock at this statement was likely to have owed less to his patient's misplaced optimism than to the unbelievable fact that Gage could articulate anything at all.

However, despite his stoic attitude and incredible initial resilience, Gage's health soon deteriorated. Three days after his injury he became delirious, showing signs of a brain infection. By two weeks, visible fungus was growing through the wounds in his skull and on the surface of his brain, and Gage became comatose. His friends and family were summoned to his bedside, and kept waiting in hourly expectancy of his death.

Yet through the valiant efforts of Gage's attending doctor, alongside the impressive healing capacity of young humans, Gage's body endured. After a month of frequent wound drainages and applications of the antiseptic silver nitrate, the fungus disappeared. By eight weeks, he was eating and sleeping well, and had begun wandering around Cavendish. In late November, two-and-a-half months after the accident, he was even well enough to return to his hometown in New Hampshire for the winter. Miraculously, it seemed Gage was going to live.

But when Gage reported back for work in April of the next year, there was reason to question his recovery after all. It was not that there were issues with his physical health – apart from developing blindness in his left eye, Gage was fully fit and functional. Instead, as his doctor remarked, it was that 'the equilibrium [. . .] between his intellectual faculties and animal propensities, seem[ed] to have been destroyed'. Where before he had been polite and respectful, he now frequently swore, quarrelled easily with his fellows, and acted impatiently and without restraint. Previously Gage had been a shrewd and persistent operator, yet he was now too distracted and disorganized to work. The railroad company, who had previously seen him as a capable foreman, refused to re-employ him. The changes he had undergone were so radical that his friends and colleagues claimed he was 'no longer Gage'.

***

While his body lived on for another twelve years following the accident, whether or not Gage himself survived is decidedly more ambiguous. When Gage's acquaintances claimed that he was no longer the same person he was before his injury, should we take this metaphorically or literally? Answering this question requires a clear understanding of what personal identity is, and under what conditions it persists.

In the last chapter, I argued that the true definition of death is the point at which a person's identity is irreversibly destroyed. While introducing the idea, I skipped over many of the philosophical and neuroscientific details required to fully flesh out what that means. This chapter will remedy that by considering the concepts of personhood, selfhood, and personal identity at much greater length.

It may seem at first that this exercise is needlessly complicated and philosophical. After all, from Gage's own point of view, there is no indication he had any doubts about his continued survival. If he thought he was still Gage, shouldn't that be enough? From an internal vantage point, concerns about whether our 'true self' persists over time seem almost laughably abstract. When remembering the tedium of sitting through high-school maths classes, or daydreaming about travelling through sunny Spain once we finally retire, it feels impossible that these collections of experiences could belong to anyone but ourselves.

Yet when observing someone from a third-person perspective, the question of identity can feel decidedly less clear cut. Meet someone when they are an awkward, high-tempered, K-pop obsessed teenager, and again forty years later when they are a late-career professional, mother of three, with keen interests in gardening and politics, and it can feel like the two are completely different people. Include the additional changes that can occur if someone develops certain psychiatric or neurological disorders, and this feeling only grows stronger.

When the changes to a person's body or mind become sufficiently dramatic, as in Gage's story, relying on our intuitions alone to judge persistence of personal identity is precarious. As we'll see shortly, making sense of identity in medical cases where people have lost all their memories, undergone radical drug-induced personality changes, or even had their brains fused together, requires a level of rigorous reasoning beyond what our everyday intuitions can handle. These are some of the complexities we will have to wrestle with on the way to developing a robust understanding of personal identity.

Analysing these real cases will prepare us to discuss whether a person could survive medical procedures that are currently theoretical but may one day be practicable. Before ever more comprehensive neural prostheses become available, let alone the possibilities of teleportation or uploading a person's mind onto a computer, it would be good to know if use of these technologies are, in principle, survivable. Specifically, it would be helpful to ascertain whether these procedures have no hope of working at all – would be merely capable of producing a dissatisfying 'copy' of you – or if they could promise you a real and meaningful chance of survival. By the time we're done, you'll be in a much better position to judge for yourself.

Before beginning though, a couple of necessary warnings:

The first regards terminology. I am going to use terms such as *person*, *self*, *personal identity*, *copy*, and *consciousness*, despite these words having inconsistent and often conflicting uses in both the general and academic literature. To avoid confusion, I will try to make my definitions as clear as possible, and to flag when other writers might use a different term. Nonetheless, if you encounter disagreement between my usage and that of others, I can only offer my apologies and ask for your consideration.

The second warning concerns the content. Those disinclined to entertain abstract discussions may occasionally find this chapter irritatingly philosophical. While I've tried to make the material as grounded and entertaining as I can, I cannot entirely avoid forays into philosophy and its bedfellows. Still, while I would encourage you to persevere, should you find yourself feeling bored enough to put the book down at any point in either this chapter or the two that follow, I'd recommend instead skipping straight to the action in Part III. This background material will still be here if you decide you need it later.

WHAT IS A PERSON?

Before getting to personal identity, we should start by defining what a 'person' even is. In a loose sense, people are entities who are both worthy of moral concern and act as agents in the world. Healthy adult humans are definitely people – we care about their welfare and consider them responsible for their actions. In Western culture, at least, rocks aren't seen as people – we don't think they have moral status nor treat them as agents. Sometimes, as with non-human animals, the case is more ambiguous.

Depending on the context at hand, different formal systems resolve this ambiguity in different ways. In a legal sense, personhood is typically afforded to beings capable of having rights and performing duties. Which beings actually meet this criteria is evaluated by judiciaries and legislatures, which in turn rely on prevailing social norms. At various times and in different cultures, legal personhood has been restricted to only property-holding adult male citizens of a specific ethnicity, or alternatively extended beyond non-human animals to include even geographical entities such as rivers.[4]

For our purposes of assessing survival through radical medical procedures, we're going to need a definition that, ideally, applies independent of any particular legal and cultural context. A candidate provided by the philosopher John Locke in 1689, and still in popular use today, holds that a *person* is 'a thinking intelligent being, that has reason and reflection, and can consider itself as itself, the same thinking thing in different times and places [. . .]'.[5,6] Unpacking that a bit, there are three key components to this definition of personhood: consciousness, self-awareness, and some sort of continuity over time and space. Let's consider each in turn.

First, *consciousness*. By the definition above, the essential starting point for deeming some being a person is that, at least some of the time, that creature has a first-person perspective. Discussing what exactly consciousness is, how it can be characterized, and which beings might possess it is a subject so convoluted and contentious that we'd best shelve it until the next chapter. For now, it suffices to say that if something is never capable of being conscious, it is definitely not a person.

Self-consciousness, or *self-awareness*, occurs when a being is not only conscious, but also aware of the fact that it is conscious. Even if a jellyfish, with its extremely limited nervous system and lack of centralised brain, does have some kind of primitive conscious experience, it is very unlikely to be reflecting on its own existence as it drifts aimlessly on ocean currents. In contrast, adult humans are capable of recognizing themselves in a mirror, and they have occasionally even been known to introspect about their own feelings and perceive that other minds exist beside their own.

Most critical for our current purposes, though, is the notion that people have some sort of *continuity over time and space*. To be a person is to be not just aware of oneself at this current point in time, but to somehow be aware of one's past and future selves. Discussing how this continuity of selfhood occurs, and in what circumstances it can break down, will comprise the meat and potatoes of this chapter.

But before we tuck in, I hope you'll excuse one more appetizer in the form of a necessary definitional clarification. Some of you may have noticed just before that I snuck in another complicated and loaded term: the notion of the *self*. If we're to discuss continuity over time by referring to a person's past and future selves, we need to be careful about what the term actually means. What exactly the self is, what properties make it up, and whether it even exists at all is what we will turn to now.

WHAT IS THE SELF?

According to William James, one of the fathers of modern Western psychology,

> In its widest possible sense [. . .] a man's Self is the sum total of all that he can call his, not only his body and his psychic powers, but his clothes and his house, his wife and children, his ancestors and friends, his reputation and works, his lands and horses, and yacht and bank-account.[7]

By this definition, the *self* is comprised of every attribute and association a particular person may possess, from their innermost thoughts to their most weakly held cultural affiliations.

Clearly, the relative importance of different attributes varies widely. Someone's key life memories, their deepest desires and overarching goals, and the physical integrity of their body are all sufficiently important that if altered they threaten the existence of a particular self. On the other hand, while someone's preferred coffee order or mattress firmness are not entirely inconsequential to their sense of self, alterations to these details are relatively minor in comparison.

This description, of an entity composed of multiple attributes with varying degrees of importance, is by no means the only way psychologists and philosophers conceptualize the self.[8] For instance, the *minimal self* refers to a state of pure existence experienced during meditation or in the transition between sleep and wakefulness, devoid of memories and self-awareness. The *narrative self* emerges as we tell stories of our past or make predictions for our future, while the *embodied self* refers to our internal awareness of bodily sensations and physical being. Some philosophers even challenge the coherence of the notion of the self, arguing it's more of a descriptively useful heuristic than a fundamental entity. There are many further variants, but I'll spare you from an exhaustive list. Suffice it to say, the definitional inconsistency of 'selves' can make for confusing reading and unavailing discussions. Still, this chapter will use the *multiple attributes* conceptualization proposed by William James, as it accords closely with most people's intuitions of what is meant by 'the self'.

As we examine this definition further, it can be useful to categorize the attributes into those that provide a self what we call a 'sense of context' and those that give it a 'sense of agency'.* A *sense of context* refers to any attributes a person feels are ascribed to them, including things as diverse as their memories, life history, body, and material possessions. In contrast, a *sense of agency* comes from those attributes that motivate and influence someone's actions, such as one's desires, goals, and preferences. To borrow from video game terminology, consider your sense of context as your character's stats, while your sense

* I am generalizing somewhat from a framework developed by the philosopher Shaun Gallagher, though it might be more accurate to say my usage is inspired by his – Gallagher uses the term *ownership* instead of *context*, and also only employs these terms explicitly in relation to how the self relates to motor actions and sensations.[9]

of agency acts like your in-game objectives. The extent to which any particular attribute contributes to a person's sense of self can differ from individual to individual, but there is generally strong agreement on the broad strokes (Fig. 5).

Let's look first at the sense of context. Of the components within

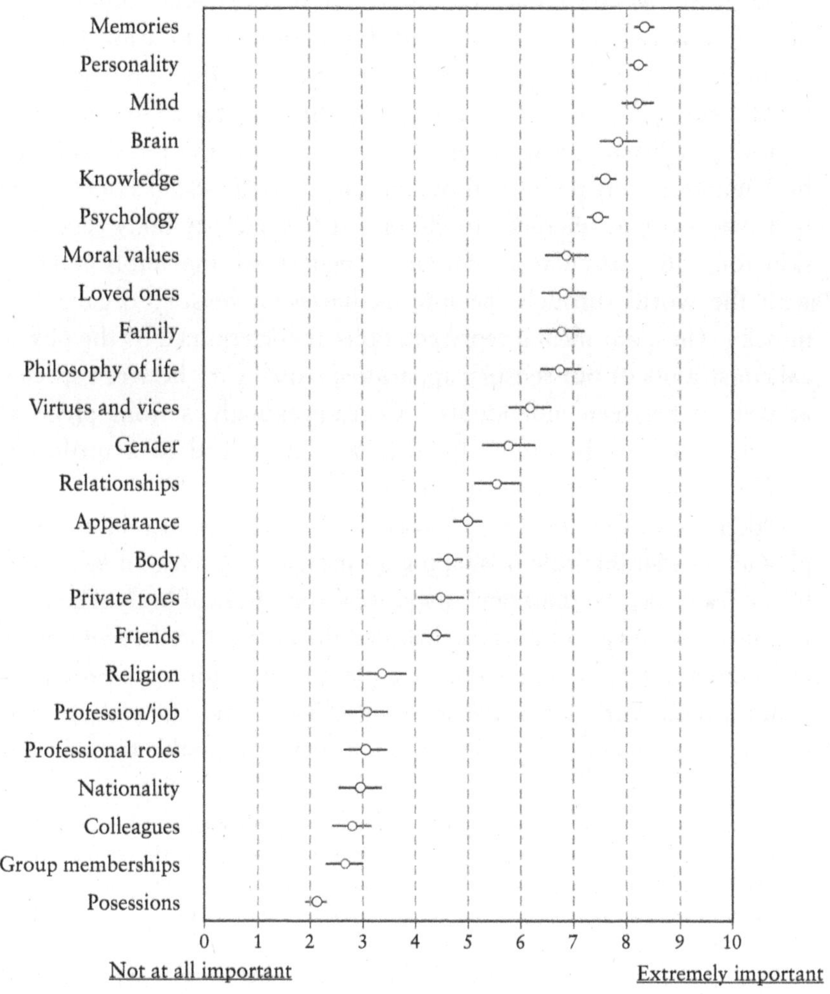

Figure 5. The relative importance of various attributes for determining a person's identity, according to a survey of 817 Americans. Modified from Fig. 7 in 'Putting Your Money where Your Self Is' by Woike et al., as per its Creative Commons 4.0 license.[10]

this category, a few stand out as particularly important. Formative experiences, such as the sense of companionship from making a best friend at school, the thrills and misadventures of obtaining a life partner, or the feeling of profound responsibility that accompanies the birth of a child, typically shape the core of an individual's memories that contribute to their sense of self. These *autobiographical* or *episodic memories* are so critical that their loss in severe amnesia or dementia amounts to a substantial destruction of one's former self. Accordingly, memories are so important to one's sense of self and personal identity that we'll later spend an entire chapter analysing them.

Additionally important to one's sense of self is the physical body, both in terms of its physiological condition and the social associations that may exist in reference to characteristics such as body type and skin tone. In particular, as embodied beings, we inevitably interact with the world through the intermediaries of sensory organs and muscles. Thus, our mental representations are determined by the physical constraints of our sensory apparatus, which vary between species as well as between individuals.* Correspondingly, serious physical traumas, such as becoming quadriplegic, may lead to a profound sense of change in one's self-perception.†

Other factors matter too, to varying degrees. Social relationships play a considerable role in shaping an individual's sense of self, even if to a lesser degree than one's memories and physical body. The feeling of community and purpose instilled through the collective prayer and community of congregants at a place of worship may provide a young person with a positive sense of religious and cultural identity for a lifetime. A child abused by a parent may feel unable to maintain

* Beyond perceiving and influencing our surroundings, other facets of embodiment matter too. The unique characteristics of one's face and voice are so deeply associated with individual identity, it is hard to imagine one without the other. Further, one's face and body can hugely determine social identity through cultural notions of attractiveness, gender ideals, and racial associations, amongst other criteria.

† The contribution of the body to one's sense of self might be most apparent when observed from an outside perspective. Consider oceanic manta rays, marine animals intelligent and self-aware enough that they potentially qualify for personhood.[11] These cold-blooded creatures have flat, triangular bodies around five metres long, and extract oxygen through their gills while cruising the oceanic expanses. Assuming that they are conscious, it probably feels rather different to be a manta ray than a human.

or trust social relationships long after the threat has vanished. Through our associated networks we may even share in the vicarious experiences of others, from the joy of a child's graduation to the pain of a colleague's project setback. And finally, while it might be uncouth to admit, one's possessions contribute too. Beyond the obvious impact of economic class, social mobility, and freedom of choice, our material reality speaks to our identity in more subtle ways as well. Advertising would certainly be less effective if there weren't people whose sense of self is at least partially defined by being the kind of person who owns the latest iPhone.

Apart from context, the other primary pillar of one's self is the *sense of agency*. One essential aspect of being an agent is having intentionality, the feeling that one can *intend* one's actions based on desires and goals. Another is to have a moral compass to steer the decisions one needs to make along the way. In particular, most people consider a person's truest self to be found in the choices one makes, both under everyday conditions and when the mettle of one's moral integrity is under stress.[12] Together, these drivers and controllers of activity are so vital to the self that a person who drastically alters their lifelong goals or ethical principles is often said to have 'become a different person'.

Despite the complex interplay between different agential forces within individuals – as demonstrated by the fact that I may both want to eat another cookie, and not want to because I am trying to consume less sugar – people still tend to report a persistent sense of self over time. In fact, this consistency even goes beyond mere individuals. Patterns of self-expression cluster to a certain degree, such that we feel individuals with overlapping desires, preferences, and abilities are in some way similar, while those with differing tastes, outlooks, and aptitudes are not. This holds to such an extent that there is some expectation that individuals who act in similar ways tend to enjoy similar things and think in similar manners. In psychological terminology, these ways in which self-expression conforms and differs in broad strokes between individuals is called *personality*.

Formally, the term *personality* refers to the patterns of behaviour and emotion that a person exhibits in response to certain situations. Some people jump at a chance to go skydiving or pursue an exciting but risky career-change overseas. Others are more content with consistency and routine, enjoying the calmness that comes with regularity and knowing things are in their proper place. While there is considerable variation between people, individuals themselves tend to be quite consistent across their lifespan in how they feel about and respond to situations.* This is true to the extent that even the temperament of infants is moderately predictive of the personality of the adults they will become, while the personality of people from their thirties onwards is strongly stable across the remainder of their lives.[13–15]

That is not to say that someone's personality describes all of what it means to be a particular person. People with very similar personalities still have different memories, different desires, and different bodies. Nonetheless, the fact that it is possible to talk about personality in a coherent sense at all, i.e. that there are any consistent psychological and behavioural characteristics of people, is decidedly useful when trying to demarcate the ambiguous contours of the self.

To sum up, by the multiple-attribute definition, a person's self is the set of properties that distinguish one person from any other person. These properties range from those of critical importance, like someone's moral compass and their autobiographical memories, to almost trivial, like their preferences for where they place app icons on their phone's home screen. We can broadly categorize these properties into the classes of context or agency, and roughly categorize different people's selves with concepts like personality. With this definition of the self in mind, we can now turn to what it means for personal identity to endure over time.

* By referring to aspects of the self in such a coarse way as *personality*, we're looking for a short description that is still useful. The problem is that there are a lot of different behaviours that could be considered part of someone's personality, for instance whether they have a tendency to daydream or doodle when bored, or how likely they are to talk to strangers at parties. Thankfully, psychologists are helped by the fact that how a person behaves in one situation is typically indicative of how one will act in another. This means reasonably accurate descriptions can be compressed into just a small number of *personality traits*. The most broadly accepted personality-trait model is the Big Five, which characterizes individuals by their *openness to experience* (curious vs conservative), *conscientiousness* (careless vs organized), *extraversion* (reserved vs outgoing), *agreeableness* (challenging vs compassionate), and *neuroticism* (sensitive vs resilient).

PERSONAL IDENTITY: THE PRAGMATIC VIEW

Philosophy is liable to get confusing, so let's check we're still on the same page. We've established that a person is a being that has the capacities for consciousness and self-awareness, and also possesses some kind of continuity over time and space. Let's imagine just such a person, and name her Shruthi. When considering Shruthi at any particular moment, her self at that time point consists of her body, goals, memories, and all the other attributes that make her Shruthi. What we still haven't covered is how the ten-year-old, twenty-year-old, fifty-year-old, and seventy-year-old Shruthi can all possibly be the *same* person. They have different memories, different goals, at least somewhat different bodies, and thus arguably different selves. What could possibly bind these different Shruthis together across time into the same person? This is the problem of personal identity.

Admittedly, for most people, most of the time, it can feel like the answer is blindingly obvious, and that all this complicated philosophical analysis is completely unnecessary. The elder and younger Shruthi talk and act the same way, like the same things, and have the same scars. They are obviously the same person. In this sense, many intuit something like the *pragmatic view*: that two individuals at different time points are identifiable as the same person if there is some combination of clearly trackable physical and psychological continuity between their earlier and later selves.

The pragmatic view appears self-evident from both a first- and third-person perspective. From the personal viewpoint of the elder Shruthi, she likely feels a straightforward continuity with her younger self, provided by the accumulated memories of all her life experiences forming a smooth transition between her younger self and now. Similarly, from a third-person viewpoint, it can feel just as easy to identify an individual over time. Both the older and younger Shruthi are physically identifiable in many of the same ways, sharing similar bodies, the same genome, the same height, and many other features. These similarities extend to the mental too, with both possessing similar intelligence, similar desires and preferences, and a very similar personality.

As such, in everyday usage, the pragmatic view is in no danger of mixing up Shruthis of any age with an Alex, Chae-Yeong, Diego, or any other person. As a result, identifying ourselves or others as the same person over time is so conventional that most of us would never have thought the matter could be up for debate.

Indeed, it's just as well that this is effortless. We'd soon be in dire straits if our present selves stopped investing efforts towards our future wellbeing, just as we'd be in deep trouble today if our earlier selves had failed to do the same. It's also important that we can easily identify our fellow citizens, as any sort of functioning social system needs the ability to recognize individuals reliably.* (We touched on this briefly in the last chapter.†)

Yet, although the pragmatic definition of personal identity holds strong everywhere from casual conversation to the convictions of our courts, the concept starts to buckle under the weight of philosophical scrutiny. There are many cases, both real and theoretical, with unintuitive and potentially unsettling implications for the tacit assumption that, no matter the circumstances, we always are who we've always been. To a large degree, these examples are uncomfortable because they violate the certainty of being able to track our own identities through a first-person perspective, and because they undermine the foundational premises of third-party identification required to make social systems function.

Moreover, if we're already worried about our definition of personal identity crumbling when confronted with contemporary clinical cases, things will only worsen when considering the needs of the future. As we're ultimately interested in assessing the prospects of using brain

* Some philosophers have even explored the idea that personal identity is primarily socially constructed, and that in the absence of communities people would not necessarily have a continuous identity.[16] Personally, I feel as though if I were marooned by myself on an island I would still maintain my personal identity, but I'm not excited to run the experiment to find out for sure.

† For example, any legal system that allocates property to an owner needs to be able to re-identify that same owner in the future. Criminal justice systems are predicated on the persistence of a person over time, in order to establish consistent connections between the individual who commits a crime, the individual who is tried for a crime, and the individual serving the punishment for that crime.

preservation to escape inevitable death through preserving personal identity, we need a clear understanding of how identity might persist or perish under any conceivable circumstances. If the pragmatic view cannot withstand the complications wrought by the following case studies, it will be our task to find a theory that holds fast where the former failed.

You aren't what you eat

Some general health advice states that one should 'take care of your body because it's the only one you've got'. This saying, in keeping with the pragmatic view, assumes a particular person necessarily has the same physical body for their entire life. But to what extent is this actually true?

To begin with, it certainly isn't the case that we are made of exactly the same atoms and molecules for any length of time. The typical person consumes about 5 kilograms of food and drink per day, and necessarily excretes or breathes out around the same volume of material. Even when restricting our view to just the mass of our cells, ignoring the additional fluids and solids that fill the in-between spaces of our bodies, this relentless turnover of our physical constituents means we replace our body mass roughly every year and a half.[17]

If we interpret the saying to mean we are 'made of the same cells', it still doesn't fare much better. An adult human is made of approximately 30 trillion cells at any one time. Though prolific in number, most of our cells are here for a good time, not a long time.[17] The cells that line your gut are replaced every few days, while red blood cells last about three months. Some of these turnover processes are a bit slower, but still substantial over time. You replace about 10 per cent of your skeleton each year, while your heart cells at only a few per cent per year. If these old cells weren't removed as new ones were made, by the time a human turned eighty, they would have accumulated about two tonnes of bone marrow and lymph nodes, as well as 16 kilometres of intestine.[18] While thankfully this cellular turnover typically occurs seamlessly without us turning into monstrous accumulations of flesh, no matter how you frame it, humans certainly aren't by any means made of 'the same cells' over time.

Sure, there are some long-lived cells with slower turnover rates, but if you pop their vintage hoods, you'll find that most of the parts inside are new. Take brain cells as an example. Most neurons in an adult's brain are never replaced, presumably because it would disrupt the memories and other information stored in their synaptic connections. But while the DNA at the hearts of these cells remains unchanged over decades, every other piece of their cellular machinery is frequently replaced.* Much as most organs constantly replace the cells within them, neurons themselves are constantly refreshing essentially all the rest of their components.

These components, called *organelles*, have particular roles that help maintain the cell. *Ribosomes* assemble amino acids into the microscopic machines that are proteins, while *mitochondria* produce energy.† Inside cells, these organelles and the molecules within them are replaced every few days.[19,20] Additionally, when looking at the synaptic connections between neurons specifically, many of the proteins used to connect brain cells are replaced on the order of days.[21] If we tried to make the continuity of personal identity dependent on having the same neurons over time, we'd have exactly the same problem as before, just shifted down a level: what makes a neuron the same neuron over time if almost all of its components are being replaced every few weeks?

Clearly basing continuity on maintaining the exact same physical components isn't going to fly. This should be expected, as the pragmatic view isn't generally concerned with the loss and gain of body parts. A leg amputation does not provide a patient with an incongruous new identity, while a kidney donation does not blur the boundaries of identity between the donor and donee. The pragmatic view is unphased by the reality that to be a biological creature is to be constantly in flux.

A more sophisticated expansion of the pragmatic definition, then, is to accept that continuity of personal identity does not require exactly the same physical constituents across all time, but can persist through

* This is also true of the enamel of adult teeth, along with some material in the lens of the eye, as was discussed in dating the age of whales in Chapter One.

† One might even refer to mitochondria as the 'powerhouse of the cell'.

the maintenance of other bodily properties. In this sense, having the same body over time is less about being made of literally the same atoms, and more about one's physical components maintaining some sort of consistent relationship over time.

One idea is that identity can be maintained even in a changing body, so long as the rate of change is sufficiently gradual and continuous.* For example, while a butterfly looks completely different from its younger caterpillar self, the two are still linked by an unbroken chain of cellular growth and replacement. Alternatively, perhaps the important thing is that there is some kind of enduring relationship maintained between body parts at a high level. The arrangement of your cheekbones, chin, eyes, mouth, and nose remain consistent enough for people to recognize you, even though the cells that make up your face are replaced on a regular basis. These relational approaches to bodily continuity seem to work a lot better, while still being in keeping with the pragmatic view.

Even so, the fact that people can undergo limb amputations, plastic surgeries, organ transplants, and other fairly radical and rapid changes to their bodies, without any question of whether their personal identity has been maintained, calls into question the importance of the body generally, as far as the pragmatic view of identity is concerned. Meanwhile, an injury to a relatively small part of one's brain, such as Gage's impromptu frontal-cortex surgery, can immediately raise doubts about the continuity of personal identity. What this shows is that the relative importance of parts of the body for personal identity is not evenly distributed, but predominantly located in the structure and function of the brain. In the end, our day-to-day evaluation of personal identity over time requires us to do one crucial thing: keep a person's mind in mind.

* The standard philosophical thought experiment brought up here is that of the Ship of Theseus. It goes as follows: 'Each year, the Athenians take a ship that belonged to the minotaur-slaying hero Theseus on a pilgrimage to Delos. After several centuries of maintenance, in which each individual piece of the ship has been replaced at least once, is it still the same ship?'

Mind the gap

Ask someone to describe what it is about an individual's psychology that makes them the same person over time, and, after they raise you an eyebrow in response to your admittedly intense question, they may list off some of the following possibilities:

- A person's identity is maintained by their experience of a continuous, unbroken stream of consciousness from one moment to the next.
- They're the same person as their younger self because they remember being that same younger self.
- They have been and will always be the same person because no matter how old they are, they tend to have very similar desires, capacities, and personality traits.
- Some combination of all of these.

As with similar attempts to define personal identity based on having the same body over time, these pragmatic answers work well enough under ordinary circumstances. However, as we consider certain neurological facts and examine some strange case studies, it'll become apparent that we'll need a more sophisticated view.

First of all, it's highly likely that no individual has ever had a continuous stream of consciousness for anything more than, at most, a few tens of hours.* Humans sleep for about eight hours every night, within which they have periods of dreamless and dreaming sleep. During the dreaming periods they are presumably conscious, albeit in a radically different fashion to normal waking experience. However, while researchers remain open to other possible explanations, it seems likely that during at least some periods of dreamless sleep there is no consciousness at all.[†,22]

* Possibly much less time than that, even, depending on whether people are still conscious during mind blanking.

† Other possible explanations for our seeming lack of consciousness include that, while we are in fact conscious, we cannot remember our experiences during periods of so-called 'dreamless' sleep and so assume we were unconscious, and that dreamless sleep involves a period of very repetitive experiences with uniform content that is difficult to describe upon waking.

Even if you suspect there is always some level of consciousness present during all periods of sleep, there are medical procedures where unconsciousness is even more assured. Individuals given high doses of general anaesthetics can be placed into a reversible coma where they show no behavioural signs of consciousness, no brain activity indicative of consciousness, and have no memory of their time under once they emerge from anaesthesia.[23] There are even surgical procedures where a person's body can be cooled down to entirely stop their brain and heart activity for short durations, as we'll discuss in greater detail in a later chapter.[24] Thus, unless we're willing to accept the possibility that we die every time we go to sleep or undergo surgery, we can dismiss the notion that an unbroken stream of consciousness or neural activity is required to maintain one's personal identity.

If not through consciousness, perhaps memory will provide a better means of explaining how someone can maintain continuity with their earlier self. One of the most famous cases relevant to this possibility is that of Henry Molaison, usually known by his initials H. M.[25,26] At the age of ten, possibly as a result of a head injury from a bicycle accident the year before, Henry developed epilepsy. By sixteen he was suffering from major seizures, and for the next decade he experienced debilitating and life-threatening epileptic attacks. His epilepsy remained stubbornly resistant to pharmacological treatment, and as a last resort, at the age of twenty-seven, he was referred for brain surgery. After discussion with a neurosurgeon, Henry agreed to an experimental operation to remove an area on both sides of the middle of his brain known to sometimes cause epilepsy, including most of his hippocampi. The subsequent surgery was successful in dramatically reducing the severity of his seizures, even though it did not manage to cure his epilepsy entirely.

However, the procedure came with a dramatic and unexpected cost. Upon waking up after the operation, Henry was unable to recall the medical staff who had been treating him, or even that he had had an operation at all. On further investigation, it became apparent that he had lost a significant portion of his past memories; while he was still capable of accurately recounting his childhood experiences, he could not remember that his favourite uncle had died three years earlier. More striking still, he was now entirely incapable of forming new memories about his life. On any given day, he did not know what he had had for lunch only half an hour before, let alone breakfast that morning. He could do the same jigsaw puzzles again and again, and read the same magazines cover to cover without ever finding them familiar. As the years and decades went by, Henry was unable to remember anything that had happened to him since that eventful day in his mid-twenties. While it may have stopped his seizures, the surgery had sacrificed Henry's ability to make a record of his life's journey.

At the same time, much of Henry's mind was the same as it always had been. His intelligence was unaffected, and, according to the opinion of his family, his personality showed no change.* He still enjoyed watching television and doing crossword puzzles. Amazingly, he was still able to acquire new skills, such as learning to draw, despite retaining no recollection of having done so. Removal of some of his brain tissue had cut the connection between his past, present, and future selves, but his childhood memories, along with his unchanged personality and cognitive abilities, at least partially linked him to his younger self.

It was as though one part of Henry was stuck in the past, unable to extend the chain of narrative events, and yet another part of him was floating into the future untethered, as he aged and learned unconscious skills. The question is, then: did severing this narrative chain leave Henry's personal identity unaffected, constitute his death, or produce something in between? What is the pragmatic view's answer to whether Henry could continue to be the same person over time despite his memory deficits? Compared to Gage, who kept his memories but lost his original personality, is Henry's survival more or less certain? The pragmatic view does not have any obvious answers to these questions.

Same same, but different

Aside from the stream of consciousness or the chain of memory, the other candidate suggested for providing someone with a sustained

* There is, however, some reason to doubt the veracity of this claim. Post-surgery, Henry apparently rarely complained of pain, hunger, or thirst, and also showed an absent libido. This lack of desire was probably due to the bilateral removal of his amygdalae.

personal identity over time is the consistency of their desires, capacities, and personality traits. This *mental similarity* of a particular person at different ages is typically extremely high, to the extent that someone's behaviour and feelings can often be reliably modelled and predicted even by friends and family who have not seen them for some time.

That is not to imply that any changes to a person's psychology at all constitute destruction or damage of their personal identity, as many shifts can be accommodated while still leaving someone's younger and elder selves overall quite similar. Some of these are slow and minor, like acquiring a new taste or shifting preferences for music genres. Others can be quicker and more profound, such as the development of sexual desire during adolescence. It's true that, in some ways, Shruthi at eighteen is quite different to Shruthi at eight: she doesn't mind broccoli as much and is now very interested in boys. Even so, she still talks loudly when excited and falls asleep while reading. As such, the consistency in personality and temperament between the two is such that the pragmatic view isn't bothered by this degree of alteration.

Sometimes, however, usually due to injury or disease, these changes can happen with a speed and magnitude that seems to exceed the acceptable bounds through which the constancy of personal identity is assured. The case study of Phineas Gage is one illustration of this. Equally dramatic changes in mental characteristics, though considerably less violent, can also be induced by pharmacological remedies for certain neurological problems.

As an example, take treatments for Parkinson's. As briefly discussed in the last chapter, Parkinson's is a progressive neurodegenerative disease that usually starts with issues controlling muscle movements before commonly progressing into dementia. The exact cause of the disease is still unknown, but the death of dopamine-producing neurons is an identified contributor. As dopamine is a neurotransmitter used by some neural circuits involved in muscle control, the decrease in dopamine resulting from the dysfunction of these neurons contributes to the symptoms of the disease. In response, symptoms can be reduced through the artificial provision of this missing dopamine with drugs that mimic the neurotransmitter, such as *dopamine agonists*.

These dopamine agonists are a great boon to many patients, but sometimes come at a cost. While dumping a heap of artificial dopamine into the brain can improve muscle coordination, it can also affect other neural circuitry that makes use of the neurotransmitter. Side effects may include drowsiness, nausea, and dramatic changes in one's deepest desires.

A small percentage of patients treated with dopamine agonists develop uncontrollable behaviours.[27] Sometimes these are somewhat amusing, such as a fishing obsession or compulsive gardening. Other times they are not so droll, such as pathological gambling or problematic hypersexuality. In one case, a fifty-two-year-old man, who had previously gambled only once or twice a year, developed a habit of waking in the night and driving to a casino where he would occasionally gamble for over thirty-six hours continuously. This same man would also perform cacophonous lawn maintenance, including blowing leaves for up to six hours at a time. His wife commented that this behaviour was 'completely out of character' and within weeks of ceasing the agonist therapy his compulsions disappeared. In another case, a similar drug led a forty-nine-year-old man to become obsessed with stained-glass window making. Less whimsically, he also developed unacceptable sexual behaviours, to the extent that his wife had to call the police on one occasion. In her words, the treatment had led her husband to undergo 'a complete transformation' and she felt she 'was married to an alien'. Just as in the previous case, after his treatment was discontinued, she reported 'I have my husband back.'

As with Phineas Gage, some of those treated with dopamine agonists had undergone sufficient mental changes to arguably become different people to who they were before, at least according to their partners. If we take this at all seriously, it entails formidable practical quandaries for the pragmatic view. Should a patient who develops a compulsive gambling habit be held liable for their debts once off the treatment? Could someone who breaks their marital commitments reconcile their infidelity on the grounds of having been a different person to the one who made the vows? The pragmatic view works well enough in everyday life, but, with tricky questions like these, it would help to have a fully robust theory of personal identity.

Kindred spirits

But before we start formalizing our definitions, let's take a look at one last neurological case. All of the previous cases described individuals whose selves were split in time to form at least two distinct versions, so dissimilar from each other it was questionable whether they were still the same person. But what about a situation where the opposite occurs? What insights can we draw from a case where two seemingly separate individuals are so similar it is ambiguous as to whether they constitute one person, two people, or an intermediate state?

Enter Krista and Tatiana Hogan, Canadian conjoined twins who are joined directly at the brain.[28,29] Each twin is able to receive sensory inputs from the other's body, as well as exert some control over the other's muscles. When Tatiana's eyes are covered, she can describe what can be seen through Krista's eyes. Krista can taste food that is in Tatiana's mouth, while Tatiana can feel pain that affects Krista's body. Both have joint control over at least Krista's right arm and Tatiana's left leg. As a collective, they are capable of walking, running, and swimming through synchronous control of all their limbs.

Enabling this joint activity is a 'thalamic bridge', a neuroanatomical structure unique to the twins that connects their thalami together (Fig. 6). In doing so, this thalamic bridge is possibly serving a similar role to that typically played by the corpus callosum, which in a typical brain consists of the nerve fibres that join the left and right hemispheres into one unified entity.

If so, this could go some way towards explaining how their intimate connection goes far beyond mere joint control over their bodies. The twins state that they are capable of communicating without speaking, a claim backed by behavioural observations from their family members. Their mother reports that their 'emotions definitely are connected. When one feels angry, the other one automatically feels angry. And I've never seen one happy without the other being happy.' No matter how good you may think you are at relating to other people's emotions, I doubt you're as empathetic as this.

Is this thalamic bridge, and the depth of shared feelings, coordination, and communication it enables, enough to define the Hogan twins as not two individuals but one self? While systematic psychological

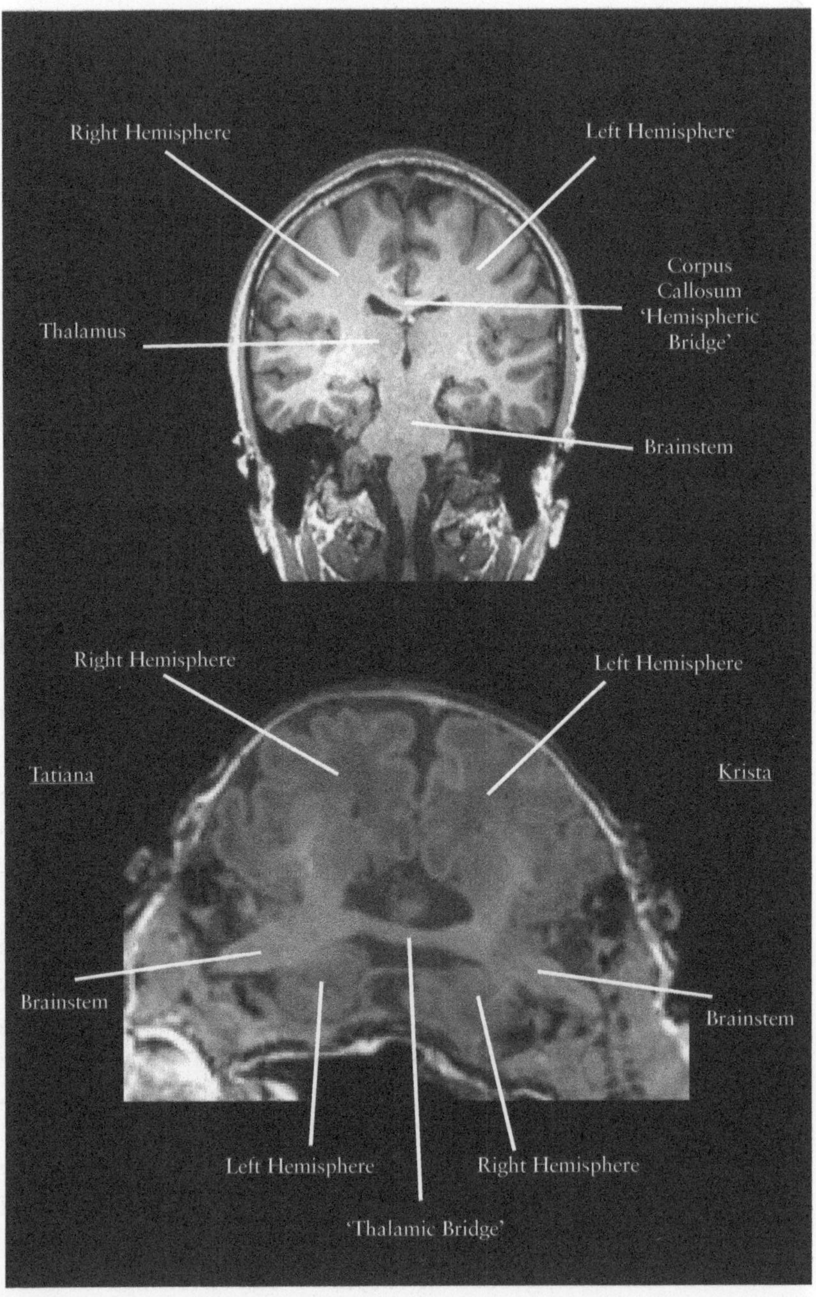

Figure 6. (Top) A front-on view of the author's brain, as imaged by MRI. (Bottom) A similar front-on view of the brain(s) of Krista and Tatiana Hogan.

and neurological observation of the extent to which the twins share mental content has yet to be published, they and their family have revealed some information publicly which might provide some hints.

Firstly, let's consider whether from their perspective they feel like separate people. The twins have provided no public statement on the matter, but some evidence for them possessing two separate streams of consciousness comes from the observation that it is possible for one twin to be asleep while the other is awake.[30] However, this is not as much of a knockdown argument for separate personhood as it may initially seem. It is fairly well known that dolphins can put half of their brain to sleep at a time. Less well known is a more recent discovery that even humans can have small regions of their brain fall asleep while an individual is still overall awake.[31] As a result, without directly asking the twins, we cannot easily make any assumptions about their subjective experiences.*

How about the attributes that comprise their self, or selves? With respect to their sense of context, they have two bodies, with the twin on each side in primary control of that body. This provides some evidence for separate selves, but weakened by the aforementioned degree of shared control and sensation. With respect to their sense of agency, things get a bit more interesting. Tatiana is reported to enjoy the taste of ketchup while Krista does not, to the extent that Krista will try to prevent Tatiana from eating it. This seems to provide clear evidence for two selves, on the basis of their differing desires and goals.

Or it would, if not for the fact that individuals frequently demonstrate conflicting desires. If a typical human can experience a firm massage as both painful and pleasant simultaneously, or feel on a bad day they would like a hug while also wishing they would be left alone, can we be sure that conflict between the Hogan twins is an absolute guarantee of separate personhood? While their clash over food preferences deviates from the typical internal tug-of-war individuals face between immediate

* Also consider patients who provide an almost opposite case to that of the Hogan twins: where communication between the brain's hemispheres is forcibly hampered through surgical destruction of someone's corpus callosum. There is also no consensus on what the experience is like for these 'split brain' patients, and whether or not the procedure results in a single or multiple streams of consciousnesses still divides neuroscientists and philosophers alike.[32,33]

gratification and long-term ambitions, it isn't quite enough evidence to confirm their identities as distinct. This is further complicated by the mother's claims that the twins' emotions are perfectly synchronized, which makes it uncertain how far their desires truly diverge.

In the end, it does not seem clear whether Tatiana and Krista are separate people. Perhaps they will one day consent to provide a clearer answer, but for now the evidence publicly available is decidedly ambiguous.

Even so, what we do know about their case is enough to push the pragmatic view of personal identity, already strained by the previously described cases, to its breaking point. If Krista commits a crime, should Tatiana be held criminally liable as well? Is Tatiana's consent also required for a medical procedure on Krista's body? Does it make a difference if the surgery is an area Tatiana can or cannot feel? To these questions, the pragmatic view is at a loss.

PERSONAL IDENTITY: THE PHILOSOPHICAL VIEWS

A reminder: because we established in the last chapter that death should be defined as the irreversible loss of personal identity, in this chapter we're ultimately trying to work out the conditions under which someone's personal identity is maintained. An everyday, pragmatic view intuits that the answer to this will always be fairly obvious, but the previous case studies make clear that an unrefined view is not always going to cut it. As we've done enough head scratching, it's now time to turn to some of the more reasoned approaches for defining personal identity.*

One philosophical position with some support is the *biological*

* There are a few formal philosophical views of personal identity that are less popular than the two that will be discussed here, but still have some proponents. The *narrative identity* view holds that people exist over time through constructing a coherent narrative about their lives.[34] The *social construction* view asserts there is no fact of the matter about personal identity except through society choosing to identify and re-identify someone as the same person over time.[16] The *phenomenal continuity* view suggests that we survive not through the continuity or connectedness of psychological

view of personal identity, which holds that a person persists over time if their later body is the same as, or continuous with, their earlier body.[*,36,37] Rather than focusing on memories, motivations, or other mental aspects, the biological view espouses that all that is necessary for a person's survival is that their body continues to exist.

There are certainly some advantages to this theory over a view that focuses on psychological aspects. It accords with the pragmatic view that each person has a unique body by which they can be identified. It avoids the seemingly unscientific questions of whether a person can be distinguished from their body, or the morally fraught one of whether a person can die even while their body still breathes. Through a focus on biological rather than psychological continuity, it bypasses the problems of whether a person is still present when they are unconscious, or whether an infant is the same person as the adult they grow into. On its surface at least, the biological view appears philosophically robust.

But the biological view's inclusiveness in ascribing survival to all situations involving bodily continuity is also its downfall.[†] We have already discussed extensively how the bodies of people are constantly changing, which makes it difficult to find a definition of 'body' that describes something that persists for any length of time. Now we have a related problem, which is developing a theory which avoids claiming a person has survived in situations where intuition would suggest they have died. Take, for example, the fact that a dying person's body continues to exist in some form long after they are declared clinically dead. Or, if we restrict the example to the case where continued biological functions are still present, consider a brain-dead body being kept on indefinite life support. Loss of function in only a single organ, such as losing a kidney, is not normally considered enough to cause a discontinuity between a body viewed at two different times. If,

---

properties like memory or personality across our selves of different ages, but through some sort of similarity between our streams of consciousness across time.[35]

* Depending on who you ask, the biological view is either closely related to or the same as the *brute-physical*, *animalism*, or *bodily* views.

† This line of argument is very much related to the discussion in the last chapter criticizing the definition of death based on 'an organism's breakdown in ability to act as a unified whole'.

likewise, the biological view doesn't offer any special treatment for the brain, our definition has a serious problem. You don't need the French Revolution to know a king can't rule without a head.

In dismissing the importance of the brain, the biological view misses most people's belief that psychological properties are the key to being the same person across time. As a result, the biological view is a minority position among both philosophers and the general public, at least in the English-speaking world. When surveyed, only 19 per cent of professional philosophers support the biological view, as opposed to at least 44 per cent who explicitly support some kind of psychological view.[38] Equivalently, a small study of undergraduates in the US found that 64 per cent of them favoured a psychological view over other positions, while larger online surveys of the general American public have also shown an emphasis on mental properties as key to personal identity.[12,39,40]

As the reigning champion of personal identity, then, at least as far as popularity is concerned, the *psychological view* deserves the most attention. The psychological view holds that for a person to persist over time there must be a particular relationship between the mental properties of the earlier and latter individual.[36] Key elements may include: that the latter individual retains the memories of the earlier one, that they hold the same moral compass, that they have a similar personality, or that there was a continuous evolution of psychological states between the earlier and later selves.

Compared to the biological view, this psychological one better matches the intuitions of most people as to when personal identity is maintained. At least for Americans, surveys indicate people believe that their identity, or 'true self', is primarily dependent not so much on their bodies but rather in their morality, personality, memories, desires, and other psychological components.[12] Similarly, in the neurological cases previously mentioned of patients suffering marked changes in their psychology, the psychological view raises significant ambiguity as to whether someone was still the same person after a mentally altering medical event. This sounds about right, as formal surveys of patients' families also suggest that substantial psychological changes pose a threat to personal identity, in a way that, for example, medical issues that merely affect mobility do not.[41] As a result, the psychological view appears the best candidate to be developed into a philosophically robust theory of personal identity.

A self-consistent view

Outside of cases of advanced dementia, the memory of elderly individuals maintains a remarkably substantial record of the lives of their younger selves. Consider the ease with which aged individuals recall their youthful escapades: rowdy play with excitable siblings, the quiet anxiety of starting one's first 'proper' job, and the countless other landmarks that constitute a life. It is true that, as the years slip by, the fine-embroidery of specific dates and names can fray and tangle a little. Yet, as we age, we retain the capacity to remember the more robust threads of experience, the essence of our pasts, with impressive fidelity. Studies assessing the accuracy of long-term memories have shown that people are more than capable of accurately remembering events years or decades later.[42–44] That is not to say that human memory for specific details is so infallible as to always be comfortably reliable in high-stakes circumstances, such as courtroom testimonies. But an overfocus on forgetting and false memories obscures the broader picture that human memory provides a remarkably good link across the lifespan.[45]

On this basis, the psychological view of personal identity can ground a person's consistent sense of self in an enduring bedrock made of core memories and other psychological properties.* Irrespective of superficial changes, a deep-seated sense of context comes from memory acting as a binder, collecting and preserving experiences over time. Alongside a person's stable sense of agency – their moral compass, their aspirations, the unique traits that define their personality – the constancy of these properties is what provides someone their consistent self across their lifespan.†

* A different approach is to try and ground the psychological view's conditions for the persistence of personal identity over time in the overlapping continuity of psychological properties across one's life, even if those properties are inconsistent between distant time points. For a discussion of why I think that approach fails, see the entry 'Psyching oneself out' in Appendix One.

† We covered the evidence for the stability of personality across the lifetime back in the 'Social stagnation' section of Chapter Two.

While humans naturally evolve to some degree over time, a considerable part of their inner world, from personality traits to their sense of life's overarching narrative, remains rooted in a common configuration. The ability of a person's younger and older selves to recognize each other, despite the passage of time, is proof of a persistent psychological foundation even as the surface expression may somewhat shift. It is this constancy of a person's mind that ensures their enduring personal identity and ultimately constitutes an individual's ongoing existence.

It follows then that as we journey deeper into an exploration of consciousness and memory, we will see how a person's unique mind is determined by the stability of the particular architecture of their brain. A point worth emphasizing is that the exact physical constituents of the brain do not matter, so long as the configuration remains the same, as is evident from natural biological turnover. Similarly, while our bodies are important for how we sense and navigate the world, as well as for sensing and navigating our emotional interiors, it is not an absolute precursor for personal identity, as shown by survivors of quadriplegia, organ donations, or amputations. Even a continuous stream of consciousness is not a requirement, as sleep and anaesthesia clearly demonstrate. All that fundamentally matters for survival is that a person keeps enough of their psychological properties intact to be able to preserve the possibility of maintaining their unique identity.

Correspondingly, once we've covered more of the details of how the structure of a person's brain maintains their psychological traits over time, we will be equipped to go through the technical details of how brain preservation can save someone's life.

But before being sure the effort of going through all that material is worthwhile, we should put our reigning champion, the psychological view, through a proper philosophical gauntlet. The neurological cases we have covered so far serve to put severe scrutiny on incomprehensive views of personal identity, and it is not completely clear that any formal view will escape unscathed either. To this end, philosophers have gone further still, devising a series of thought experiments that test the robustness of theories under extreme conditions. If the validity of a theory of personal identity is a matter of life and death, as it is practically speaking in situations I'm about to describe, then we want to be pretty damn sure that the theory is correct. Should the psychological view withstand the scenarios to come, then the prospect of brain preservation will look all the more promising.

***

Imagine that, during an otherwise routine medical appointment with your doctor, they break some disturbing news. One of your recent medical tests has come back indicating that you are in the early, asymptomatic phase of Alzheimer's disease.* They inform you that you won't notice symptoms for decades yet, and that your memory is currently functioning as expected for someone of your age. Unfortunately, though, the test is highly reliable, and they guarantee you that by your early eighties you will suffer from full-fledged dementia.

However, your doctor continues, there is some good news. Recently, nanotechnological breakthroughs have led to a treatment that can fully prevent neurodegenerative diseases. It works as follows: a patient receives an injection of nanobots that travel through their bloodstream, cross the blood–brain barrier, and spread throughout the nervous system. Once in place, the nanobots enter every neuron and spread themselves throughout the interiors of the cells. At this stage, if a neuron is still healthy, they remain dormant. However, should they detect a decrease in the function of the neuron, the nanobots awaken. Upon activation, they start to carefully replace the biological components of the neuron with synthetic versions. Critically, they do this while maintaining the exact functional properties of the neuron, and ensuring the synaptic connections to its neighbours remain precisely the same.

The process occurs gradually, with 5 per cent of neurons expected to be replaced at ten years after the initial treatment, 40 per cent at thirty years, and approximately 100 per cent at sixty years. Patients in the initial clinical trials, performed in those at risk of early-onset

* Something like this is a disturbing reality for those who find out they have certain gene variants. Those who have two copies of the Apolipoprotein ε4 gene variant have around fifteen times the odds of developing Alzheimer's disease compared to those with the more common versions of the gene.

dementia, reported that the process was completely unnoticeable and that they suffered absolutely no side effects.[46]

Eager to avoid dementia, and assuaged by these previous trials, you consent to the treatment. The doctor gives you the injection and tells you to obtain a scan every few years to track the progress of the nanobots. Each time you receive the new scan you marvel at the increase in the percentage of your brain that is now synthetic. You don't feel any different, and your friends and family haven't noticed any changes. As far as you or anyone else can tell, you remain the same person you've always been.*

According to the psychological view, there is no doubt that you would survive this treatment. The process of gradual neuron replacement is similar to the continuous turnover of cells and subcellular components that already occurs in natural, biological brains. There would be no alteration of your memories, no change to your personality, no shift in your subjective experience. Whether the replacement was 5 per cent, 50 per cent, or 100 per cent complete, there is no moment at which you would cease to be. While the technology required is still fantastical by today's standards, replacing a biological brain with a cyborg one is the logical endpoint of the neuroprosthetics already in use and under development. Accordingly, the psychological view's position that you would survive this procedure accords with popular intuition. Let's pick a harder test next.

***

The year is 2077. Earth and Mars are now intertwined communities with a constant stream of people transiting between them. You, as a regular commuter, have found the novelty of space flight ebbing away. Instead, the thought of spending three months in the claustrophobic confines of a spacecraft leaves you with a profound sense of

* Assume for the moment that your consciousness is completely unaffected by this process, though we will interrogate that assumption in the next chapter. This scenario is based on one described by David Chalmers, where he explores its implications for consciousness as well as personal identity.[46]

ennui. So, when news of a faster, revolutionary mode of travel reaches your ears, a surge of relief and anticipation sweeps over you.

A few weeks later, you find yourself in front of a gleaming cylindrical chamber at your local TeleX station. A screen mounted beside the entrance explains how the device functions. First, it instantly scans and dematerializes a person at the atomic level, recording the exact position and energy state of every component of your body. Next, all this information is beamed at light speed to a receiving station on Mars. Upon arrival, a materialization chamber draws upon its energy reserves and uses the newly arrived information to rapidly recreate the person who entered the original chamber. At the end of all this, under an hour after stepping into the original chamber, the user is free to step out onto Martian soil.

Once the video finishes, you swipe the screen to accept the terms of service, and step into the quiet chamber. Settling onto the single chair in the centre of the room, you see the door you entered through slide back into place. A calm voice commences the countdown: 'Three, two, one . . .'

—

You're startled to attention with a sudden jolt, like a piercing alarm has woken you from a foggy daydream. The chamber door reopens, and you rise to exit. You find yourself in a terminal almost identical to the one you left behind, but for a cheery 'Welcome to Mars!' banner hanging from the ceiling and a red landscape beckoning through the windows. You check the time, and note it has been a mere forty minutes since you first entered the TeleX station. A smile creeps onto your face; you could definitely get used to this.

***

This kind of teleportation scenario, popularized in science fiction by *Star Trek* and in philosophy by the writings of Derek Parfit, tends to elicit responses that can be divided into two opposing camps.[47] The first camp, those who would willingly embrace any technology that could forever eliminate the drudgery of traffic jams, delayed trains, and economy-class flights, reports a feeling of wonder. In contrast, the second rejects the idea out of hand, explaining with fear that using such a teleporter would be a form of suicide.

Those in the second camp, who are worried that teleportation might entail death, are likely to claim this would occur during the dematerialization process, either due to destruction of the person's body, a break in their stream of consciousness, or both. While initial apprehensiveness is reasonable, on reflection we will see that almost everything we have covered in this chapter so far speaks against the validity of these concerns.

Firstly, it is hard to argue that the dematerialization and rematerialization of a person's body during teleportation entails death while simultaneously claiming that the natural turnover of one's cells does not. Or, viewed another way, compare this case to the previous nanobot scenario, where your biological neurons are progressively replaced with synthetic counterparts. This time, though, instead of neuron replacement happening gradually over years, imagine it sped up to occur in months, days, seconds, or even nanoseconds. If you accept that a person survives in the gradual replacement case, why should they die if the replacement is sped up to occur arbitrarily fast? Whether replacement happens over fifty years or fifty picoseconds, afterwards you would still feel the same, your friends and family would recognize you as the same, all your psychological properties would be preserved, and nothing about your self would be lost.[48] This logic suggests that if eating and breathing doesn't slowly kill you, then the teleporter shouldn't either.

Secondly, we've already covered how breaks in the continuity of consciousness are probably routine during sleep and anaesthesia, and definitely occur during certain surgeries where people's bodies are cooled and their brain activity completely ceases. If you're the same person who wakes up in the morning as who went to bed at night, or who emerges from a surgical procedure where your heart and brain were stopped entirely, then why wouldn't you be the same when you step into and out of the teleporter?*

* Admittedly, this scenario is different in that it simultaneously combines replacement of one's physical body with a break in the continuity of consciousness. Even so, it is equivalent to other situations where I imagine everyone's intuition would be that a person has survived. Imagine a scenario where someone is held deeply anaesthetized

Still, I sympathize with the reticence of those who fear the teleporter. Currently existing modes of transportation do not bear any resemblance to being incinerated and reformed, and the proposal of just such a method is understandably disconcerting. Even so, I would encourage those who are disturbed by the idea to reflect on whether their discomfort comes solely from a place of solid philosophical objection, or if instead there's influence from a prejudice against unfamiliar technology. My strong suspicion is that, in a society that made regular use of teleporters, people would very quickly become entirely accustomed to them, just as most of us are no longer scared of cars, planes, or rockets.*

However, there is one further objection often raised that cannot be as lightly dismissed. Some people are concerned that, rather than suicide being necessary for teleportation, almost the exact opposite might occur. To explain just what they mean, let's look at one final scenario . . .

***

It's 2079, and teleportation is now the standard for your monthly commute between Earth and Mars. Today, much like every other travel day, everything has been proceeding predictably. You arrive at the terminal, enter the chamber, and settle into your seat. The door slides shut, you hear the gentle countdown, and experience the weird jolt from mind-blanking, just as you've come to expect.

Yet this time, something is different. The chamber light flickers, and the door remains shut. After a few confusing moments, a voice sounds from an unseen speaker.

'On behalf of TeleX, I offer our deepest apologies. It appears that the teleporter you just used was one of our new prototypes, which had been accidentally installed due to a labelling error. Rest assured

---

in a medical coma for years, while still being provided nutrients via a nasogastric tube. After several years, once they have replaced essentially all their original atoms and molecules with new ones, they are allowed to emerge from the coma. Here, they have undergone the same conditions as with the teleporter: in the time that they have had a break in the continuity of consciousness, their entire body has been replaced. If a person in this scenario would survive, why not through teleportation?

* In a similar vein, transplants of kidneys, hearts, and other organs are also now routine and do not trigger such concerns.

that safety is of utmost importance at TeleX and that the device has functioned perfectly. There is no need for concern, as your body has securely materialized at our receiving pod in Mars as per usual. However, our new model does work a little differently from the teleporter you're used to. This new version retains the core scanning-and-sending function, but with the added improvement of being able to perform non-destructive scans. This means that, in addition to successfully materializing on Mars, your body on Earth has also remained fine and functional rather than being dematerialized. We apologize, however, for a technical issue: the new model is not yet properly integrated into our terminal system and there has been an error with the door-opening command. We'll have you out of there in just a minute.'

For a moment you are dazed, staying seated on the chair while absorbing this unexpected turn of events. Then a startling thought grips you: 'When the door opens, will I see Earth or Mars outside?'

Maybe the earlier version of the teleporter doesn't transport you, so much as it kills you and then creates a mere 'copy' of you at the end. This worry is made clearest by imagining duplication scenarios like the one just mentioned, where an individual in a second location is created while leaving the original in the first location unaffected. If there's a version of you on Earth, and a version of you on Mars, which one is the 'real' you?

To work through the question, let's first consider what it would even mean for a 'copy of you' to exist. As per this duplication scenario, such an entity would have a physically identical body to the 'real you', down to the atomic level, along with the same personality, the same memories, all of the same psychological properties. At the same time, there are some ways in which it would differ from the other, 'real' version of you. Obviously, it would have to be in a different location. It would be made of different atoms, albeit all in the same arrangement as the original version of you. Most critically, going forwards from the moment of duplication, it would have a different stream of consciousness from you, meaning it would start to have different experiences and accumulate memories that you would not feel were your own. Surely, if you can't experience what your alternate version feels, then it must be beyond doubt that the other being is just a copy?

In the interest of keeping things clear through this potentially confusing thought experiment, let's explicitly spell out all the options for what might have happened regarding personal identity in this duplication scenario. Assuming the terms *real* and *copy* are reliable, logic dictates four possibilities:

1. The version on Earth is the real you, the version on Mars is a copy.
2. The version on Earth is a copy, the version on Mars is the real you.
3. Both the Earth and Mars versions are copies.
4. Both the Earth and Mars versions are the real you.

I don't think Option Two is held by anyone, so we're probably safe to dismiss it out of hand. Option Three is similarly implausible – it is unclear why making a duplicate of someone should affect the metaphysical status of the original individual. That leaves us with Options One and Four.

For those who believe only one of the individuals can be the real you, Option One is the likely choice. If asked to provide reasons why, the following claims might be offered: the Earth version is the original body, made of the same physical material as the body before the duplication event; the Earth version also has a stream of consciousness that started before the duplication event, while the Mars one only came into existence after being created. If only one version can be the real you, the Earth-based original seems the obvious one to choose.

But, even if that's the choice that feels right, we've already invalidated the reasoning used to support it. As we established at several earlier points in this chapter, being made of the same physical material is irrelevant to questions of personal identity. The unbroken continuity of a stream of consciousness is also irrelevant if you have any belief that we can survive from one day to the next. It is thus unfair to privilege the Earth version with the prestige of being 'real'. After all, both individuals feel they have a continuous stream of consciousness with their previous self, as both recall stepping into the teleporter, feeling the jolt of the scanner, and listening to an apology message. Before the chamber door slides open, uncertain as to which planet they are on, their streams of consciousness have been subjectively identical.[49] Overall, then, it is logically inconsistent with our earlier findings to claim the Mars version is a 'copy' while the Earth version is the legitimate you.

What are we to decide, then? We could follow this chain of deductive reasoning through to its logical endpoint, and accept that both the Earth and Mars versions are somehow simultaneously the real you. Or we could baulk at this obviously false conclusion, and believe an error in reasoning must have been made somewhere along the way. Let's consider both alternatives in turn.

A franchise opportunity

If we accept that both the Earth and Mars versions have equal claims to be the real you, then a *branching* event has occurred. There are now two individuals, with two distinct streams of consciousness, who have branched off from the same earlier self. As both have the same memories, personality, and other psychological properties as the single earlier self, either one then counts for the survival of that person over time. Just as a single fertilized human egg can develop into two distinct identical twins, so too would a TeleX duplicator enable one individual to become two.

Accepting this answer prompts a new question: if both the Earth and Mars individuals are the same person as their past self, then are they also the same person in the present? Put another way: when, if ever, do the individuals corresponding to the separate branches actually become two separate people? On this question, philosophers' opinions differ.

One view is that it would happen instantly at the creation of two separate streams of consciousness. As soon as experiences and memories start to accumulate for the individuals separately of each other, then there are two different people, even if the two do share a common past. The advantage of this view is that it fits with the intuition that a person in the present cannot be in two places at once. Its disadvantage is that it seems to cut against a psychological view of personal identity grounded in a consistent sense of self.

Previously, I argued that two individuals are the same person if they bear a sufficiently strong degree of psychological consistency. Here, there are two individuals that are psychologically the same in every single way, save for an arbitrarily small set of different experiences and memories, and yet the claim is they are different people. Some argue that the two individuals must be two different people, on the grounds that a single person may never have even an arbitrarily small number of experiences or memories allocated to the same timestamp. Even so, because this position implies that a single second of divergent experiences will create two different people, while a lifetime's worth of mental growth and change need not, it seems hard to make the claim without undermining the foundation on which the psychological view is based.

An alternative view is that although there are now two bodies with two separate streams of consciousness, for at least some time going forwards, they are still the same person. This might feel less intuitive, but it is easier to argue for from the psychological view's perspective. Until a substantial amount of time has passed, the two individuals overwhelmingly share the same personality, memories, intelligence, and all the other psychological characteristics that define a person. Given this is the same criteria we use to define two individuals as the same person across time, why not use it the same way to define two individuals across space? As philosophers have pointed out, this would require conceptualizing a person as the sort of entity that can be in two places at once, which would make us metaphysically similar to books, songs, and databases.[50,51] As odd as this seems, it might still be the most palatable view to hold when trying to devise a coherent theory of personal identity in the face of conflicting intuitions.

Yet, as far as survival of the original pre-duplication person is concerned, it doesn't really matter which opinion is correct. Whether or not the duplicates comprise one person or two people going forwards, neither view challenges the survival of the pre-duplication person. Be it on Earth, Mars, or both planets at once, the continued existence of the pre-duplicate's desires, moral beliefs, personality, memories, and all other psychological aspects of their self, enables the original person to live on.

***

At this stage, I am sure that at least some of you, dear readers, will take the alternative approach of believing I have made at least one major error in reasoning somewhere along the way. If you are sure in your conviction that a person can never branch into two people, or certain someone can only ever be in one place at a time, as some philosophers say they are, then that implies I must have made a mistake somewhere in my argument.[52,53]

I am definitely sympathetic to this point of view. At the very least, I accept that the upshot of my claim is extremely odd compared to the everyday, pragmatic view of personal identity that we use in ordinary life. It implies that, under certain theoretically plausible future scenarios, there could be two co-existing versions of ourselves both legitimately claiming to be us. This violates our usual sense of psychological unity with our past and future selves. It also challenges our social frameworks around personal responsibility. If one branch of a person commits a crime, can the other also be held accountable? In a democracy, should each branch get one vote, or is a single vote spread across them all? These possibilities are more than absurd enough to call my reasoning into question.

Even so, I do not think these concerns are strong enough to justify discarding the psychological view of personal identity. While the view entails some weird possibilities in science-fiction scenarios, it doesn't suggest logically inconsistent outcomes. As discussed in this chapter and the previous one, it accords better with our intuitions on what is important for survival than any other proposal. In particular, framed either in the current fashion or through the previously explored concept of information-theoretic death, it provides a consistently applicable answer to what conditions constitute a person's survival. Whether lost in the body of a brain-dead patient, or transmitted in a jaunt through a hypothetical teleporter, a person lives or dies through the existence of their mind.

In my own defence, while I've been walking through the potentially unsettling implications of the teleportation and duplication scenarios, the psychological view still commands considerable popular support even in the face of these thought experiments. When members of the general American public are surveyed on the duplication scenario I described above, around 75 per cent of them respond that both the Mars and Earth versions count as the real you.[40] Admittedly, this is a higher percentage than professional philosophers, who on a related survey provided a relatively even 35:40:25 split between 'real you', 'copy', and 'other'.[38] But, taken together, the surveys indicate substantial, and possibly even a clear majority, of public support for the psychological view.[10] In the search for a rigorous theory of personal identity, then, most would agree that the psychological view is our best candidate.

WHERE DOES THIS LEAVE US?

Okay, enough of the science-fiction scenarios. Let's see how the psychological view handles the real neurological test cases for personal identity we covered earlier in the chapter: Phineas Gage with his permanent, tamping-rod-induced personality change; the Parkinson's patients with their temporary, pharmacologically induced equivalent; Henry and his perpetual amnesia; and the brain-fusion case of the Hogan twins. While keeping in mind that the publicly available information about any of these cases is much sparser than required to give a thorough answer, here are my best guesses:

The drug- or injury-induced personality changes in the case of Gage and the Parkinson's patients are sufficiently large to turn them partially into different people. But, in the absence of memory loss and other psychological changes, these alterations are insufficient to clearly warrant the term *death*. Certainly, in the cases of the Parkinson's patients given dopamine agonists, they cannot have been dead according to an information-theoretic standard, because the personality changes were reversible once taken off the drugs. But, at least temporarily for these patients and possibly permanently in the case of Gage, there was at least a partial loss of identity compared to who they were before. If we were to describe personal identity as a chain, we could imagine this as though a new cord of separate material had been added on where the original chain left off, before reverting to the former cord in the case of the Parkinson's patients.

Henry's retention of most of his pre-surgery memories means that his earlier self certainly survives, but at the same time his ongoing amnesia ensures that any theoretical post-surgery selves cannot. This could be imagined as the end of a chain floating in suspended animation; the length is still intact but unable to grow. Assuming he suffered no personality or other psychological changes, as his family initially claimed, then the pre-surgery person presumably continued to survive and find expression in his future self.* But, because they cannot be recorded into autobiographical memory, the status of his post-surgery selves is more ambiguous. Perhaps they are akin to short-lived duplicator branches: flickering into existence for as long as his intact working memory would allow, then gone forever. Or perhaps it is better to think of his identity as surviving in an unusually unchanging sense, unaffected by the years of memory accumulation that normally occur with age.

In the absence of more information, the Hogan twins remain a mystery. If they have different desires, different streams of consciousness, and different sets of memories, then they are two different people, albeit with more in common than any other pair who've ever existed. But if it's more the case that they think in unison to the point of being one agent, and that there lives a single current of experience and memory in their thalamically bridged brain, then they are but one person. Whether there are two chains in parallel, or one single interlocked weave, cannot be determined without closer observation.

These cases are all so bizarre precisely because they are rare exceptions to the rule that personal identity is extremely stable across the vast majority of a person's lifetime. Much as we rarely contemplate how our livers and kidneys are keeping our bodies alive so long as they are functioning properly, the very strangeness of these cases highlights the ease with which under healthy conditions our brain maintains our personal identity. Breakdowns of these neural structures and functions are so intriguing and unsettling precisely because they pose real threats to our ongoing existence.

Speaking of threats, it would be remiss of me to not touch briefly on concerns around the moral, legal, and social implications of embracing this psychological view of survival. Fully addressing these concerns is well beyond the scope of this book, so I shall keep it short.

* As previously stated, there are strong reasons to be dubious of the family's claim that Molaison remained entirely unchanged. See Lichterman's review of the case for more details.[25]

Firstly, it's important to note that a creature does not have to be the same person over time, or even a person at all, to still have moral relevance. My guess is that a cow is probably minimally self-aware, and to a large degree lives entirely in the moment, unconcerned with its connection to its past and future selves. But if a cow is at all conscious – if it can feel joy when eating fresh spring grass or pain when bitten by a buffalo fly – then despite its lack of personhood its experiences still matter.

Secondly, those who might seek to avoid justice for past social or criminal offences on the basis of 'I was a different person then!' will obtain little comfort from this view. Neurological cases suggestive of someone permanently becoming a different person typically involve substantial brain damage. Unless offenders can provide evidence that they are psychologically incongruous with their former selves to the extent of unrecognizability, there is no escape from responsibility to be found in the psychological view of personal identity.

However, there is great comfort to be found in the implications that the psychological view holds for the feasibility of survival through brain preservation. In fact, later in the book I will demonstrate that even if you find the psychological view of personal identity uncompelling, there are still means by which brain preservation could enable your survival. But particularly from its viewpoint, so long as a person's mental properties can be maintained, no matter how, then they continue to survive. If, when dying, you choose to be preserved through a procedure that can safeguard the brain structures that retain the multitudes of your being, replete with your memories of childhood summers, your unique way of interacting with the world, and all the other important aspects of your self, then you are guaranteed the possibility of eventual revival. Not a descendant of you. Not a mere copy of you. In as strong a sense as you survive naturally from day-to-day and year-to-year, the psychological view holds that it is the true, real you who would live.

To understand the technical details of how any medical procedure could ever hope to indefinitely preserve psychological properties, it will help to first cover the natural means by which human brains provide a person's persistence over the years. In two chapters' time, we'll walk through how the neuroscientific mechanisms of memory do just that.

Before we get to how the brain enables survival over time, however, it would be good to grasp how psychological properties shape someone's subjective experience at any given moment. Exploring the theories of how we are conscious in the present will help shed light on how we can recall our past experiences. It will also greatly help to have already covered this topic when we later discuss the means by which someone may eventually be revived from a brain-preserved state. Accordingly, although we've just spent a chapter on personal identity, it's time to get even more personal still. *How, and why, does it feel like something to be you?*

5
What Is Consciousness?

Without consciousness, it may hardly matter whether you live for another five years or another five hundred. In all that time there would be nothing it would be like to be you.

Anil Seth, *Being You*

The left half of TN's visual world vanished when he suffered his first stroke. He'd barely had time to adjust when a month later another attack took the remainder of his sight. Together, the injuries destroyed the region of his brain responsible for receiving inputs from his eyes, known as the *primary visual cortex*. As a result, after fifty-two years of sunshine, motion, and colour, TN was now blind. Although his eyes technically still functioned as well as they did before, nothing was left at the other end of his optic nerves to consciously interpret their signals.

As a doctor himself, TN would have known it is extremely rare for a brain injury to be expansive enough to fully destroy the primary visual cortex and render a patient blind, while simultaneously being limited enough to not damage large sections of the rest of the brain, leaving them dead or significantly intellectually disabled. Thus, he was likely unsurprised when a group of researchers asked him if he would be a participant in their studies to further collective understanding of the neuroscience of vision.

With TN's consent, the research team lined up a battery of behavioural tests and brain scans, aiming to ascertain the extent of his impairments and identify the anatomical changes that caused them. Over the course of these investigations, an intriguing finding emerged.

Despite TN's lack of conscious visual perception, it seemed some information entering his eyes might still be subconsciously steering his behaviour. His empathetic discernment of other people's mood was better than could be expected from just auditory cues, as if he could somehow still read the emotions on their faces. While he used a cane to feel out the path in front of him while walking, his ability to avoid impediments, even before his cane brushed against them, exhibited an uncanny precision. Although TN had no visual sense of the world, he was doing a surprisingly good job of navigating through it.

Intrigued to explore the limits of TN's unexpected abilities, the scientists devised an unconventional experiment. One day, they brought him to a corridor and asked him to lay aside his cane. Although TN couldn't see it, an obstacle course filled with miscellaneous office detritus lay spread out before him. As they explained to him the task at hand, TN felt more than a little nervous. He reminded them that he could not see, and was liable to trip over something and injure himself. But when one of the researchers assured TN that they would shadow him closely the entire way, ready to catch him at the slightest sign of a stumble, TN begrudgingly agreed to the experiment. The pursuit of scientific advancement does sometimes require a blind journey into the unknown; though, to be fair to TN, it isn't usually quite so literal.

The initial moment of truth came with the first obstacle, a dustbin strategically positioned in the middle of the path. With bated breath, the observing scientists watched as TN, three steps from what appeared to be an inevitable collision, sidestepped to the left and shuffled past. The researchers were stunned. His successful evasion of the next bin was equally remarkable. As he proceeded through the maze, he smoothly transitioned to the opposite side of the corridor, circumventing a tripod on his left. In a triumphant finale, TN dodged a document tray and an assortment of boxes and made his way to the finish line at the end of the corridor. The research team broke out in spontaneous applause.

Countless previous studies had established the critical role of the visual cortex in conscious vision. But TN was adamant about his lack of visual experiences, and the brain scans were unequivocal about the extent of the damage he had suffered. Somehow, seemingly paradoxically to TN and researchers alike, here was the first documented case of a blind man who could 'see'.[*,1–3]

***

This phenomenon, where people report possessing no visual experiences while simultaneously behaving as though they can see to at least a limited degree, is known as *blindsight*.[4,5] Individuals with blindsight are genuinely surprised when informed of their performance on visual tasks, and are often suspicious they're just making repeated lucky guesses. Despite this, as TN and others demonstrate, blindsight patients can succeed at a variety of visual tasks, including pointing at objects, tracking motion, and even unassisted navigation. What blindsight demonstrates is the existence of a potentially treacherous gulf between the inferences we make from someone's behaviour, and the distinct reality of their subjective experience.

Interest in this kind of dissociation between behaviour and consciousness has recently been pushed into the mainstream by the rise of artificial intelligence. As of 2023, the Turing test has already been given a run for its money. ChatGPT can hold conversations, Stable Diffusion can produce beautiful artworks, and MuZero can play games from chess to Pac-Man. It is easily imaginable that, before long, machines will exist that can equal or surpass humans at any conceivable task. Yet, even so, the question remains as to whether these synthetic entities will ever be able to perceive the content they manipulate. The extent to which our intrinsic experiences are shared – experiences like appreciating the precision of a well-crafted argument, feeling compelled by an arrangement of clashing colours, or becoming entirely absorbed in a game of chess – is already hard enough to establish with our fellow humans, let alone our computers.

Even before artificial intelligence recently thrust the question of consciousness into the public spotlight, the importance of unspooling its mysteries has long been apparent to neuroscientists and philosophers. Consider patients stuck in persistent vegetative states, unable to

* You can watch a video of TN successfully navigating such a gauntlet here: https://www.youtube.com/watch?v=GwGmWqXoMnM

communicate in any fashion. Are they quietly enjoying something like a vague but pleasant dream, suffering silently in their beds, or feeling nothing whatsoever? Or think of the fellow creatures with which we share our world, from the tiniest insect to the mightiest whale. Are they merely biological automatons, reacting to their environment but experiencing nothing? Does subjectivity creep in somewhere in the great chain of being, maybe at the level of a worm or a mouse? Or does consciousness permeate everywhere and reside in all things, sparking like a match when cause meets effect? These questions are far from indulgent philosophizing – our efforts to improve the welfare of any creature, human or otherwise, depend on knowing just what they can experience.

To take a slightly less lofty tone, the problem of understanding consciousness is also fairly salient to our immediate concern of assessing the feasibility of survival through brain preservation. Just why this is the case is put particularly clearly by the neuroscientist Anil Seth, who in his book on the science of consciousness asks his readers to imagine being given the following choice:

> Imagine that a future version of me, perhaps not so far away, offers you the deal of a lifetime. I can replace your brain with a machine that is its equal in every way, so that from the outside, nobody could tell the difference. This new machine has many advantages – it is immune to decay, and perhaps it will allow you to live forever.
>
> But there's a catch. Since even future-me is not sure how real brains give rise to consciousness, I can't guarantee that you will have any conscious experiences at all, should you take up this offer. Maybe you will, if consciousness depends only on functional capacity, on the power and complexity of the brain's circuitry, but maybe you won't, if consciousness depends on a specific biological material – neurons, for example. Of course, since your machine-brain leads to identical behaviour in every way, when I ask new-you whether you are conscious, new-you will say yes. But what if, despite this answer, life – for you – is no longer in the first person?[6]

It's not that this thought experiment poses any threat to our confidence in being able to preserve a person's personal identity. As we'll see in a couple of chapters, this can already be guaranteed with existing preservation techniques. Rather, the issue is that Seth's worrying scenario bears an uncomfortably strong resemblance to some of the means by which a person who has chosen preservation might hope to one day be revived.

We'll delve into the specifics later in the book, but the speculated future means of reviving someone from a preserved state are much more involved than the present-day equivalent of allowing them to emerge from anaesthesia. To give a brief overview, in addition to the straightforward approach of rejuvenating someone's original biological body, there are other techniques future medical practitioners might wish to consider. They may want to take advancements in neural prostheses to their ultimate conclusion, and fully replace a person's damaged brain and body with sturdier robotic counterparts. Alternatively, they might believe the best treatment is to 'upload' a person's mind into the digital cloud, enabling them to move as freely in virtual worlds as they once did in their original, physical form. Or perhaps they will develop techniques entirely beyond our current capabilities and as yet unknown to modern science.

The problem is, if any of these proposed treatments fail to ensure the perpetuation of an individual's consciousness, then no matter how sophisticated they might be, they offer no hope of survival. Accordingly, we need to know just how afraid we should be that some future treatment may fail to preserve a person's first-person perspective, even if it does perfectly maintain their outwardly observable behaviour. And, in order to assess wisely, we first need to understand the current theories of how traditional, biological human brains give rise to consciousness.

I imagine it will come as no surprise when I warn you that we will not complete this chapter with a full understanding of consciousness and how it fits within a material world. No-one has yet dispelled all the relevant mysteries, and any researcher who claims otherwise has yet to convince the majority of their colleagues.

But that does not mean scientists and philosophers can offer no meaningful insights on the subject, nor that there is no consensus at all on any of its facets. Centuries of philosophical thought, and particularly the last few decades of neuroscientific research, have substantially improved our understanding of the link between mind and flesh. And fortuitously, as we'll soon see, very little of this knowledge can be used to argue that our unique, first-person perspectives could never be revived from a state of preservation.

THE SCIENCE OF SENSES AND SOULS

First things first, let's clarify what we mean when we say someone is *conscious*. Sometimes the term is used to mean 'sensitive to one's surroundings', at other times to indicate a capacity for 'deliberate, purposeful thought'. But, from our own personal perspectives, the most important meaning is one that defines consciousness from an intrinsic viewpoint. To be precise, within the context of this book, when I say that some creature is *conscious*, I mean to suggest that there is 'something it is like to be that creature'.[7]

Imagine seeing the redness of a strawberry, feeling the warmth of the sun, or enjoying pride in a job well done. These sensations point at what it *feels like* to be something. You can delineate these experiences of *feeling like* by contrasting them with their absence: what it felt like to be yourself before you existed, what it is like for TN to 'see' objects in his path, or what it is like to be anything without the faculty to perceive, like a stone or a chair. It is subjective experiences, these senses and feelings, that provide the bedrock which grounds any discussion of consciousness.

The subjective experiences of what it is like to see red, taste chocolate, or feel pain are sometimes formally referred to as *qualia*.* This terminology helps to distinguish subjective experiences, or qualia, from the things out there in the world that evoke them, called *stimuli*. Keeping this distinction in mind is critical, as it's easy to confuse a stimulus for the experience it elicits. For example, a typical human experiences qualia of 'redness' when shown certain spectra of visible light, such as you might when looking at a strawberry. Yet qualia of redness can just as easily occur when a person is dreaming, with no physical stimuli

* To be pedantic, *qualia* more properly refers to the properties of experiences, such as the 'redness' of seeing red, or the 'painfulness' of feeling pain, rather than the experiences per se. If you have no idea what I'm talking about when making this distinction, don't worry about it. It won't matter for this chapter.

present. While particular stimuli and qualia typically go together, a perusal of visual illusions or a dalliance with hallucinogenic drugs will quickly disabuse one of the notion that this always has to be the case. In fact, if you've ever wondered whether your 'red' might be your friend's 'green', then you've already contemplated just how philosophically complex the distinction between stimuli and qualia can be.[8]

The complications only compound from here. For the sake of our sanity, we usually assume that our fellow humans are conscious and experience the same qualia as ourselves when presented with the same stimuli. But what about other creatures? To take a classic example from the academic literature, consider how it may feel to be a bat.[7] When flying through caves or hunting for insects, bats navigate their environment by chirping and then listening for how the noise reflects off their surroundings. This echolocation involves sound, so maybe from a bat's perspective it feels like listening, albeit with an incredibly sensitive ear. But bats use echolocation in a manner akin to vision, so it could be that echolocation for them feels more like sight does for humans.* Then again, nothing mandates that their subjective sensations are equivalent to ours, so perhaps it feels completely unimaginable to be a bat. Or maybe they aren't even conscious, and being a bat feels like nothing at all. How are we supposed to tell?

One might hope that a sufficiently detailed understanding of the brain – human, bat, or alien – would reveal where and how a mind is rendered out of meat. But, counterintuitively at first, pursuing this solution only appears to bring more problems to light. From initial introspection, it seems quite dubious that the ethereal stuff of qualia – colours, tastes, thoughts, and feelings – could be made of the same physical stuff as brains. How could it possibly be the case that our psychological reality, our conscious experiences, can be explained entirely by the composition of the sticky wad of mindless atoms that forms our physical body? This is the *mind–body problem*, and attempts to solve it have been ongoing for centuries.

A notable early approach was that of the philosopher René Descartes,

* Amazingly, some blind humans have also learned to echolocate, typically by making mouth clicks. Blind people can become good enough at this to accurately navigate their surroundings, even to the point of being able to safely ride bicycles.[9]

who in 1641 published the first modern formalization of the intuition that feelings and the physical are fundamentally distinct. In doing so, he claimed that the mind and the body are two metaphysically separate substances, a stance now called *dualism*.* Dualism holds that physical properties, such as mass and charge, exist in the domain of material substances, while consciousness is a property of an immaterial substance. As a bonus to this philosophical position's intuitive nature, dualism is also naturally compatible with the religious belief that a soul provides the essence of a person.

But, intuitive as it may be, dualism faces some daunting issues. For one, it appears unable to explain how a desire to move one's arm could ever result in the contraction of one's muscles. This problem with causation was noticed almost immediately, with Princess Elizabeth of Bohemia, a contemporary correspondent of Descartes', writing to him in 1643 to say, 'Given that the soul of a human being is only a thinking substance, how can it affect the bodily spirits, in order to bring about voluntary actions?' What she was asking by this was: how can our reason and will be immaterial, if producing an action is inherently physical?

Consider how we might wish to move our arm to pick up a strawberry. If our soul can somehow transmit this desire into our muscles, and be affected in turn by the sensation of grasping the fruit, then the soul interacts with the physical, and there must be some physical trace for us to find of this bi-directional relationship. This is a problem for those who would insist that a soul is indeed an entirely immaterial entity and thus not subject to physical forces; if so, they cannot then explain how the corporeal phenomena of movement and sensation could ever be affected by the machinations of one's soul.

As a result, the soul is either physical in at least some capacity, and thus subject to traditional scientific investigation, or its explanatory power is dubious, and it is thus likely irrelevant to explanations of consciousness. Neither of these possibilities are compelling arguments

* Specifically, *substance dualism*, as opposed to *property dualism* which holds that only physical substances exist but that some materials may also have mental properties. My apologies to the philosophers among my readership for not exploring the difference in the main text. For the sake of simplicity, I'm going to stick with just using the term *dualism* without clarification.

for dualism and, perhaps unsurprisingly, the theory's popularity has waned over the centuries.*

As alternatives to dualism, a whole host of other solutions to the mind–body problem have been proposed. *Idealism* holds that if we can't see a way for the mental and the physical to interact, but we know from our own first-hand experience that mental things definitely exist, then perhaps what we commonly assume to be external physical reality is in fact just an extension of our minds. Alternatively, maybe there is an objective physical universe, and all material things within it, from electrons to galaxies, inherently have some degree of conscious experience. This generous position is known as *panpsychism*. Or perhaps the mental and the physical, if viewed correctly, could be shown to actually be the same thing, each providing a co-equal description of the fundamental nature of the universe. This is the theory of *neutral monism*. Any or all of these theories might seem scarcely credible at face value, and each has serious outstanding problems that prevent them from being widely adopted. Even so, all have reputable defenders, and any could yet turn out to be a component in a complete explanation of consciousness.

By far the most popular alternative to dualism, however, among both philosophers and scientists is *physicalism*: the belief that consciousness is somehow equivalent to, or emerges from, the same material stuff that comprises the rest of the universe. While dualism might be the most intuitive at first glance, motivation for physicalism abounds once one considers all the ways that interactions between physical objects affect consciousness. Damage to someone's brain, such as a stroke that causes blindsight, demonstrates that material changes can radically alter a person's subjective perception of the world. Psychoactive molecules, from the caffeine in coffee to the LSD in tabs of acid, produce effects on subjectivity ranging from subtle to profound. Even if it seems our desires and sensations are far removed from the physical realm, in fact our subjectivity rests on an intricate house of cards built from chemical

* Descartes attempted to provide an explanation for brain–soul interaction by claiming that the immaterial soul somehow still exerts an influence on the brain through controlling the flow of animal spirits through the pineal gland. In actuality, the role of the pineal gland is to produce hormones, such as the sleep-wake cycle regulator melatonin.

interactions, the precariousness of which reveals an unequivocal link between the psychological and physical domains.

In parallel to this line of argument, physicalists also point out that the standard laws of physics have otherwise done an excellent job thus far of describing everything else we've observed in the universe. The scientific method, typically combined with the assumption that all phenomena are physical, has had a remarkable track record of improving human understanding for the past few hundred years. In light of this, supporters of physicalism suspect that consciousness will eventually be shown to be compatible with a fully material world.

Exorcizing the ghost in the machine

Yet suspicions offer no guarantees, and there are still reasons to be sceptical of purely physicalist theories of consciousness. Remember Anil Seth's offer to replace your decaying biological brain with an unaging artificial one, but without assurance you will continue to enjoy a first-person perspective? Although the thought experiments are not exactly the same, the concerns expressed in that scenario are very similar to those explored in an alternate thought experiment about zombies. Just as zombies in fiction chew on the physical material of human brains, the zombies in this thought experiment mangle certainty in the physicalist nature of the human mind.

Instead of the usual brain-eating variety, however, this scenario involves a different kind of zombie that is a much tamer creature. It acts like a normal person, talks like a normal person, and as far as an outside observer can tell is fully indistinguishable from a normal person, no matter how sophisticated their investigative techniques might be. Indeed, a *philosophical zombie* is exactly the same as a normal person, all the way down to the atomic level, except in one respect: it lacks any conscious experiences, or any first-person perspective. A philosophical zombie version of myself would still write papers, state that pizza was delicious, and wince in pain when pricked with a needle. But while a philosophical zombie appears to be a normal person from the outside, there is nothing it feels like to be one on the inside. The argument goes that if philosophical zombies are conceivable, let alone possible to create, we have cause for concern regarding physicalist theories of consciousness. The specific reason why is as follows:

Imagine that, one day, future neuroscientists can provide a perfect description of the input–output behaviour of the brain. Showing someone *this* particular stimulus reliably causes *that* particular pattern of neuronal activity, which inevitably leads to *this* particular behaviour, and so on. The enigmatic clockwork by which people remember, describe, plan, are motivated to action, and sense their environment has been fully disassembled by comprehensive neuroscientific understanding of the brain. And yet, no neuroscientist has discovered where in the brain to find colours, tastes, moods, or any of the other qualia that constitute our inner experience. The depths of neuroscience have been plumbed, but the inner cave of consciousness could not be found.

How to surmount this concern – that even a complete physical description of the brain might fail to provide an explanation of consciousness – was termed the *hard problem* by the philosopher David Chalmers.[10] Its hardness is apparent in comparison to comparatively 'easier' problems such as how humans can focus their attention, record memories, or transition from sleep to wake. While difficult to answer, these questions are all amenable to the standard neuroscientific tools of brain imaging, psychological experimentation, and computational modelling. In contrast, the hard problem threatens to remain stubbornly resistant to even the most advanced technology. As a result, there is presently no guarantee that philosophical zombies could not exist, and so there are still worries that a physicalist explanation of consciousness may yet fail.

To be clear, not all researchers accept the challenge presented by the hard problem. Questions of whether philosophical zombies are a conceptually coherent possibility, and thus whether the hard problem is a genuine concern as opposed to a dismissible misunderstanding, continue to divide philosophers.

But the fact that there is any uncertainty at all is enough to be unsettling. If there is truly an explanatory gap between qualia and their physical explanation which we never learn how to bridge, then it may forever be impossible to know if any creature is conscious no matter how complex its behaviour may be.[11] This is uncomfortable, as it would be decidedly more satisfying to have surety in whether one's friends, pets, or AI assistants are conscious or not. But most pressing of all are when the questions have life-or-death stakes, as they do when considering methods of revival from brain preservation.

It is perhaps reassuring, then, that despite hard problems and the ravages of zombies, physicalism is still the most popular position for philosophers and is almost ubiquitous among neuroscientists.[*,12] To a large degree, this is because, while theories like dualism have little explanatory power, physicalism, combined with an experimental approach, already has a solid track record for revealing the mechanisms of what were once deeply mysterious phenomena.

Take life, for example. Nowadays, scientists can describe how an orchestra of complex chemical reactions and interactions transforms an oily bubble filled with molecules into a living cell. But before the nineteenth century, the notion that biological creatures shared the same elemental composition as inanimate objects was unthinkable to many. In a parallel to dualism, some early researchers proposed that living creatures must contain a 'vital spark' which animated them, allowing them to take otherwise inert chemicals and imbue them with animal spirits. A compelling argument for this was that, at the time, living creatures could produce organic compounds that no chemist could, such as the nitrogen-containing urea found in animal urine. This seemingly miraculous capability was taken as evidence for *vitalism*, the idea that living things were governed by fundamentally different principles to inanimate matter.

But, as science progressed, the foundations of vitalism began to crack. As chemists discovered how to artificially synthesize urea, and as biologists began to control and recreate the physical processes occurring within cells, the evidence for a vital spark was snuffed out. In the end, clever experiments and careful theory demonstrated that the mystical essence of life was reducible to the mundane material world. The aim of physicalism-inclined neuroscientists is to conduct experiments and develop theories that erode the hard problem, just as biochemical discoveries dissolved vitalism.

* However, there is disagreement as to whether currently known physical phenomena are sufficient to explain consciousness, or whether there are new fundamental discoveries in physics required first.

Correlation hints at causation

In an effort to achieve this goal, the last three decades have seen a dramatic rise in the activities of consciousness scientists.[13,14] In particular, 1990 saw the publication of a seminal paper by Francis Crick, one of the co-discoverers of the structure of DNA, and the neuroscientist Christof Koch.[15] Their article argued that to understand the physical basis of consciousness, it would be helpful to be able to isolate what physical changes in the brain were reliably indicative of changes to a person's experiences. They noted that this activity would not be trivial to identify, as much of the happenings in the brain have little or nothing to do with consciousness, such as the brainstem activity that regulates one's heart rate and body posture. Still, if neuroscientists could just find a method to isolate the brain activity responsible for experiences away from the rest of these unconscious neural processes, studying this circuitry of consciousness might provide invaluable hints towards a robust physicalist theory.

A key suggestion made by Crick and Koch regarding potential experimental methodologies was that scientists should try to find a way to induce a participant's subjective experiences to change even while keeping their environmental conditions completely constant. If participants could be placed in a situation where their experiences would vary even while being presented with unchanging stimuli, researchers would know that any changes occurring in the participant's brain would have something to do with consciousness, rather than irrelevant unconscious processes.

Fortuitously, an experimental setup to obtain this outcome can be achieved by taking advantage of stimuli that can be perceived in two distinctly different ways. For example, imagine looking at a line drawing of a cube (Fig. 7 a). Even as the drawing remains exactly the same, the square that appears to be the front of the cube can shift, with people typically flipping between the two experiences every few seconds. Images like these are known as *bistable* stimuli.* Another related paradigm involves simultaneously showing two different and incompatible images to each eye individually, such as a face only visible to

* Other common examples include the duck/rabbit and face/vase illusions, which are also fun to look up online if you haven't seen them.

a

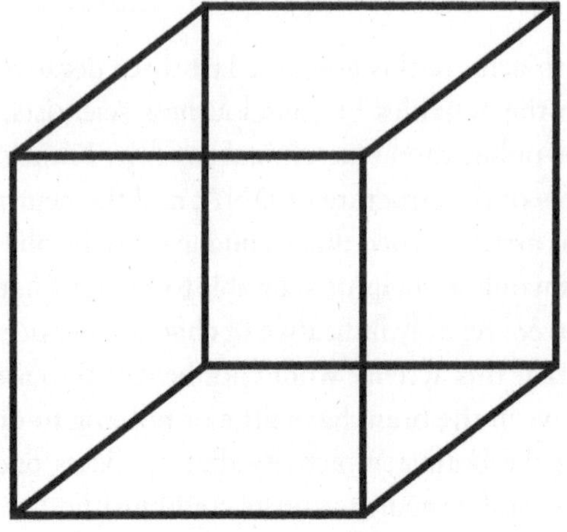

b

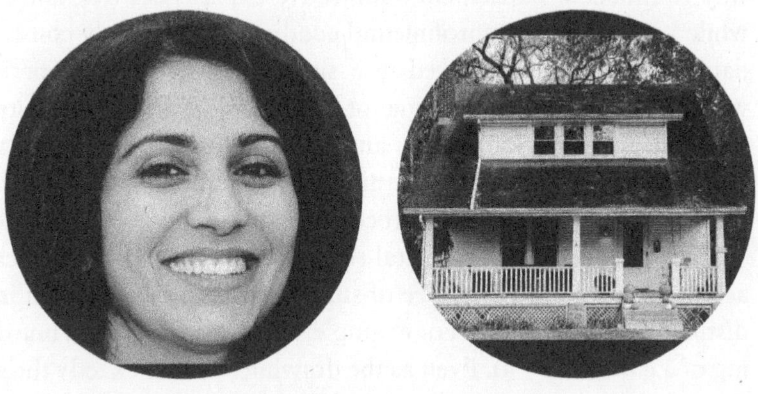

Figure 7. a) This line drawing of a cube can appear so that either the bottom-left or top-right square is the front of the cube, the one facing out of the page. b) In binocular rivalry, where the face stimulus is presented to only someone's left eye, while the image of the house is presented to only their right eye, a person will perceive only one of the stimuli at a time. You can try this yourself, though it won't work as well at home as it would with a laboratory setup. If you still want to try, read all the following instructions first, and then give it a shot:

the left eye with a house only visible to the right (Fig. 7 b). Observers presented with these conflicting stimuli do not experience some sort of face-house hybrid. Instead, they see a face for a few seconds, then transition to the house, then back to the face, and so on, continuously flipping back and forth. This setup is called *binocular rivalry*, as it is as if each eye is fighting for the stimulus it can observe to be the one that elicits a conscious experience.

If an experiment using either the bistable stimuli or binocular rivalry technique is combined with a way of recording brain activity, such as EEG or MRI scans, then it should be possible to isolate the brain activity responsible for changes in visual experience away from the rest of our incessant unconscious neural processes. With this proposal, Crick and Koch initiated the search for the *neural correlates of consciousness*. Several decades of research later, neuroscientists have a treasure trove of results from both neural correlates experiments and other, newer techniques.

While experimentalists have been busy collecting this data, theorists have not hesitated to propose a plethora of creative physicalist theories of consciousness. In fact, there is now an overabundance of theories, ranging from the modest suggestion that subjectivity results from how we control our attention, through to the more outlandish idea that consciousness depends on quantum mechanical effects in the cellular skeletons of neurons.[16] Imaginative thinking is normally

---

First, find a place to set this page down flat. Next, curl your hands up (or position two toilet rolls) as though you were pretending they were imaginary binoculars, and bring them to your eyes. After that, close your left eye, and position your head and hands so that your right eye can see only the house through the tube of your right hand. Then close your right eye and perform the same procedure with your left eye and hand, while being careful to not move your head or right hand. You may have to have your hands almost on the page to get this setup to work. You may also have to angle your hands (or the toilet rolls) inwards towards each other. Once complete, open both eyes, and let them relax and unfocus so that the two stimuli appear to overlap into one circle. You should now sometimes see a face, sometimes a house, with your perception transitioning between the two every few seconds.

thought of as the prerogative of artists, but when trying to unravel the enigma at the core of ourselves, neuroscientists and philosophers have been remarkably adventurous.

Even so, the hard problem continues to loom over all these proposed solutions. So far, no-one has convinced the research community that they have succeeded in solving it and proving that philosophical zombies are logically impossible, and so, for now, the potential for a complete dissociation between feelings and the physical remains worryingly conceivable. As a result, an assurance that revival therapies for brain preservation will one day be feasible hinges on the yet-unresolved establishment of a physicalist basis for consciousness.

But it's still far too early for scientists to be walking away and admitting defeat. Vitalism may have seemed difficult to disprove in the early nineteenth century, but from our vantage point of the twenty-first, it is trivially easy. To see if any physicalist theory might warrant optimism in neuroscience's equivalent eventual success, let's walk through a few of the currently leading candidates for how mere matter might give rise to the mind.

IS CONSCIOUSNESS A FUNCTION?

When confronted with the prospect of soulless zombies, devoid of experiences yet passing indistinguishably among the rest of us, the most popular class of physicalist theories elects to simply deny the possibility of their existence. Instead, the doctrine of *functionalism* asserts that any creature capable of performing consciousness-related functions must necessarily have accompanying conscious experiences.[17] According to functionalism, if a creature is capable of sensory perception, cognitive processing, behavioural control, or other related functions, then its possession of corresponding feelings and thoughts is beyond question.

To provide a painfully explicit example, imagine the throbbing pain you would feel if you burnt your finger on a hot pan. Accompanying the pain comes the knowledge that your finger has been damaged. The series of mistakes you made that led up to this point are seared into your memory. Until it heals, you will avoid touching objects with your still-tender finger, changing your behaviour to prevent the damage from being exacerbated. A functionalist would argue that this combination of sensation of bodily damage, explicit thinking about what went wrong and how to prevent it next time, and behavioural changes to compensate for your injury, could not possibly occur without an accompanying feeling of pain.

The generality of this approach becomes interesting in its application to creatures very different from ourselves. Take an octopus, for example. These alien-looking, eight-legged sea creatures have a nervous system markedly unlike our own. Instead of having one central brain containing most of their body's neurons, octopuses have substantial collections of neurons in each tentacle, meaning each leg has in effect its own 'mini-brain'. Given these distinctions from human anatomy, should the implication be that octopuses cannot feel pain as we do when they scrape a sucker as we might stub a toe?

If you are confident that animals are conscious, then you are likely to find a functionalist account of consciousness appealing. Despite their anatomical differences, pain-related functions appear just as present in these cephalopods as they are in humans. Octopuses withdraw their tentacles from noxious stimuli so as to limit the damage they sustain. They learn to actively avoid situations where they have been hurt before. They even rub their injured tentacles and seek out pain relief drugs if available.[18] According to functionalism, then, there are strong grounds to argue that octopuses can suffer just as we can.

Formally, this inclusive feature of functionalism is known either as *multiple realizability* or *substrate independence*, in that the same functions, and hence conscious experiences, are realizable with different physical substrates. Multiple realizability implies that a creature can be conscious whether it is made of flesh, silicon, or something completely alien, so long as it possesses the right functions. There is no chauvinistic privileging of human brains – anything that could walk, talk, and think as well as we could, no matter what it was made from, would have the right to claim a first-person perspective just as meaningful as our own.

But hold on. It can't be as simple as 'if it looks like consciousness then it is consciousness', right? Wouldn't this contradict the evidence that functions like sight and conscious experience of visual perception can dissociate, as shown by TN and his blindsight? Aren't the experts still deeply sceptical that it feels like anything to be ChatGPT, despite the AI's impressive language capabilities? Does functionalism suggest that TN is a liar and ChatGPT deserves human rights?

Not quite. While functionalism asserts that at least some functions are indicative of consciousness, it is not so inclusive as to suggest that any behaviour at all necessarily entails subjective experience. For example, consider that simple creatures such as bacteria are capable of sensing their environments, while some plants and fungi are even capable of elementary communication with each other. Functionalists do not see these behaviours as synonymous with consciousness, nor grounds to grant subjectivity to all living things, but instead reasons to be more restrictive about what capacities count for consciousness.

Consider again the case of TN. It's true that, despite the substantial damage to his primary visual cortex, TN maintained the ability to navigate his environment. But a focus on only his retained abilities belies the severity of his debilitating functional losses. After his strokes, TN could no longer walk into a supermarket and know what items were on the shelves. He could not learn new skills from watching instructional videos, or draw a sketch of his upcoming plans. He had no trust in whatever unconscious visual abilities he had remaining, as he had no sense of his own performance on tasks requiring sight, nor a direct way to know if he was succeeding or just making lucky guesses.

On this basis, functionalists do not feel forced to accept that blindsight demonstrates a dissociation between functions and experience. Instead, they assert that consciousness depends more on the presence of deliberate and introspectively available abilities, such as being able to describe your favourite food to someone by drawing them a picture of it, than it does on more basic and instinctual capacities that merely allow one to avoid walking into walls.

We can come at this from the opposite direction too. Functionalists contend that some disabled humans who are chronically unresponsive may still have a first-person perspective, so long as they have some key functions remaining. For example, take cases of patients suffering from locked-in syndrome, a condition where individuals become completely paralysed and unable to move or speak.[19] While some of these patients retain the ability to communicate by moving their eyes in distinct patterns, others cannot muster even this, losing all ability to affect the world. At a casual glance, these patients appear entirely unresponsive, with unclear evidence as to whether they retain an inner mental life. However, functionalists contend that this does not matter if more sophisticated tools can discover that the critical capacities for consciousness remain within them still.

To reveal whether a conscious mind persists within the bodies of some unresponsive patients, scientists have combined cleverly designed psychological tasks with imaging of brain activity. In one illustrative study from 2010, patients were asked a series of yes/no questions while lying in an MRI scanner.[20,21] In place of verbal responses, the participants were asked to imagine performing one of two distinctive activities. As an example, one patient was asked 'Do you have any brothers?' and instructed to visualize playing tennis to indicate 'Yes,' or to instead imagine walking from room to room in their house to indicate 'No.' Because the two different tasks activate distinctly different brain regions, the experimenters could take the pattern of brain activity observed after a question was asked as indicative of the participant's response.

Out of a set of twenty-one patients who were otherwise fully behaviourally unresponsive, two individuals showed a pattern of brain activity that reliably tracked the correct responses to the investigators' questions. The findings presented strong evidence that these two patients were still capable of imagining, planning, and communicating, even if their bodies would no longer obey their commands. According to functionalists, these remaining abilities are highly suggestive that these verbally unresponsive individuals remain conscious.*

This viewpoint certainly aligns with the widely held notion that some functions are much more critical to consciousness than others. On the one hand, basic reflexes, while integral to survival, are probably not so important. Neither does it mean much to instinctually recoil from threats if one is unable to introspect on one's state of mind and provide some report of one's train of thought. On the other hand,

* As we'll see shortly, though, functionalism is not the only theory that would still ascribe consciousness to these patients.

the ability to learn novel tasks, such as to ride a bike or play the piano, is suggested to be a critically necessary capacity. In particular, voluntarily controlling behaviour – choosing our words, setting our goals – is much more indicative of a conscious mind than the primitive processes responsible for maintaining posture or regulating blood pressure. But if this is so, the question remains: if only some are relevant, how do we sift out those specific functions that lie at the root of consciousness?

Fame in the brain

One of the most prominent neuroscientific theories of consciousness, sitting within the broader functionalist camp, believes it has an answer to which functions are critical. Specifically, *global workspace theory* holds that the key to consciousness is the ability for information to be made available to many different cognitive processes simultaneously. According to this view, consciousness is not to be found in the self-contained, closed-loop neural circuitry that raises one's heart rate when standing after sitting. Instead, it arises from the highly interconnected brain regions that enable you, when presented with a piece of chocolate, to evaluate how delicious it looks, articulate how it stimulates your hunger, and remember who gave it to you, all at once. At least, such is the claim of the theory's most prominent developers, the scientists Bernard Baars and Stanislas Dehaene.[22,23]

To provide some background, global workspace theory finds its motivation in the question of how, out of all the different sights, sounds, somatic sensations, and other stimuli that we are constantly bombarded with, our brains select the particular content we are conscious of at any given time. For context, we are entirely unconscious of most of the functions to which our brains are dedicated. We are almost completely unacquainted, for example, with the activity that regulates our breathing, body posture, heart rate, and digestion. In fact, at any given time, we are aware of only a tiny proportion of the deluge of information flooding our senses. What then determines which pieces of sensory information, among all the multitude of candidates, are temporarily elevated to the throne of conscious experience?

Again, well-designed psychological experiments, combined with recordings of brain activity, can give us insight into what is going on. Take one study published in 2018, where researchers trained monkeys to report when they saw a stimulus, while simultaneously recording activity in multiple regions of their brains.[24] On half the experimental trials, the monkeys were presented with a faint, difficult-to-detect, circular stimulus. In the remaining half, no stimulus was shown at all. The monkeys were instructed to correctly identify whether the stimulus was present or absent, and given a juice payment to reward them for their efforts when successful.* By carefully calibrating the contrast of the stimulus, the researchers could ensure the monkeys would frequently fail to detect the circle, even on trials when it was present and they were looking straight at it. This clever experimental design meant that presence of the stimulus, and the monkey's awareness of that fact, could be completely dissociated, as any trial could fall into one of four conditions: stimulus present and detected, stimulus present but unseen, stimulus absent and correctly noted as missing, and stimulus reported present when it wasn't really there (Fig. 8). With this setup, the researchers could ascertain what brain activity was associated with awareness of the stimulus, by considering trials where the circle was present, but only sometimes seen.

Let's consider first what they found regarding brain activity in the primary visual cortex, the region in the back of the brain that is the first point of call for information making its way from our eyes and into our minds. On trials where the stimulus was present, compared to those when it was not displayed, there was always detectable activity in the primary visual cortex. Intriguingly, this activity was observed whether or not the monkey reported seeing the stimulus. This meant that primary visual cortex activity, while indicative of a stimulus's presence, gave no indication by itself of whether or not the circle ever entered conscious perception.

These findings were in stark contrast to recordings made further forwards in the brain. In the prefrontal cortex, a region commonly considered to possess 'higher-level' functions, activity was detected

* Researchers have ascertained that other suitable incentives to motivate behavioural-task performance include softcore pornographic images of other monkeys.[25]

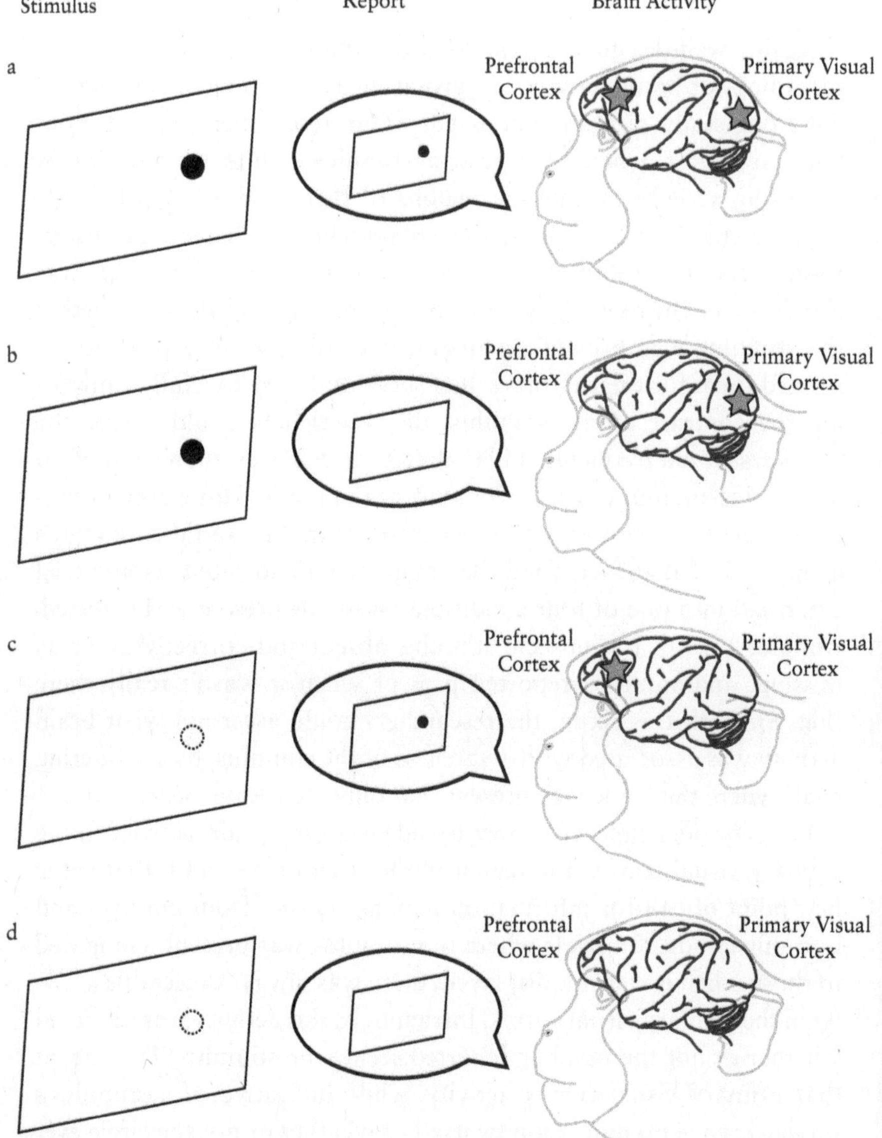

Figure 8. A difficult-to-see stimulus is presented only on some experimental trials, with the monkey trying to correctly report whether the stimulus was present or absent.[24] a) When the stimulus is present, and correctly identified as such, activity is present in both the primary visual and prefrontal cortex, as marked by the star symbols. b) When the stimulus is present but not detected by the monkey, activity is present in the visual cortex but absent in the prefrontal. c) In contrast, when the stimulus is absent but reported as present, activity is seen only in the prefrontal cortex. d) When the stimulus is absent and correctly reported as such, no activity is detected.

only on trials when the monkey reported seeing the stimulus.* Importantly, this occurred even on 'false alarms', trials where the stimulus was reported as present even when it had not been displayed. Considering these two findings together, this experiment showed that activity in the prefrontal cortex tracked a monkey's reports of awareness, while that in the primary visual cortex did not. Assuming this is accurate, the next question is: why might the functions of the prefrontal cortex be especially linked to consciousness?

Global workspace theory argues this is because activity in the prefrontal cortex is particularly indicative of a phenomenon called *ignition*. Ignition is defined as an event where a certain piece of information moves beyond local brain areas that support only limited functions and becomes 'globally broadcast' throughout the entire brain.

Take the example above of a monkey being shown a hard-to-see circle. If the stimulus information only makes it as far as the primary visual cortex, ignition does not occur, meaning the stimulus is not consciously detected and thus cannot drive the monkey's behaviour. But when that same information reaches the prefrontal cortex, and enters the monkey's awareness to the extent that it can be used to teach the monkey to perform a task for a delicious juice reward, then ignition has occurred.

To bolster their argument that ignition reliably corresponds to conscious experience, proponents claim the notion is not just useful for explaining simple stimulus detection, but also in more complicated settings too. For example, consider a participant in a binocular rivalry experiment as discussed earlier. Why is it that at any one moment, this person might be seeing a house instead of a face? Global workspace theorists argue that the answer lies in which particular stimulus is being broadcast at any one time.

To dive further into how this works, let's return to our trusty experiments where brain recordings are combined with psychological tasks, this time with a binocular-rivalry design.[26,27] This particular setup is ideal for searching for the neural correlates of consciousness, as it can

* More properly, this should be 'above baseline activity'. There's typically always some degree of activity happening everywhere in the brain, however, the question is how the pattern changes when one switches between different tasks and activities.

expose the specific brain activity that changes only on the basis of whether it is the face or house that is currently being consciously perceived.

So what have these studies found? Firstly, work in this vein has revealed that whether one sees the face or the house at a given moment is not determined by something as simple as one eye getting switched off or on. Again, neurons in the primary visual cortex seem to care little for changes in conscious experience. Only 20 per cent change their activity based on whether the house or the face is currently reported to be perceived, with the activity of the rest bearing no observable relationship with consciousness (Fig. 9).

Once more, a correspondence between subjective experience and brain activity becomes more apparent when moving forwards from the primary visual cortex into brain regions less directly connected to the eyes. In a broad set of areas, including the prefrontal and inferotemporal cortex, more than 50 per cent of recorded neurons altered their activity depending on whether it was the face or the house that was currently being experienced. As with the previous study, global workspace theorists claim the changes in these areas indicate which stimulus is currently undergoing ignition, allowing information about it to be broadcast throughout the entire brain.

With those studies as background, we can now be more specific about exactly what function global workspace theory alleges is synonymous with consciousness. The theory claims that the key ability is the capacity for otherwise unconscious sensations to enter a 'global workspace', where information becomes broadly available to the brain's various functional capacities. This global workspace depends on neurons distributed across many brain areas, allowing integration of information from the more specialized subsystems that control sensory perception, memory recall, and evaluative judgements, while also distributing said information to other functions like memory formation and the control of voluntary actions. According to the theory, it is this workspace that is identifiable with consciousness, with whatever information is being broadcast within it at a particular time determining a person's current conscious experiences. In the end, the reason why humans are only conscious of a small proportion of the information assaulting our

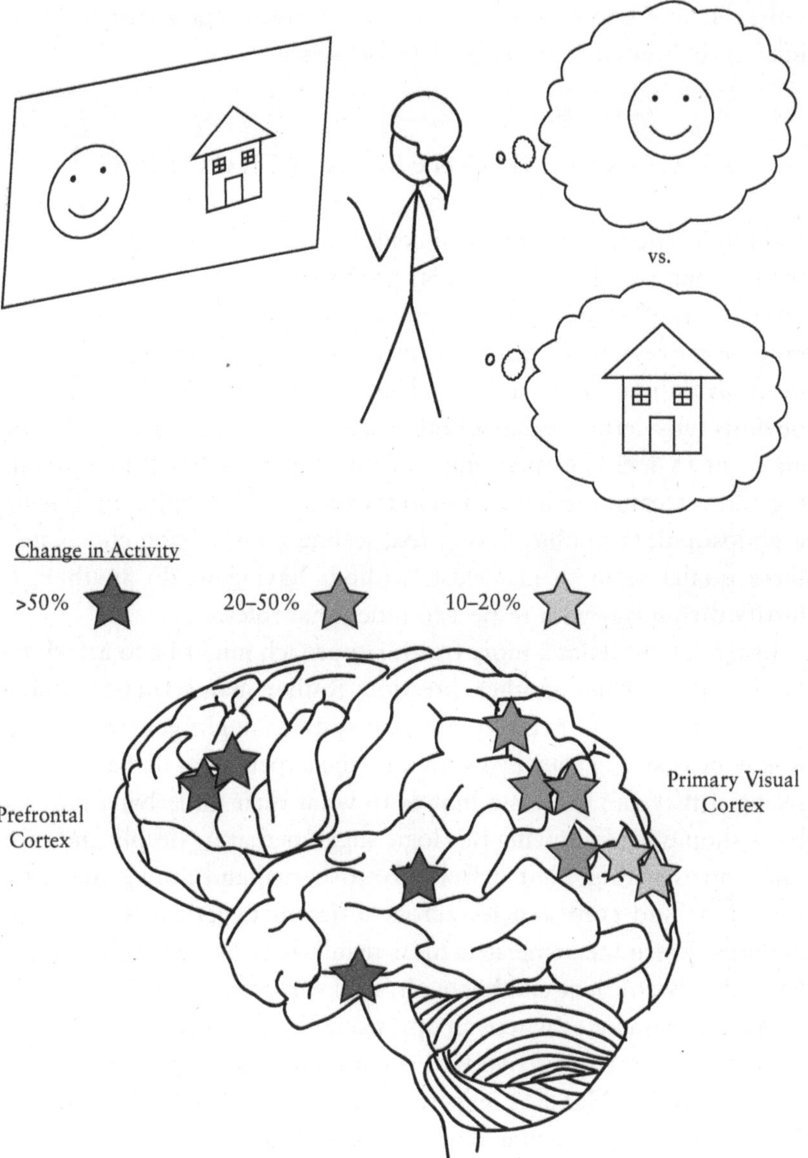

Figure 9. During a binocular rivalry experiment, the proportion of neurons whose activity is affected by a switch in conscious perception varies across brain regions.[26]

senses at any one time is that it is a necessary consequence of the inherently limited capacity of the workspace.

IS CONSCIOUSNESS A STRUCTURE?

Although functionalist views of consciousness like global workspace theory comprise the most popular group of ideas at present – held by around a third of philosophers and a plurality of neuroscientists – as far as some researchers are concerned, the doctrine starts from fundamentally dubious premises.[*,12,42] These sceptics hold that it's not at all obvious why certain behavioural or cognitive functions should cause an agent to 'feel like' anything, nor that there is any obvious advantage for a creature to have conscious experiences as opposed to being a philosophical zombie. Seeing red, feeling pain, tasting chocolate – these qualia seem to just exist, without having to do anything to justify themselves with respect to functional roles.

Instead, they claim a more fruitful approach might be to attack the hard problem from another direction. Rather than trying to analyse why the functions of certain physical systems might generate qualia, it may be easier to start by examining the experiences themselves and seeing if they can give us a hint as to what their underlying physical basis should be. Following this logic suggests that by deeply and carefully introspecting what it feels like to be us, and noting down the variations and consistencies across different experiences, we could perhaps determine some structural regularities of qualia that would be suggestive of their candidate physical substrate.

For an example of where an approach like this has worked before, we can look to the discovery of the physical basis of genes.[28] In the 1860s, Gregor Mendel's experiments on pea plants showed that flower colour, petal shape, and other traits could be inherited as discrete units. These discrete units, labelled genes, were described well before their physical basis was understood. It wasn't for another forty years that experiments were able to show genes had something to do

* For criticisms of functionalism generally and global workspace theory specifically, see the 'Once more, with feeling' section of Appendix Two.

with chromosomes, and another forty years after that before they were linked to specific sequences of DNA. The phenomenon of inheritance was characterized first through deduction, to be followed only later by an understanding of its physical basis.

The hope of the *qualia structure* research programme is to make use of the same process for consciousness as was previously applied to genetics.[*,29–32]. Except, this time, instead of botanical drawings and gardening equipment, the tools of choice are introspection and similarity judgments.

To understand the methodology of the qualia structure research programme, imagine you are participating in a binocular rivalry experiment while simultaneously listening to some music. Your main focus is probably on how your visual experience is switching back and forth between a face and a house, while you might also be aware of a melody playing in the background.

Already, from this simple observation of your mental state, there is information about consciousness to be gleaned. Firstly, let's remember that you can never experience the house and face simultaneously in the same place and time, let alone some kind of house-face hybrid. This reveals that visual experiences are *definitive*, in the sense that you cannot visually focus on more than one entity at a time. Secondly, consider how instead of your perception of the music being entirely disconnected from your visual experiences, your consciousness contains both concurrently. In this sense conscious experiences are *unified*, in that different aspects of an individual's perspective at any one time are all integrated together, rather than experienced separately.

In other cases where the nature of our subjective experiences is hard to determine through introspection alone, experiments where participants judge the similarity of different qualia can provide another avenue to characterizing consciousness.[33] For example, if you ask a person to explain directly what 'redness' looks like, they are likely to look at

* This programme has been articulated in various forms and with various names by different researchers, with some of the other prominent names being *neurophenomenology* used by Varela, *objective phenomenology* by Lee, and *neurophenomenal structuralism* by Fink and Lyre. While each of the terms refers to a project with a somewhat different methodology, they mostly agree on the same underlying principles and approach.

you in confusion. However, ask them to systematically report the similarity between 'redness', 'pinkness', 'greenness' and many other colours, and they would likely have no issues. Analyse the resulting data, and you will reveal that the relationships between colour experiences can be characterized by a sphere, with grey located at the centre, white at the top, black at the bottom, and with the unique hues of red, yellow, green, and blue located at ninety degrees apart from each other on the equator.* Barring certain practical limitations, this kind of experiment to reveal *qualia structures* can be applied to any sort of experience that a person may possess.

So, let's assume that the structures of consciousness can be revealed by introspection and similarity judgments, yielding a description equivalent to a trait-based definition of genes. If this can be established, then what physical substrate might provide the equivalent for qualia structures that DNA plays for genes?

Informing ourselves

A suggestion provided by the neuroscientist Giulio Tononi is that consciousness is identical to any physical structure that contains the right kind of information. His idea, named *integrated information theory*, attempts to develop this proposal into a formal framework.[34] The theory starts by suggesting certain characteristics of consciousness are so immediately obvious through introspection that they can be known with no further justification, i.e. axiomatically. One example is the *axiom of existence*, which, much like Descartes' 'I think, therefore I am,' asserts that experiences exist at all. Another is the *axiom of information*, which says that each experience is specific and different from other experiences, such as how an experience of redness is different from one of orangeness or greenness.

With this proposed characterization of qualia in hand, Tononi's next step is to go looking for candidate physical substrates that bear a resemblance to consciousness. As is apparent from the theory's

* This is a simplification – perceptual colour spaces are likely far more complicated than the commonly used three-dimensional red-green, blue-yellow, black-white models initially indicate.

name, his preferred candidate is *integrated information.* Since that term is about as transparent as a glass door in a steam room, let's clarify what he means by *information* and how it can be *integrated.*

My home city of Melbourne has notoriously unpredictable weather; even if it's currently raining, it may well be sunny in an hour. On any given day it may rain, hail, shine, or all three in short succession. When I'm at work, staring at my computer monitor, it's hard for me to know what the weather is outside. Yet once I look out through the window and see rain clouds, my uncertainty evaporates, along with any desire to venture out of my apartment. The view gives me *information*: interpretable data that informs me of the particular state of the world out of a set of possibilities.*

That is information, but what does it mean for such a thing to be *integrated*? Well, consider how, either naturally or by design, pieces of information can sometimes be related to each other. To stick with mundane but relatable examples pulled from my physical surroundings, consider how in my bedroom I have both an air conditioner for the summer and a portable heater for the winter. Let's further imagine that, with the luxuries of modern technology, I have programmed the air conditioner to come on automatically when it's over 25°C and the heater when it's under 16°C. But unfortunately, due to my flawed human nature, I have made a mistake,† and set the air conditioner to cool the room down to 15°C. Were I to do this, I would have inadvertently created a cycle. First, the air conditioner would cool the room down and turn itself off. Next, the heater would notice it is too cold, switch itself on, and heat the room up. In response, the air conditioner would notice it is too hot again, and resume its previous efforts. As my power bill skyrocketed, the room itself would have entered a stable (though expensive) feedback cycle of heating and cooling.

Now, normally, examining whether a device is on or off at one location doesn't necessarily inform you about the activity of another

* The example I give here is more similar to a classical Shannonian view of information, while proponents of integrated information theory prefer to analyse what they call 'intrinsic information'. The two concepts are related but not identical – see the references for more detail.[35]

† Really not at all hard to imagine.

device somewhere else. But because of the way I've accidentally connected the activity of the heater and air conditioner in this scenario, the two devices are now acting as part of a single system. In this system, one appliance being on means the other device must be off. As a result, together the air conditioner–heater system has *integrated information* not present when looking at each device individually.

While this is an admittedly simplistic example, Tononi postulates that there is a natural connection between each of his proposed axioms about qualia and characteristics of integrated information present in the brain. Consider again the axiom of information, which asserts that experiences are always specific, such as seeing a face instead of a house. This axiom aligns well with what we saw in the binocular experiment – that it is impossible to visually perceive more than one entity at a time. Tononi suggests that this is connected to how information always specifies a single state out of a limited set of possibilities, such as heater on and air conditioner off, as opposed to the other way around. Or consider another of Tononi's axioms, the *axiom of integration*, which claims that individual qualia experienced in combination fuse into 'broad' qualia which are unitary and irreducible, such as how we experience the audio and video of a movie not as two discrete, simultaneous processes of listening and watching, but rather as one inseparable experience. Tononi contends that this corresponds to how a system with integrated information is unable to be reduced to the state of its individual components in isolation, such as how either the heater or air conditioner considered alone cannot explain the behaviour of the air conditioner–heater system.

With that preliminary description out of the way, let's walk out of the temperature-controlled environment of our previous example and steel ourselves for the inclement conditions of real-world situations. Rather than home appliances, neuroscientists are generally interested in assessing the integrated information present in any system they believe might be conscious, be that a human brain, an octopus's tentacle, a supercomputer, or anything. To do so, they first need to identify the individual units that make up the system, and next determine the different states those units can take. In a human or octopus brain, the obvious candidates to examine would be neurons, which at any time point may either be active or inactive. For a different system, like a computer, the units might be digital switches, which can either be in an ON or OFF state. Once the system has been specified, the neuroscientists then need to make observations of how the states of its units evolve over time, such as by taking recordings of how a brain's activity changes over an hour. From this data, it becomes possible to calculate the level of integrated information present in the system.

There are roughly three possible outcomes from this analysis procedure when applied to any particular system.

The first is that, at any time point, the state of each unit in the system appears to be random, with the activity of one unit having seemingly no influence on that of any other. This is what we would expect to see if we took random recordings of bits of brain activity from multiple people and lumped them together into one set – the neural activity in one person's brain would have no detectable influence over the neurons of a different individual.* As these random relationships do not specify any information, we can conclude that the system viewed overall is not integrated.

The second is that for every observed time point, all of the units have exactly the same activity, such as if a set of digital switches were wired together into a single light switch. This boring entity has no integrated information, as the whole system is essentially reducible to just one ON/OFF unit.

The third and most interesting case occurs when the evolving states of the individual units is best described only when viewed in the context of what all the other units in the system are doing. For example, if the activity of a neuron in a particular person's brain appears random when viewed in isolation, but can be shown to influence, and be influenced by, their other brain cells when viewed as part of a larger system, then the person's brain possesses a large amount of integrated information.

Now that we have a more concrete idea of what integrated information actually is, let's examine the practical implications of integrated information theory's core claims. One of its most notable suggestions is that the more integrated information a system has, the more

* A much more interesting question is what this analysis would show for individuals with fused brains, such as the Hogan twins.

conscious it should be. To check whether this is true, one could experimentally measure the integrated information present in the brains of people who were awake, asleep, anaesthetized, or who had other alterations to their level of consciousness.

Unfortunately, for a variety of technical reasons ranging from ethical constraints on obtaining invasive brain-recordings from humans through to the enormous computational costs of analysing the required data, these experiments are challenging to perform directly. However, it turns out that proxy measures for integrated information are reliably able to distinguish individuals who are awake or dreaming from those anaesthetized or in dreamless sleep.* In turn, this suggests that integrated information does indeed correlate with level of consciousness.[36] Additionally, this human data is bolstered by results from experiments performed in the much simpler brains of flies, where researchers are more straightforwardly able to demonstrate that integrated information is lower in anaesthetized than awake states.[37]

Yet despite these compelling empirical findings, there are many who still baulk at integrated information theory's philosophical implications.† Remember, anything in the entire universe, be it a human, a bacterium, or even a simple thermostat circuit, is supposed to be conscious if it has any integrated information at all. While this supposition is already somewhat panpsychist, it might not be too worrying if the amount of integrated information a physical system possessed always lined up with our intuitions about how conscious that system should be. Problematically, this is not always the case.

According to the theory, a large enough grid of digital switches, arranged to perform simple multiplication calculations, could have more integrated information than a human brain.[38] While some are willing to accept that maybe such a grid really would somehow have feelings far greater than our own, many others interpret this as strong

* For the methodological details of how this was done, see the 'Measuring integrated information theory' section of Appendix Two.

† For more detail on the strengths of integrated information theory's approach to linking specific qualia to specific integrated information structures, as well as a longer exploration of criticisms of the theory, see the 'Integrated information theory: Strengths and weaknesses' section of Appendix Two.

evidence against integrated information theory, at least in its current formulation. So, just as early-twentieth-century scientists initially thought genes were encoded in proteins rather than in DNA, it may well turn out that looking for consciousness in integrated information isn't quite right, even if the overall qualia-structure research programme may still be on track.

Ultimately, the success of the qualia-structure programme will depend on how well its adherents can demonstrate a link between experiences and structures that aligns with our pre-existing intuitions. Despite the aforementioned concerns regarding integrated information theory, there are a significant number of prominent academics who believe something like its approach will one day achieve a solution to the hard problem, even if not quite as many as those hedging their bets on a functionalist approach. Still, be it the qualia structure methodology or the functionalist framework, the research community has yet to proclaim any theory a winner.

THE CONSENSUS ON CONSCIOUSNESS

For now, then, the problem of why material things like the firm grey jelly inside our skulls should ever give rise to subjective experiences remains a hard problem for physicalist theories of consciousness. Functionalist theories might posit that consciousness arises from information broadcast to multiple brain functions at once, but struggle to explain why it should feel like anything to be a global workspace. Integrated information theory, the most developed candidate for identifying consciousness with some physical structure, has both questionable starting assumptions and unintuitive conclusions. Each of these theories still has a chance, but none yet commands the consensus of the community.

If that wasn't dissatisfying enough, I regret to inform you that none of the alternatives can claim to be doing any better. Though I've focused on a few of the most popular theories among consciousness researchers, they are far from the only ideas out there. Some of those I've not discussed are quite popular. One such group are the higher-order theories, which claim that consciousness occurs when representations of stimuli like a house or face that exist in some brain region, say the visual cortex, in turn get meta-represented somewhere else in the brain, such as the prefrontal cortex. Other propositions can call on far fewer supporters but still demand some respect. The theory that consciousness arises from quantum mechanical effects inside the sub-cellular skeletons of neurons has very few adherents, but when one of those followers is the Nobel Prize-winning physicist Roger Penrose, it is difficult to dismiss out of hand. Until the community rallies around a likely winner, almost no theories can be counted out of the race.

Amongst this plethora of theories, the field of consciousness research is not short of suggestions for how to make the hard problem more tractable. Anil Seth, the neuroscientist whose artificial-brain scenario was quoted at the opening of this chapter, believes a focus on experimentally explaining, predicting, and controlling aspects of conscious experiences will eventually make the hard problem easier. One encouraging development in this regard is the recent explosion of research into how our experiences are determined less by what stimuli are out there in the world, and more by the incessant predictions our brains make about what they are going to be presented with next. This idea is called *predictive processing* and may turn out to provide a general description of how the brain works.[39] Another promising path is to focus on conscious states that have been stripped back to the bare minimum, as can occur during deep meditation, as a simpler starting point than tackling the full richness of consciousness at once.[40] These and other actively ongoing research projects cut a trail by different means, and together will hopefully reveal a final path forward in the coming years.

But, despite these efforts, fears remain that the hard problem will never be solved. These concerns are substantially bolstered by a paper from 2021, which outlined how physicalist theories of consciousness can never be experimentally proven or falsified unless one is willing to accept drastic changes to our current models of physics.[41] Yet, even here, the depressing conclusion of the paper is tempered by its suggestion that non-experimental methods remain available. In particular, there still exists the possibility for theorists to one day derive from first principles how and why certain functions or physical structures correspond to consciousness, guided by hints from scientific findings.

In any case, there certainly has not been enough work done, empirically or philosophically, to be giving up hope just yet. Two centuries ago, we had no better idea how matter became life than gesturing to some 'vital spark'. Today we routinely read, write, and edit the very code of life itself on an industrial scale in every pathology centre and vaccine factory. In the fullness of time, there is reason to hope that one day our internal geographies will look as familiar to us as any classroom map of the Earth on which we live.

The implications for revival

Okay, time to get back on track. Pondering the mysteries of the universe might be fun for some of you, and possibly exasperating for others, but either way we should return to why we're discussing consciousness in the first place. Hard problems aside, the real question we're concerned with is the feasibility of methods of revival from a medical procedure like brain preservation. In the coming chapters we're going to examine what the prospects are for all sorts of strange medical technologies, from the stem cell and prosthetic implants of today's medicine up to the future possibilities of fully machine brains and mind-uploading. Should we have some hope that these new devices might leave our consciousnesses unscathed? Or would making any modifications to our decaying biological brains only doom us to zombiehood?

Based on everything we've looked at this chapter, I think optimism is justified.* Notably, I take comfort not only from my own analysis of the theories, but because the opinions of the research community suggest that subjective experiences should exist in many more places than just the brains of today's humans. The following data comes from a survey of consciousness researchers conducted over 2018–2019.[42] Seventy-eight per cent of them reported that it was likely that bats were conscious, while 83 per cent said the same for octopuses. Their beliefs

* I mean, I would say that, though, given I've written this book . . .

around which creatures could have feelings and experiences was not limited to animals with biological neurons either: 67 per cent thought that some machines could likely one day be conscious, if not already, while only 12 per cent thought this was unlikely. Even David Chalmers, who articulated the hard problem of how consciousness could ever be tied to physical things, has said 'I think the default attitude should be that both biological and nonbiological systems can be conscious.'[43] On this basis, while the neuroscientific community has not yet been comprehensively surveyed on what they believe our survival prospects are through technology from implants to uploads, reading what they have said so far suggests that a substantial chunk would deem survival feasible through at least some revival techniques.

The reason why consciousness researchers are ready to ascribe consciousness to all sorts of biological and machine brains other than just standard human ones is that most theories of consciousness are at least somewhat substrate independent. Functionalism is completely agnostic to the physical material that a mind is made of, so long as that substance is capable of fulfilling the right functions.* In contrast, integrated information theory does care about the physical properties of systems that are candidates for possessing experiences, denying consciousness to those that lack integrated information even if they act intelligently. Despite this restriction, though, there is no requirement that integrated information is limited to biological neurons. In summary, none of the most popular theories discussed in this chapter deny consciousness in principle to current animals or future machines.

But just because an animal or machine might be conscious does not mean that they feel things the same way we do. Correspondingly, when we worry about what future medical technologies might do to our consciousnesses, we might be more concerned with alterations to our experiences than an outright loss of feelings altogether. Even with

* There are a few philosophers who believe that some of the functions required for consciousness involve metabolic processes that would be incredibly difficult to replicate outside of biological creatures.[44] Even so, that's not an argument that it can never be done, just that more functions are required than might be suggested by something like global workspace theory.

standard human brains, there is already the question of whether what I see as 'red' might be what my friend sees as 'green'. Perhaps a person fitted with extensive brain implants, or with their mind uploaded into the cloud, would have experiences completely alien to our own?

Again, the most popular theories suggest this is unlikely, at least without deliberate efforts to alter a person's experiences. The core premise of functionalism is that mental states depend only on the functions that some physical system can perform, implying that if functions are kept the same then so will the 'what-it-feels-like' properties. Integrated information theory explicitly states that qualia are equivalent to structures of integrated information, so as long as these structures are recreated, a person will feel the same regardless of what physical material their brain is made from.*

This does put some restrictions on what future neurosurgeons could do with a person's brain without altering their experiences, as we'll cover in a couple of chapters' time. It would be best for any brain implants or replacements to maintain the same functions and possess the same information structures as the original brain. Many philosophers and neuroscientists would also suggest the person should be *embodied* in the same way, meaning that they possess a biological, robotic, or virtual body that is functionally equivalent to the one with which they started. Get all these things right, though, and the chances are high that someone would keep their unique first-person perspective despite all sorts of material changes to their brain.

So, while the hard problem of consciousness is yet to be convincingly solved, none of the currently prominent theories pose a threat to the prospect of survival through brain preservation. This is a relief, because if we imagine a capacity for consciousness is possible in systems unconstrained by the decaying brains we've been provided through human genetics, we can return to our former, and comparatively 'easy' problem, of explaining how our brain enables our personal identity to persist across time. Critical to our survival is that we each have a stable way of experiencing the world from our own

* Again, for more detail on integrated information theory's approach to linking specific qualia to specific integrated information structures, see the 'Integrated information theory: Strengths and weaknesses' section of Appendix Two.

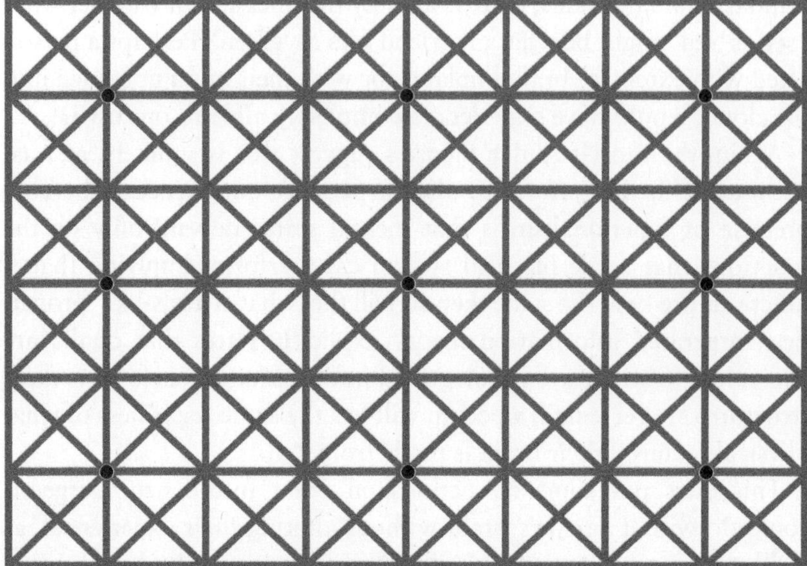

Figure 10. As a reward for reaching the end of what I think are the book's two most conceptually challenging chapters, I wanted to share with you my favourite visual illusion. The grid above contains nine black dots, but it is impossible to see more than a few at a time. This simple image is enough to provoke in me a profound sense of the limitations of human perception and the degree to which we construct our experience of reality with only a rather loose connection to the objective physical world. It's based on a variation of a Hermann Grid published in 2000.[45]

perspective, shaped by our personalities and our previous experiences. How is it that our constant psychological properties, our memories in the broadest sense of the word, bind a person's past, present, and future experiences together? Thankfully for our survival prospects, this problem of memory, which we'll turn to next, is very different from explaining consciousness, and one that neuroscientists have already substantially solved.

6
What Are Memories?

Memory is the glue that binds our mental life together.
Nobel laureate Eric Kandel, *In Search of Memory*

'I hear some music.'

Electrode in hand, Wilder Penfield paused momentarily for the operating-theatre nurse to register the location. 'Stimulation Site 23,' the nurse confirmed. Methodically, he gently touched the same spot once more.

'I hear music.'

Again, Penfield paused for a moment. He wanted to be sure that the response was really due to the electrode, and not simply a coincidence of timing. After a few moments, and unseen by the patient, he pressed the electrode to her brain one more time.

'I hear the music again. It is like the radio.'

The patient was D. F., a twenty-six-year-old woman who had suffered from seizures since she was six years old. Like many patients with epilepsy, D. F. experienced a recurring sensation before her seizures called an *aura*. Epileptic auras can feel like almost anything, including buzzing sounds, flickering lights, smells that aren't there, a sense of déjà vu, or all manners of other unusual experiences. For D. F., her seizures were reliably preceded by an odd sensation in the centre of her chest. However, her current auditory experience, of a phantom radio playing music in the operating theatre, was nothing like her usual auras. Something else was going on.

The neurosurgeon, Wilder Penfield, was an expert in treating epilepsy. He had determined that the cause of D. F.'s seizures was probably an abnormality in the right side of her brain, somewhere in an area just above the ear called the *temporal lobe*. Penfield believed that surgically removing the abnormal tissue would have an approximately 55 per cent chance of curing or greatly diminishing her seizures. In 1951, with few anticonvulsant drugs available, surgeries like this offered an effective treatment option for patients like D. F.

Routine as the procedure might have been, this was still no ordinary operation. In this kind of surgery, outcomes are improved if the patient takes on a much more active role than usual. In particular, although local anaesthetics are used to ensure that patients like D. F. will not feel any pain, they remain wide awake throughout the entire procedure, ready to perform their duties as their surgeon's most critical assistant.

What Penfield needed D. F.'s help with was knowing how her sensations shifted as he went about the operation. Over the course of his career, Penfield had become highly acquainted with the ways in which electrically stimulating a point in a patient's brain could cause a change in their subjective experience. Apply an electrode to the postcentral gyrus, and they might feel a tingling in their hand. Touch another spot and they may be compelled to bend their leg. Most usefully, from a clinical perspective, stimulating the brain of a patient with epilepsy in just the right location can sometimes induce them to experience their pre-seizure aura. By combining subjective patient reports with the surgeon's observations of stimulation sites, the exact location of an epilepsy-inducing brain abnormality can be deduced and removed in order to reduce a patient's seizures.*

'I hear it.'

By this point in the operation, Penfield and D. F. had already found a location in her brain that, when stimulated, brought on the warning feeling in her chest. Adjacent to it, on the underside of her right temporal lobe, Penfield had spotted some abnormal looking tissue, which he surgically excised. At this current stage, he believed he had likely eliminated the source of D. F.'s seizures. Still, thoroughness required that he check the surrounding areas.

Penfield left the electrode in place at site 23 for a little longer, and D. F.

* It also means neurosurgeons can identify regions critical for bodily control and sensation, and try to avoid removing those where possible.

started to hum. He asked her what the song was called, but, although it felt very familiar to her, she couldn't remember its name. After a few more seconds, though, the operating theatre nurse piped up: she recognized the tune from the radio as 'Running Along Together'. Somehow, through artificial cortical stimulation, a melody had been brought back into D. F.'s mind.

As fascinating as this was, further stimulation gave no indication that this site was associated with her pre-seizure auras. Finally, after checking one last adjacent area, Penfield was satisfied that the major part of the surgery was complete. He began to patch up her open head, first by sewing closed the thick membrane of her dura, then weaving her skull shut with steel wire, and finishing by stitching her scalp back together. Operation complete, Penfield told D. F. he'd check in on her later, and started to prepare for his next patient.

—

Twelve years later, in 1963, Penfield published a report summarizing the surgeries he had performed over the past twenty-five years. In the course of approximately a thousand operations, he had seen forty notable cases where electrical stimulation had sparked sudden memory recall. One patient experienced a striking memory of giving birth. Another relived a visit from their niece and nephew to their home. There were flashbacks to family arguments, distinct recollections of childhood experiences in émigrés' countries of origin, and even one person for whom brain stimulation caused her to vividly recall Rembrandt's painting *The Night Watch*.

D. F.'s surgery was detailed in case number five, in which Penfield remarked upon two notable findings. Firstly, that stimulation of a site near her first temporal convolution had caused her to recall a distinctive tune from the radio. Secondly, and most importantly, that in the twelve years since her surgery she had lived a seizure-free, 'happy, normal life'.[1–3]

***

By the mid-twentieth century, through the work of Wilder Penfield and others, it became evident that the dark archives of our brains could be artificially stimulated to retrieve stored memories and bring them back into the light of consciousness. Contemporaneous case studies, such as that of Henry Molaison and his amnesia, further strengthened this notion by demonstrating how memory recall and storage depends on the physical integrity of our brains.

These findings did not come as a complete surprise. Earlier case studies, such as that of the unfortunate Phineas Gage, had long since demonstrated the dependency of a person's psychology on the delicate structure and function of their brain. Taken together, the compilation of these early investigations, while far from deciphering the fundamental neuronal-level circuitry of how memory functions, set the stage for modern neuroscientific memory research. And, thanks to these earlier pioneers, neuroscientists of the early twenty-first century have now developed a remarkably sophisticated understanding of how our brains enable memories to be formed, stored, and recalled.

But before we walk through the electrifying details of how brains record a lifetime of experiences, it's worth briefly recapping the material we've covered these past few chapters. Our overall goal has been to understand the circumstances under which a person survives. We've established that a person endures by virtue of the ongoing existence of information that constitutes their personality, memories, desires, and other psychological properties. So long as this information persists between a person's younger and older selves, they continue to survive. Or, to put it another way, the destruction of this information beyond a certain critical point results in the loss of a person's personal identity, which is to say, their death.

What we have not discussed until now are the physical means by which a person's psychological properties persist over time. When you recall the layout of your childhood home, what is it about the structure of your brain that enables you to do that? How is it that the child who donates their pocket money, and later the adult who volunteers for Doctors Without Borders, is able to maintain a consistent neural structure that compels them towards kindness? To put it generally, how do we keep our memories, beliefs, morals, dreams, and desires – the very essence of ourselves – intact across our lifespans? By focusing specifically on the biological mechanics of memory, we will shed light onto how these psychological properties are maintained more broadly.

In recent years, neuroscientists have made rapid progress in understanding the nuts-and-bolts of how brains create, maintain, and use memories. Particularly since 2012, a biomedical cornucopia of advanced tools, including lasers, viruses, neural implants, and genetic engineering, have vastly improved scientific descriptions of the relevant neurobiological mechanisms. The work is not yet finished, and there are still processes that are not completely described or understood. But there is vastly more consensus on the mechanisms of memory than those of consciousness, and the remaining issues to be worked through pose no challenge akin to the hard problem. Be it the neural circuits which form records of specific episodes from our lives or the neuroanatomical contributors to our more general psychological character, neuroscience is now able to provide a substantive description of how the stability of our brains ensures the cohesion of our minds.

DISTINGUISHING 'WHAT WAS' FROM 'WHAT COULD HAVE BEEN'

Before getting into the details of human memory, it's worth flagging a point of confusion you may not even know you had. How is it that '256 gigabytes of computer memory', 'immune memory of SARS-CoV-2', 'geological memory of ancient atmospheric CO_2 levels', and 'remembering one's high-school graduation', can all be valid uses of the word *memory*?

In the most general sense, memory is data that is accessed and interpreted at a time after it was generated. Think of a camera recording the light that falls on its sensor at a particular time, storing it in a hard drive to be played back in the future. Or consider the bones left behind by a poor dinosaur that became stuck in some mud 100 million years ago. When eventually uncovered, this fossil provides an anatomical record of the long-deceased animal. In a similar fashion to remembering an internet banking password you created a year ago, both examples demonstrate data being accessed and interpreted after a delay.

But if memory is just delayed data access, this just pushes the question down a level: what is data? This can best be explained through some examples. Consider rolling a six-sided die, where any of the numbers one through six could be the eventual outcome. If the die comes up 'five' after being rolled, then recording 'five' in that instance becomes a piece of data. Alternatively, imagine your friend has given you a box of assorted chocolates. Before you open it, you suspect it could contain caramels, peppermints, Turkish delights, or any other of the many possibilities that exist for chocolate-covered sweets. After you open it, you have data on what the specific chocolates actually *are*, rather than your best guess as to what they *could be*.*

To be precise, *data* is the record of which event, out of all the many possible states of affairs, actually happened. For example, atmospheric CO_2 levels are around 420 parts per million as of 2023, and were lower in the recent past. Accordingly, it's plausible that atmospheric CO_2 levels from 1,000 years ago might have been somewhere between 100 and 400 parts per million. Yet, after examining Antarctic ice cores, you would obtain data that the specific level was around 280. Or, to use another example, I might guess that tomorrow's temperature will be somewhere between 15 and 25°C, but come tomorrow I'll have data on what the actual temperature is. To put it another way, data is that which turns the potential into the precise.

A formal account of how data is created, transmitted, and quantified is provided by *information theory*, a discipline concerned with developing methods for efficient and error-free data storage and transfer. If you're grateful you can use the same cable to stream movies that your neighbour uses to download videogames, or that your mobile phone can function in close proximity to others without suffering interference, then you have information theory to thank.

These information-theoretic conceptualizations of data and memory provide a helpful foundation for ideas we'll cover later in the chapter, so it's worth our while to spend just a few paragraphs on the topic. To stop this from getting too abstract, let's ground the concepts by considering how they apply to the functioning of a video camera.

For someone to take a recording of their surroundings, several events must occur in sequence. First, light has to bounce off objects in their environment and enter through the lens of their camera. Next,

* And, in my case, delight if caramels are present.

the light must be focused onto a grid of light-sensitive sensors called photodetectors. Lastly, those photodetectors convert the intensity and colour of said light into a digital signal. Critically, it is the potential for these photodetectors to distinguish between different patterns of light that gives the camera the ability to collect data.

While a typical phone camera has a sensor with around 12 million colour-sensitive photodetectors, for simplicity's sake, let's limit our imaginary camera to a grid of 64. To further reduce complications, let's pretend that, at any given time, each of these imaginary photodetectors can register only one out of two possible states, either black (no light) or white (light). Altogether, even this extremely simplified camera could distinguish between a total of 18 billion billion – or 18 quintillion – different images (Fig. 11).*

Now that we've designed our imaginary video camera, let's install it somewhere useful: inside the vault of a bank, to allow a security guard to surveil the area for intruders. The camera feeds the data it collects into a monitor in the guard's office, which provides a display of the situation in the vault. If the monitor's design specifications ensure it can display every image that the camera can detect, this means that at any particular moment the monitor is showing a single, specific image out of the quintillions it could potentially be displaying.†

But now imagine that, instead of the vault camera being directly linked to a display, it is adjusted so that its data is instead written into a hard drive. Rather than being displayed on-screen momentarily and then lost forever, the data is stored for future replay at some later

* An 8 x 8 grid contains 64 photodetectors. ON/OFF = 2 different states. Two different possible states for each of the 64 photodetectors = 2 x 2 x 2 ... = 2^{64} = 18,446,744,073,709,551,616 total possible images the camera can capture.

† By the way, it's worth noting that *data* and *information* are not exactly the same thing. To clarify, imagine that one day a thief hacks into the vault camera and reprograms it so that its photodetectors start to report random values. In effect, the camera is now randomly selecting an image to transmit out of the quintillions of different images it can record, but these images no longer correspond to reality. In fact, the vast majority of them will look like static noise. As a result, while the camera is still transmitting *data*, this data is no longer interpretable. Because this data does nothing to reduce the guard's uncertainty about what is happening in the vault, it does not constitute *information*, and is thus useless.

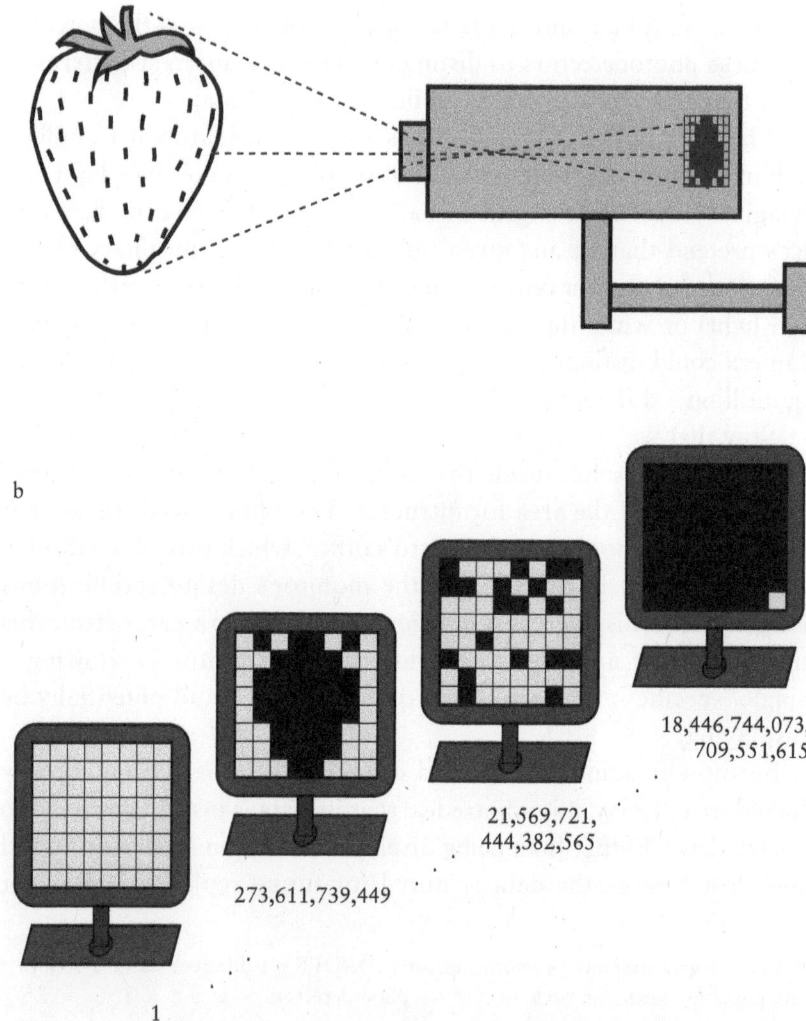

Figure 11. a) A camera can distinguish between different scenes by sensing different patterns of light that fall onto its sensor, comprised of a grid of photodetectors. b) Even for our simplified camera with a sensor made of an 8 x 8 grid of binary photodetectors, there are still around 18 quintillion different images it can distinguish. The pattern of light falling onto the camera sensor determines the particular data displayed at any one time. The vast majority of possible states look like random static.

date. As a result, the scenes from the vault have now been entered into memory.*

Even though I call both 'memory', I don't mean to imply that neural and computer-data storage work in exactly the same way. Rather that, at an abstract level, the fundamental principles describing memory are the same no matter the substrate involved. A computer retrieving a record of which cat photo to show next, out of all possible images its monitor can display. A squirrel remembering which tree they buried their acorns next to, out of all the trees in its territory. A human recalling which location they left their car in this morning, out of all the spots in the parking lot. Whenever data is used to specify a particular past, out of all the possible worlds that could have been, it constitutes memory.

With that general overview of memory, data, and information out of the way, I can now point out that we actually already encountered these concepts earlier, though I didn't acknowledge it at the time. Remember the alternate name for a definition of death based on the loss of personal identity, *information-theoretic death*? This event occurs when there is no longer any information to specify a particular person, with their unique personality and memories, from the set of all people who could ever possibly exist.†

* It is also worth emphasizing that if someone wishes to replay this video recording at a later date, it is critically important that the computer they use knows that the data in memory originated from a camera, as well as the specifications of the range of images that camera could capture. Without this, there is no way for the computer to tell whether the data corresponds to images, audio, text, or any other kind of information. This is why JPEG, MP4, TXT, and other computer file type names exist. Even though the underlying storage medium is ultimately all zeroes and ones, the file types ensure the data is interpreted correctly. In much the same way, a string of G's, T's, A's, and C's mean nothing unless one knows they are supposed to correspond to a genetic sequence, and characters written on a stone tablet are meaningless unless one understands the language from which they come. If there's no way for data to be correctly interpreted at some later date, storing it in memory is pointless.

† We also employed these concepts when examining the integrated information theory of consciousness. This theory assumes as an axiom of information that a conscious being always possesses a specific subjective experience at any particular time, out of the set of all possible experiences they are capable of possessing.

REFLEXES, INSTINCTS, DESIRES, AND OTHER EVOLUTIONARY MEMORIES

Biological creatures, born into a world filled with promise and danger, benefit from hints on what to expect. Fortunately, the best strategies for survival do not completely change with each generation. As a result, an animal inheriting implicit knowledge of the rewards and hazards of its environment will start its life with a marked evolutionary advantage over those to whom every aspect of the world comes as a complete shock.

It is no surprise, then, that all animals begin life with some degree of a head start. Human infants do not have to learn to breathe; the inherent knowledge of how to extract oxygen from the atmosphere comes hardwired into their brainstem from the get-go. Chickadees can skip music school; the neural circuits controlling their calls are innately encoded in their tiny bird-brains. There may be plenty more to learn across the lifespan, but all creatures start life already possessing a huge amount of the information they require to survive.

Because they provide an organism with some indication of how to deal with the environments they'll likely find themselves in, the genes that confer these advantageous abilities are a kind of *evolutionary memory*. Don't take this in the spiritual sense that people are somehow able to directly re-experience moments from the lives of their ancestors. Instead, I mean that the information in our genes provides an implicit memory of the evolutionarily successful strategies our ancestors used to overcome the challenges of their environments.

Natural selection provides the means for forming these evolutionary memories. The process starts with random mutations, in which related organisms are provided with slightly different variants of genes. Should an environment apply selection pressure of some kind, only those gene variants conferring the most advantageous abilities will continue to exist. For example, the ancestors of mice may initially have had random preferences for different kinds of scents, but the presence of predators would have 'taught' the mouse species to avoid the smell of cats over successive generations.

The biochemistry of DNA enables evolutionary memory storage.

In humans, this data is maintained with remarkably high fidelity. When genes are passed down from parent to child, mutations only occur once in every 100 million letters of genetic code, or about sixty times in total per child.[*,4]

Recall of evolutionary memories occurs in every way genes can influence an organism's traits, from how they digest food to whether they hibernate in the winter. But, for our purposes, the most interesting way in which evolutionary memories influence behaviour is in their control over the design, development, and function of a creature's nervous system, i.e. their *neurophysiology*. Out of all the ways in which neurons could interact with each other, and out of all the neural circuits that they could be configured to build, our genes provide guidance on which specific options have historically been proven to work well.

To provide a classic example, I want you to once again imagine you've just touched a hot pan. If you've ever accidentally done this, and had your hand quickly recoil before you were even conscious of what had happened, you've experienced the *withdrawal reflex*. You were never taught to do this, the reflex came already installed when you were born. This evolutionary memory is stored in the genes that regulate nerve and muscle growth, formed over multiple generations of selection for animals that avoided destroying their appendages. The withdrawal reflex serves as a simple example of a neural circuit implementing the recall of an evolutionary memory, so let's run through how it actually works.

When your hand touches the burning pan, the heat is immediately detected by the *sensory neurons* of your skin. These neurons possess a network of delicate filaments that weave themselves between your skin cells. Covering these filaments are temperature sensors, which when heated above a safe threshold, activate the sensory neuron.

Once activated, sensory neurons relay a danger signal to the next player in the chain: an *interneuron*. Think of an interneuron as a middleman. It receives messages from a group of sensory neurons and decides whether the message is urgent enough to pass on. If just one sensory neuron reports feeling heat, the interneuron might

* Humans are normally described as having a (haploid) genome of 3 billion base pairs, but because we inherit a copy of each chromosome from each of our parents, most of our (diploid) cells actually contain 6 billion base pairs.

disregard it. But if several sensory neurons sound the alarm simultaneously, the interneuron registers the urgency and sends the message forwards.

Finally, we have the *motor neurons,* which form the end of the line for any neural circuit. They are the ultimate point where processed information is transformed into the act of moving, or not moving, a muscle. In the painful case of touching a hot pan, the motor neurons of the withdrawal reflex prompt muscles to contract, swiftly pulling your hand away from the burning surface (Fig. 12).

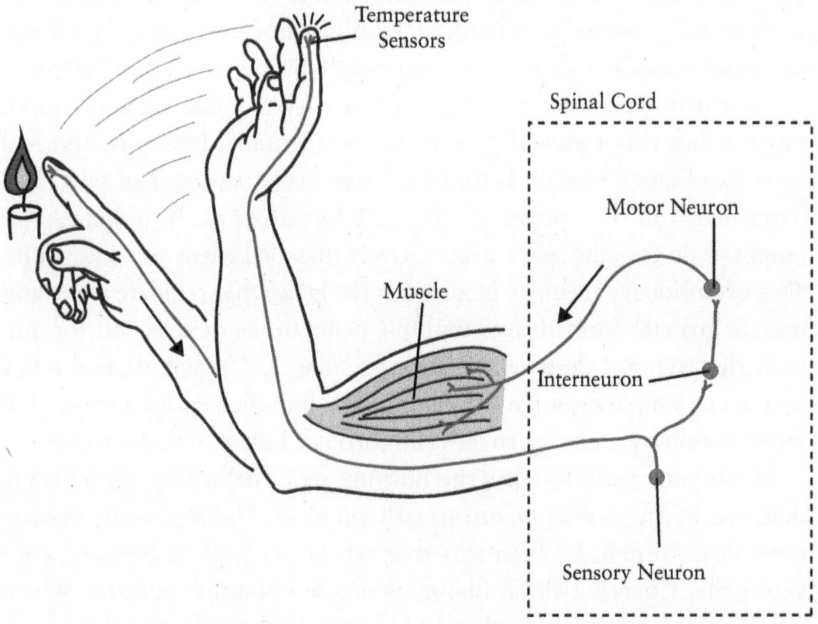

Figure 12. The implementation of the withdrawal reflex. Damaging heat is first detected as input to the sensory neurons embedded in the skin. This signal travels up to the cell body of the sensory neuron. If the inputs to the sensory neuron reach a certain threshold, it sends an electrical impulse to an interneuron. In turn, this interneuron may send a signal to a motor neuron. If motor neurons activate, they can cause muscles to contract, resulting in the withdrawal of the arm from the source of damaging heat. Amazingly, all this can happen in the spinal cord alone, without the brain ever having to get involved.

With this high-level description of the withdrawal reflex, we're now in a better place to comprehend how it actually operates down at the microscopic, neurophysiological level.

First of all, let me clarify how a sensory neuron actually receives information from its environment, or how an interneuron picks up signals from its upstream neighbours. Whether it's a sensory, motor, or any other kind of neuron, all of these specialized communication cells collect information through networks of filaments called *dendrites*. The word means 'related to trees' in Greek because, just like a tree's vast network of boughs and leaves, dendrites branch out from the neuron's cell body to capture illuminating stimuli from their surroundings.

On the surface of these dendrites are miniscule gates called *ion channels*. Think of these channels as sensitive switches that respond to specific triggers, like leaves to sunlight. When activated – perhaps by temperature in one instance, or by chemicals in another circumstance – these switches open, allowing electricity to flow into the neuron. If enough of these ion channels open at once, a significant current-surge occurs. Should this electrical influx surpasses a specific threshold, the neuron 'activates', signifying it has crucial information to relay to its downstream neighbours.

This signalling process starts with the neuron sending an electrical impulse down its *axon*, essentially a large wire extending out from its cell body.* Axons branch and connect to multiple neurons downstream, in some circumstances over a thousand times. At the end of these axon branches, where the activated neuron reaches out to its neighbours, are connections called *synapses*. When the electrical impulse reaches these synapses it causes the release of chemical messengers, termed *neurotransmitters*. These chemicals bridge the tiny gap between neurons, transmitting information to the next cell in the chain.

Barring minor differences, pretty much all neurons work in fundamentally the same way. They collect sensory information through their branching dendrites, covered in the sensitive switches that are ion channels. While some ion channels are triggered by external stimuli like heat and others are switched on by contact with neurotransmitters, all

* The electrical impulse is formally called an *action potential*.

function by converting sensory inputs into electrical currents.* If sufficient current passes through these ion channels, then a neuron will transmit – or, less formally, *fire* – an electrical impulse. When this impulse reaches the ends of a neuron's axon, it causes the release of neurotransmitters into synapses. These chemicals are then detected by the dendrites of the downstream neurons, and, with the message having been passed on, the process can begin again (Fig. 13).

Now that we have this deeper neurophysiological understanding, let's review the withdrawal reflex one last time. You accidentally touch a hot pan with your hand. Temperature-sensitive ion channels on the dendrites of sensory neurons embedded in your skin detect the heat and allow electrical current to enter into their cell bodies. These sensory neurons fire electrical impulses down their axons and towards their synaptic connections with interneurons, the next cells in the circuit. On the other side of these synapses, the dendrites of the interneurons collect the information transmitted by sensory neurons. If the neurotransmitter-sensitive ion channels present on these dendrites are sufficiently stimulated, these interneurons will also fire an electrical impulse, which subsequently activates their downstream motor neurons. These motor neurons then force muscle cells to contract within a few hundred milliseconds, moving your hand away from the hot pan before you even notice you've been burned.

To return to our original topic, and to help make clearer how this is genuinely a kind of evolutionary memory, consider how the circuit could have been configured differently. If there were fewer synaptic connections between the sensory neurons and the interneurons, more sensory neuron activity would be required to generate the withdrawal response. This would mean that the pan would have to be hotter, or you would have to touch it for longer, before your reflex would kick in. Alternatively, instead of connecting the motor neurons to muscles

* Worth noting here is that both the heat- and neurotransmitter-sensitive switches are more formally known as *receptors*, which is a general term for sensors on the surfaces of cells that are sensitive to the presence of some external stimulus. Also, as an additional complication, not all receptors work directly by gating the flow of electrically-charged ions through the cell membrane. While that is certainly the case for the receptors known as ion channels, other receptors termed *metabotropic* have more complicated and indirect effects on the flow of electricity through neurons.

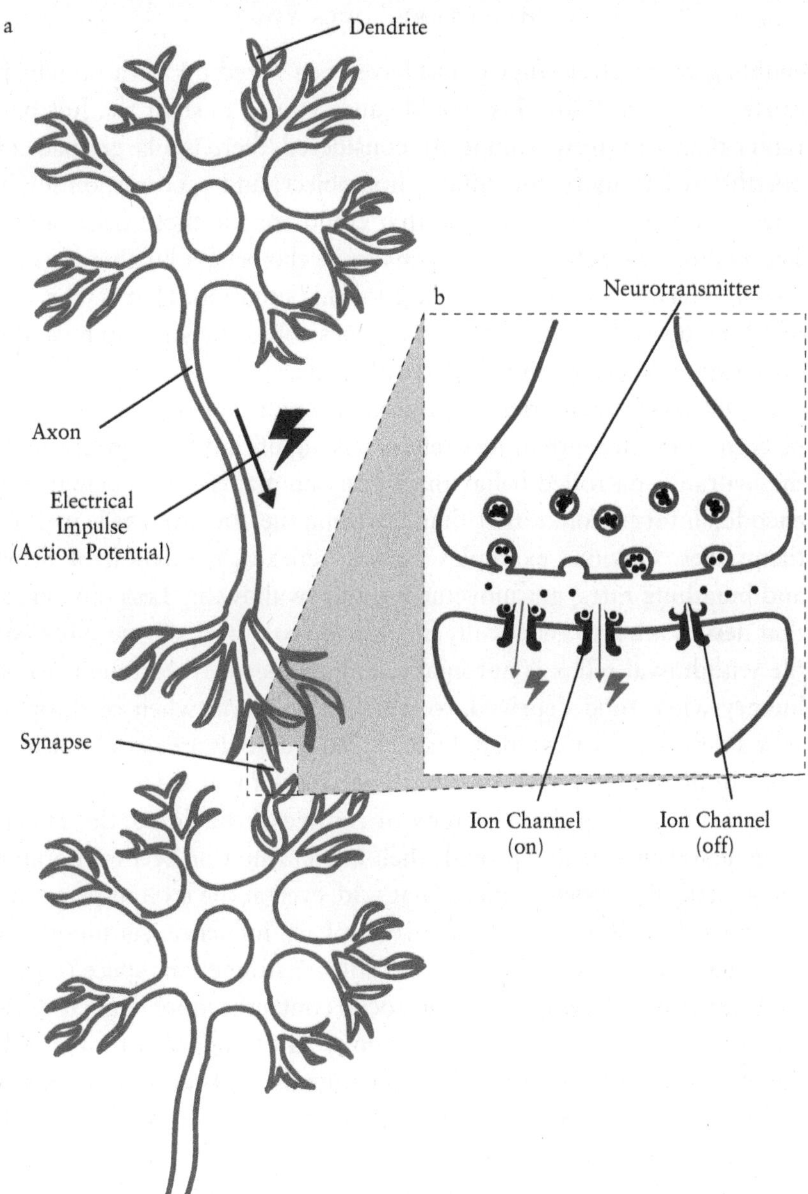

Figure 13. Neuronal signalling. a) Two neurons connected by a synapse. If an electrical impulse is created in the upstream neuron, this leads to the release of neurotransmitters at the end of its axon branches. This signal is detected at the dendrites of the downstream neuron. b) Neurotransmitters released from the axon terminals of the upstream neuron can 'switch on' the ion channels of the downstream neuron. This allows current to flow into the downstream neuron.

enabling contraction, they could have been wired up to those which cause extension. If so, this would cause you to push at the hot pan rather than withdraw from it. All considered, there is a large space of possible reactions to touching a hot object, and a correspondingly huge number of neural circuits that could encode those behaviours. The withdrawal reflex just happens to be the behaviour that natural selection has determined as the best for this situation. That is why, out of all the possible circuits that your genes could encode, you have the evolutionary memory of this particular one.

Evolutionary memories, expressed through neurophysiology, can be seen in far more than just reflexes. A significant proportion of all the neurally controlled behaviour of any animal is due to genetically encoded information, rather than anything the creature has learnt for themselves. Obvious examples include reflexes, regulation of heart and breathing rates, gut movements, and swallowing. Less obvious is that desires are also genetically determined to a large degree. Much as the withdrawal reflex is automatic, nobody needs to be taught to be hungry when food deprived, to want to be warm when cold, or to seek safety when threatened. Instead, these core desires are built into basic brain circuitry and come preloaded when you are born.

As we ascend up the hierarchy of complex behaviours, the underlying neural circuits that provide their implementation become notably less genetically predetermined. That said, even at the level of personality traits there remains a clear evolutionary influence. As unique as every person is, natural selection has still constrained the space of possibilities. A human wired to avoid social contact is more likely to miss out on the survival benefits a community can bring, even though isolation is a common preference in other animals like bears or platypuses. Similarly, a person with no sexual desire will likely have fewer children, someone with no boredom may ignore useful opportunities, and one constantly angry may get themselves killed in a fight. Even before acquiring any specific memories of their own, genetic memory of what has previously worked well ensures humans are typically wired to be hungry, horny, curious, creative, social, and self-preserving.*

* That is not to say everything about a person's psychology comes genetically predetermined. Even identical twins, who share exactly the same genetics, are not so

For our purpose of trying to understand how a person's mental attributes are stable across their lifespan, however, it doesn't matter if particular properties find their origins in a person's genes or in the environment in which they live. Instead, the key point to note is that once the slate is written on, it is not easily wiped away. In some ways this is trivially obvious – people do not forget how to breathe or swallow over time, no matter how many other memories they accumulate. But it holds almost as true for more complex aspects of our psychology. Once the underlying neuronal circuitry has developed, people do not randomly switch their personalities as time progresses, nor easily lose their core memories and beliefs. Instead, through the stable neurophysiology of our brains, we implicitly remember how to be ourselves from month to month and year to year.

The best demonstration of how this psychological consistency is maintained is given by considering components of personal identity that are formed entirely through environmental influence, yet become highly stable across the lifespan once created. I am, of course, at last talking about what is traditionally labelled *memory* in the narrower, psychological sense: the ability for an organism to acquire, store, and recover information based on its own personal lived experience.

Next, we will go beyond the preset settings provided to us by our evolutionary ancestry, and come to understand how memories from within a person's lifetime can be created and retained. Because if we can comprehend the neurophysiological methods for ensuring the long-term

---

psychologically indistinguishable as to be the same person. In fact, it is through comparing identical twins to their fraternal counterparts that we have historically even been able to analyse the degree to which our behaviours are not entirely determined by our genes. Because twins of any kind usually share the same household, school, and other environmental factors, but only identical twins have the exact same genes, examining how much more psychologically similar identical twins are than their fraternal equivalents can provide an estimate of the degree to which psychological traits are influenced environmentally versus genetically. It turns out that across all the ways people can have traits that differ from each other, about half the variance is due to genetics and half due to the environment.[5] When constraining our view to personality traits alone, such as how agreeable or neurotic someone might be, the proportions appear to be around 60 per cent environmental influence versus 40 per cent genetic. In contrast, when looking at the variance in height between different people, 80 per cent is explained by genetic differences, 20 per cent by environmental ones.

stability of memories, we will be able to see how these same mechanisms are made use of more generally to ensure the stability of beliefs, morals, and all of a person's other psychological properties. When we're done, we will at last achieve an understanding of the physical means by which personal identity is maintained across the lifespan.

LEARNING FOR OURSELVES

Being endowed at birth with reflexes, instincts, and predispositions gives a young animal a great head start in life, but even better is for them to be able to use those gifts as a jumping off point for adapting to the specific environment they find themselves in. You may have generic evolutionary memories of a desire to eat and how to swallow, but it still helps to learn exactly which fruits are nourishing rather than poisonous in your particular habitat. This kind of adaptive learning within an individual's lifetime is where neurophysiology shines, enabling animals from worms to humans to learn the peculiarities of their particular environment among the myriad they could potentially encounter.

There are many different kinds of activities an animal needs to learn in order to successfully interact with its environment, and there is a corresponding diversity of different kinds of memory. Embodied beings that we are, we need to learn procedural skills, like how to walk or ride a bicycle. As hungry animals, we need to accumulate facts about what kinds of plants and animals are edible, and where they can be found. But for self-aware, social creatures such as ourselves, we place a particular importance on our ability to remember events that happened at particular times and places in our lives.

Be it the exhilaration of a first date with your future life partner, or the relief that comes with handing in a resignation from an awful job, there are episodes that are especially salient in our memories. Appropriately, then, mental records of these events are formally referred to as *episodic memories*. Humans are able to remember a staggeringly large number of distinct episodes from their lives, and many other animals also show a capacity to recall events that occurred in a particular time and place. For this to be possible, brains must somehow be capable of storing and retrieving information on enormous numbers of distinct events that happen across our lives. Here we'll explore how the neurophysiology of the brain enables exactly that.

Updating the index

The first thing to understand is how an episode from our lives leaves a trace in our brains. The ways in which a network of neurons is altered by the creation of a memory is called an *engram*, and is defined by four features.[6] First, an engram corresponds to a specific change to brain structures due to a specific experience. Second, the information stored in these structural alterations must have the potential to be later retrieved and expressed in behaviour. Third, the experience that triggered the engram formation, and the content that is stored, must be mutually related. And fourth, the engram must be able to exist in a dormant state between creation and retrieval, potentially for years.

Explaining how an episode from our lives is recorded for later recollection requires some consideration of what was occurring during the original experience of an event. This is what we explored in the last chapter, where we covered the theories around how brain structures and activities give rise to consciousness. To recap briefly, neural correlates of consciousness research suggests that what makes any given moment of experience different from another is the particular pattern of activity present in various regions in the cortex. For example, seeing a face involves subtly different patterns of activity in parts of the visual cortex compared to when viewing a house, while playing tennis would engage completely different regions still. This suggests that in order to form an episodic memory of these experiences, the brain must have some way of recording which patterns of activities, in which neural circuits, were taking place during the original events.

The most plausible theory for how the brain normally creates these records is suggested by cases in which the capacity is absent. Remember how Henry Molaison became incapable of forming new memories after brain surgery to treat his epilepsy? This was primarily due to removal of both of his hippocampi, usually referred to with the singular *hippocampus*.* This seahorse-shaped brain structure, located underneath the bulk of the cortex in each hemisphere, receives connections from most of the brain.† These connections provide it with information about what activity is happening in the cortex at any given moment. On this basis, *hippocampal indexing theory* proposes that neurons in the hippocampus are constantly keeping a record of which cortical circuits are active at any given time.[8]

This is not to say that the hippocampus stores a complete record of the activity of each and every neuron in the cortex. Instead, the idea is that it creates an *index* of the activity, i.e. an indicator of which cortical circuits were active at a particular time rather than a full record of all the actual activity that took place within them. Critically, in doing so, the index specifies which cortical circuits would have to be reactivated in order for a specific memory to be recalled.

Going beyond human cases studies like that of Henry Molaison, subsequent animal studies have honed in on the details of the hippocampal circuitry that enables index formation. In order to do this, neuroscientists have needed a way to observe what occurs in the brains of laboratory rodents before, during, and after they develop a memory, ideally one linked to a clearly observable behaviour. Fortunately for scientists, rodents have at least one particularly distinctive mannerism: they stop moving and freeze if they find themselves in a dangerous situation.

This freezing behaviour enables an experimental paradigm called *contextual fear conditioning*. With this setup, a rodent can be trained to freeze in a particular environment through exposure to an unpleasant stimulus, typically a mild electric shock to their feet. Critically, the same mouse can be trained to freeze in environment A, while continuing to behave normally in a different environment B. If indexing theory is correct, neuroscientists should be able to identify the specific hippocampal index formed during the scary experience of environment A. Ideally,

* To be more precise, it was actually due to a removal of a large portion of his medial temporal lobes, not just his hippocampus. Other regions removed included parts of the piriform, entorhinal, and perirhinal cortex, as well as the amygdala, subiculum, and anterior parahippocampal gyrus.[7]

† The hippocampus takes its name from its shape: the Greek *hippo* ('horse') and *kampos* ('sea monster').

they should even be able to use this isolated index to manipulate the mouse's fear memory, perhaps through forced recall or erasure.

Neuroscientists have achieved exactly this kind of artificial memory manipulation in recent years, with the first key breakthrough experiment published in 2012.[9] While Wilder Penfield had previously managed to induce artificial memory recall only haphazardly, neuroscientists can now do so deliberately and specifically. Explaining just how the 2012 study initially managed it is a tad involved, so bear with me.

To force the recall of a fear memory formed in environment A, the researchers needed some way of identifying which hippocampal neurons were used to form an index of the event. To do so, they made use of a tool that could tag which neurons were active when the mice received their foot shocks. To be more specific, the method consisted of inserting artificially modified ion channels into the neurons that were firing around that time.

Achieving this tagging procedure was not as simple as just observing which hippocampal neurons fired during fear conditioning, and then afterwards injecting those specific ones with modified ion channels. In fact, the genetic instructions to make these artificially modified ion channels had already been injected into a large proportion of all hippocampal neurons two weeks earlier.* However, these instructions were designed to be initially inactive, only triggering the production of the special ion channels if two specific conditions were met.

The first condition was that a particular drug had recently been fed to the animals. This ensured the ion-channel tags would only be produced when the researchers wanted them to be, around the time of the foot-shock event.† The second condition was that the neurons had to

* The genetic instructions had been delivered inside a volume of non-replicating virus injected during a neurosurgical procedure. Now, normally viruses are parasites that inject their genes into a host's cells and use the intracellular machinery to create more copies of themselves. However, we can turn the tables on viruses by genetically manipulating them to insert genes of our choosing rather than just those which would create more copies of the virus. This is a very useful technique in the biomedical sciences.

† I'm simplifying, as, in reality, it was the other way around. The mice were actually fed a drug which continuously *suppressed* the production of the artificial ion channels, until just before the fear-conditioning event, when the drug was removed from their

have been recently active. This meant that even when the drug was fed to the mice in the hours before the fear conditioning event, only those neurons in the hippocampus active around the time of the foot shocks would become tagged. If both of these conditions were met, these active neurons would start to make the special ion channels, providing a tag for the putative memory index.

The question the scientists wanted to ask next was, 'If the same neurons in the hippocampus that were active when the animal experienced a foot shock are artificially reactivated, will the animal recall the memory and freeze?' To test this hypothesis, they needed some way of forcing the tagged neurons to fire at the researchers' command. Thankfully, the required setup was already complete.

Aside from tagging the putative memory index, another reason the artificially inserted ion channels were special was because they had been modified to switch on in the presence of blue light. This technique, known as *optogenetics*, meant that this specific population of neurons could now be forcibly reactivated at a time of the experimenters' choosing.* By using fibre-optic cables that had also been implanted into the brains of the animals at the same time as their previous injections, it would now be possible to test the indexing hypothesis directly (Fig. 14).

For the reactivation test, the mice were placed in a completely different environment B, with markedly different sights and smells to the environment A in which they had originally been shocked. Upon initial arrival in environment B, they would freely explore, nap, or perform their usual grooming behaviours. However, when a blue laser at the other end of the fibre optic cable from their hippocampus was turned on to shine light into their brains, the mice would abruptly freeze. Presumably the mice suddenly remembered the shock they had experienced in environment A, just as D. F. had remembered a song

---

diet. Once the drug was removed, they could now produce the artificial ion channels in neurons that were actively firing during the foot-shock events, where previously this would have been suppressed by the presence of the drug.

* *Opto* ('optical') + *genetics*. The genetic code to make a light-sensitive ion channel originally comes from green algae. They use the ion channels to move in response to sunlight.

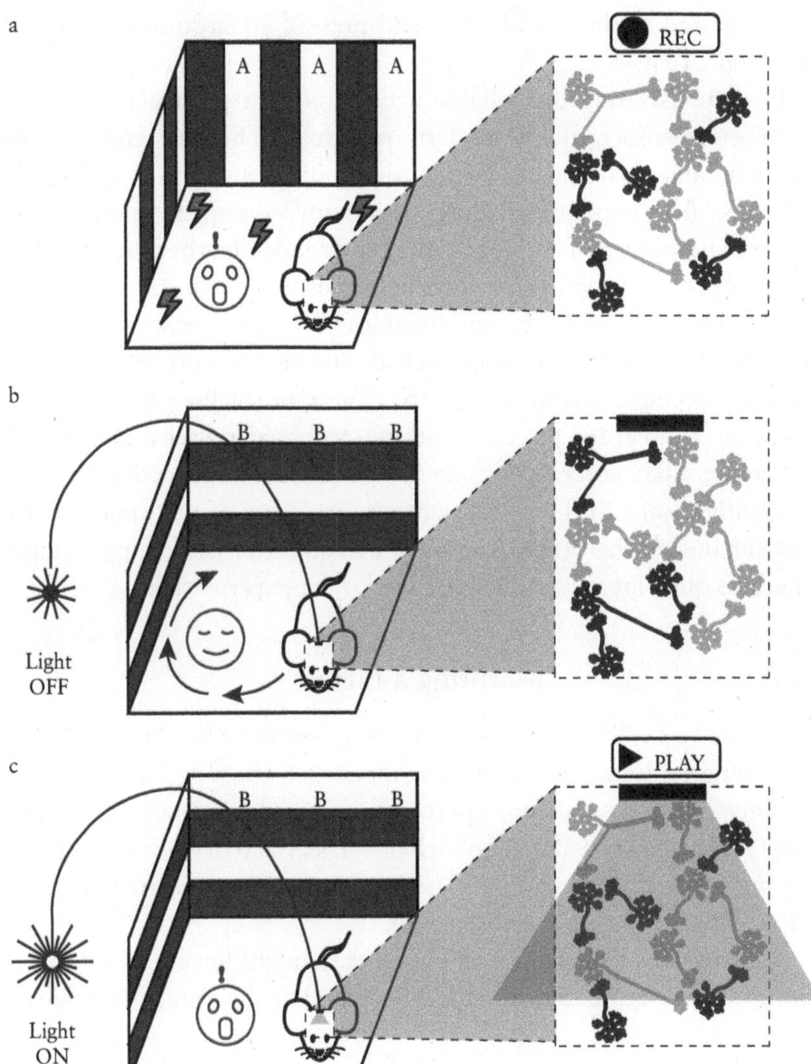

Figure 14. a) If a mouse receives an unpleasant stimulus such as a foot shock in environment A, the subset of neurons in its hippocampus that are currently active will strengthen their connections with each other. This forms an engram which provides a memory of the event. b) While the mouse is now scared of environment A, it will still feel safe in a different environment B. c) Even though the mouse is safe in environment B, it will recall its unpleasant experience in environment A if the engram formed during the foot-shock event is artificially reactivated using optogenetics.

from the radio when Wilder Penfield pressed an electrode to cortical location 23.

In demonstrating the reliable activation of a particular and pre-specified memory, these modern researchers became the first to identify and manipulate a neural circuit constituting a specific engram.* This experiment, along with many subsequent ones, suggest that the hippocampus is indeed constantly indexing the cortical activity that provides our conscious experiences.[10,11]

In doing so, the hippocampus enables new experiences which are in some way similar to older ones, such as returning to a previously visited location, seeing a picture in a photo album, or smelling the scent of a lover on a discarded piece of clothing, to act as retrieval cues which trigger an index entry to become active. Because this reactivation subsequently results in the cortex reproducing some of the same activity present during the original episode, activation of these hippocampal engrams quite literally results in a kind of 're-experiencing'.[†,12]

Maturing a memory

What we've explored so far explains why someone like Henry Molaison could no longer form episodic memories after his surgery. In the absence of the hippocampus performing its indexing role, there is no way to lay down a record of what cortical activity is taking place during particular episodes, and hence no way to reactivate this activity again later during memory recall.

But hold on! Particularly astute readers might have noticed something doesn't quite add up. If you remember the details of Henry's

* In order to check their results were not spurious, they also had a series of control experiments. One control group of mice that went through all the same procedures except for receiving the foot shocks in context A did not freeze when the blue light was turned on in context B. Another control group that was not injected with the virus but went through all the rest of the same procedures, including receiving foot shocks in context A, did not freeze in B when the light was turned on. Given these controls, by far the most plausible explanation of the results was that the researchers had succeeded in artificial memory recall through engram manipulation.

† For more details on how this retrieval process actually works, see the 'Pattern separation and pattern completion' section of Appendix Three.

case, there was a discrepancy between his inability to form new episodic memories and his capacity to retrieve old ones. While Henry became unable to form new memories of experiences that occurred after his surgery, he was still able to recollect events from his younger school days. Given he could still recall these old experiences despite having no hippocampi, surely there must be more than just the hippocampus when it comes to long-term memory storage and retrieval?

Indeed, Henry's retained capacity to recall memories from his youth suggests that episodic memories must gradually become retrievable by the cortex alone. One theory for how this works is that the high-fidelity, context-dependent memories initially formed in hippocampal engrams are somehow converted to a more abstract record conveying the gist of the memory, which is then transferred to the cortex over a period of weeks to months.[11,13] As an example of this process in progress, reflect on how more recent episodes from your life tend to be precise and detailed, such as 'I bought bananas from Sammy's Supermarket on Tuesday,' but then gradually shift to become more general and abstract, as in 'I remember shopping at Sammy's Supermarket once.' This process, which ensures that information is retained over long periods of time, is referred to as *memory consolidation*.*

Although it would be straightforward if consolidation worked simply by slowly transferring engrams from the hippocampus to the cortex over time, this turns out not to be the case. Instead, a study from 2017 discovered that these memory records are actually created in both locations at once during initial memory formation.[13] Rather than the engram being transferred between brain regions, what occurs is that the cortical engram becomes more important for recall over time, while the hippocampal engram slowly degrades.†

* More specifically, the process of transferring the dependency of memories from the hippocampus to the cortex is known as *systems consolidation of memory*, as changes are required to take place at the 'systems' level of the brain, rather than just on a local synaptic scale.

† In speculating on why the brain runs parallel systems for engram formation, it helps to look at the ways in which hippocampal and cortical engrams are similar and different. Both are created by the strengthening of pre-existing synaptic connections between a subset of neurons active during an initial memory formation. Both can be used to artificially force memory recall by means of optogenetics. However, in the first few

As the initially 'silent' cortical engrams slowly mature into circuits that can be used to retrieve memories, they gradually become independent of the hippocampus. Importantly, once matured, these cortical circuits can be stable over the years required to retain life-long memories.[14] However, while memories can survive hippocampal destruction once this process is complete, these cortical engrams cannot mature in the hippocampus's absence.

This maturation process is suspected to be dependent on an interplay between the hippocampus and cortex that takes place during sleep. Sleep has long been known to be important for memory, and some evidence suggests that rhythmic electrical activity in the hippocampus as we slumber somehow supports the consolidation process.[15] Notably, disruptions of sleep, or even merely disrupting the electrical rhythms normally present during sleep, can impair long-term memory storage. A particularly striking phenomenon is that sequences of hippocampal neuronal activity initially observed during memory formation are 'replayed' during sleep, in a process that is highly suggestive of specific information about recent memories being reinforced. Whatever the exact maturation mechanism turns out to be, the outcome is that once-silent cortical engrams become usable for memory recall.

Keeping all this material in mind, let's consider why natural selection has designed a brain that runs two parallel systems for recording episodic memories. I should caution you that this part is informed speculation. While neuroscientific research in this area has progressed incredibly quickly in the past decade, it has yet to provide all the required information for a definitive answer.

---

days after a memory is formed, they differ in one particularly notable way. If an animal is exposed to natural retrieval cues while a memory is still young, such as a return to environment A, only the hippocampal engram neurons will initially become active. Although reactivation of this hippocampal engram will subsequently lead to the cortical activity required for memory recall, this initial silence of the cortical engram is a notable point of difference.

Another major divergence between the two is that initially silent cortical engrams slowly become sensitive to natural cues, while the response of hippocampal neurons shows the reverse pattern. Hippocampal neurons lose their responsiveness to natural cues after two weeks, with some evidence suggesting this is due to a reset of the strengths of their synaptic connections.[13] This periodic clearing of data stored in the hippocampus thus makes it unsuitable for long-term storage of episodic memories.

Some neuroscientists, myself included, guess that one of the roles of the hippocampus is to provide an index of recent events, on the order of days-to-weeks, that initially stores a large amount of context and detail. If elements of these events continue to recur during this time period, the index will be repeatedly reactivated and the corresponding memory strengthened.* This repeated hippocampal engram reactivation induces its cortical counterpart to consolidate, enabling a more abstract and gist-like version to be triggered by natural recall cues. With responsibility for this memory now handed over to the cortex, the hippocampus gradually resets the strength of its connections over the next few weeks, effectively making space for new memories to be formed.† Any hippocampal engrams that do not get reactivated before the data is cleared, presumably because they store only boring and unimportant events, fail to consolidate their cortical equivalents, and are thus forgotten.

Altogether, if this theory were true, it would explain three important features of memory. Firstly, lots of recent memories are stored, as it's often unclear at the time of memory formation which will end up being important in the long run. Secondly, through repeated reactivation, important memories can become consolidated and stored life-long. Thirdly, unimportant memories are forgotten, ensuring they don't waste storage space and potentially cause interference through inappropriate associations.‡ For a mouse, man, or any other animal that would benefit from remembering what has happened in its environment, but only has limited brain space in which to store information, such a system would be greatly advantageous.

* But also, if the initial event is sufficiently emotionally salient, such as finding out you are allergic to a new food and ending up in anaphylactic shock, then the need for reactivation might be skipped and the memory can be burned into your brain on the basis of a single occurrence.

† As always in science, though, the real story is not quite this clear-cut. Some studies have shown hippocampal damage can impair memory retrieval for certain remote memories, particularly those involving spatial navigation.

‡ Catastrophic interference, or catastrophic forgetting, is a phenomenon observed in artificial neural networks where learning new information can cause abrupt and dramatic losses of previously stored information. This can occur for a variety of reasons, but one cause is the storage capacity of some memory device becoming saturated, resulting in it starting to overwrite old information. If the equivalent occurred in a biological brain, it would be less than ideal.

THE BRAIN'S BUILDING BLOCKS

Up until this point, I have been flippantly asserting that memories can be stored in 'synaptic connections between neurons' without really explaining what these connections are or how they work. I mentioned earlier that they have something to do with ion channels and neurotransmitters, but left it at that. Now that we have a general idea of how memory storage works, it's worth being more precise about the exact details of how neurophysiological data is stored.

Every data-storage medium has a basic physical unit of memory, whether it is a vinyl record, a computer hard drive, or a brain. When playing a vinyl record, the sound that is produced is determined by the shape of the path a needle takes as it moves through a groove in the record. The storage capacity is limited by the width of the grooves – the narrower the grooves, the more music you can pack onto the record. With an old-fashioned computer hard drive, the basic units are micrometre-sized 'magnetic domains' embedded into a disc.* Each of these domains acts as a tiny magnet that can be pointed forwards or backwards, and the direction of each of these microscopic magnets determines whether a 0 or 1 is recorded at each position. The storage capacity of the hard drive is ultimately limited by the size of these magnets – the smaller they can be made, the more data can fit onto the drive. As we'll see shortly, the basic unit for brains has something to do with synapses.

What makes some physical thing a 'basic' unit of data storage is that you can alter its materials without affecting the data it represents. For example, the grooves of a musical record can be made from vinyl, shellac, or many other substances – the molecules don't matter, so long as the route the needle takes remains the same. Or consider the tiny magnetic domains that define individual bits of memory on a hard drive, themselves made of a few hundred grains of iron oxide crystals. These grains could be replaced with other crystals, or switched out for

* As of 2023, solid-state drives are becoming increasingly common compared to magnetic-disc hard drives. Solid-state drives work by storing data in a special kind of 'floating-gate transistor' rather than in magnet orientations.

different magnetic materials entirely, without affecting what data the hard drive was storing. In contrast, physical changes made above this basic level can lead to data losses. Scratch a new groove into a record, or run a magnet over a hard drive, and the data stored will inevitably change.

We do not yet know exactly what the basic unit is for data stored neurophysiologically. As I doubt you'll be surprised to learn, this is because neuroscientists do not currently understand the brain as well as engineers understand hard drives. That being said, the past decade of neuroscientific research has brought a lot of clarity as to what the most primitive elements probably are for memory storage in the brain.* In the words of many of the leading neuroscientists whose studies we have been exploring, 'There is a clear consensus on where the memory engram is stored – specific assemblies of synapses activated or formed during memory acquisition.'[16]

These neuroscientists feel confident in their claim because of observations of what happens to synapses before, during, and after a distinct memory is formed. Let's walk through these observations, and see if we too will end up confident in our understanding of how memories are stored neurophysiologically.

Prior to acquiring a new memory, the neurons in the hippocampus and cortex that will create its corresponding engram are already synaptically connected to each other. No new neurons need be created, nor must neurons connect to neighbours from whom they were previously isolated.† Instead, it is the strength of pre-existing connections that will change to allow new data storage.

Wholly new connections are not required because they have already been made: during gestation, infancy, and childhood, each of your developing neurons connected to thousands of others across your brain. When they formed links with their neighbours, they did not generally do so via only a single synapse. Instead, each neuron often created many synapses with each of its downstream partners. However, at least at first,

* Particularly aided by the advent of optogenetics and two-photon microscopy.

† Whether or not new neurons are actually created at all in the adult brain, and whether this has anything to do with memory formation, is still a hotly debated area of research as of 2023.[17,18] Either way, they're definitely not obligatory for memory formation.

a large proportion of these connections are what are called *weak* or *silent*, meaning that the activation of an upstream neuron does not have much influence on those downstream. It is the strengths of these weak and silent connections that will change during memory formation.

Be it a foot shock, a lottery win, or any other memorable experience, the formation of a corresponding engram can be implemented physically in two ways: the pre-existing silent synapses can change in size, or the number of synapses that connect the two neurons can change.[*,20] These processes are known collectively as *neuroplasticity*, and we'll consider each in turn.

As a reminder, an individual synapse typically allows a signal to be passed from the *presynaptic* neuron's axon to the *postsynaptic* neuron's dendrite. Neurotransmitters released from an axon terminal open ion channels embedded in the postsynaptic neuron, which allows current to flow into the downstream cell. What is critical for learning and memory is that the strength of these individual synapses can be altered, which ultimately results in changes to the magnitude of these current flows. The more the presynaptic neuron influences the postsynaptic neuron, the more current flows inside and the more likely the postsynaptic neuron is to activate.

It turns out this level of influence is modifiable by the timing of activity between the presynaptic and postsynaptic neurons. If a postsynaptic neuron reliably becomes active at the same time as one of its many different upstream presynaptic neurons, then any synapses that connect the two can become *potentiated*. This means that the strength of the current flow occurring at these synapses increases compared to before they were potentiated. The way this is achieved is that coincident activity in the pre- and postsynaptic neuron induces the postsynaptic neuron to insert more ion channels into its synapses.

This can happen at already active synapses, in which case the current flows produced at that synapse become stronger. It can also happen at previously silent synapses, in which case a current flow can

* That is not to say these are the only physical processes involved in memory formation, just that they are the primary ones. As an example of a non-synaptic change involved in some kinds of memory formation, changes in myelination are thought to be involved in at least some kinds of motor learning.[19]

now be generated where before none would have occurred at all. This means the release of the same amount of neurotransmitter from the presynaptic neuron will now induce a bigger current flow into the postsynaptic one. Because the influence of the upstream neuron over its downstream counterpart is made more potent as a result, the synapse is now said to be potentiated (Figure 15).

Potentiation can also occur through the formation and stabilization of new synapses between already connected neurons. To make sense of this, it is necessary to distinguish between two different levels of synapse maturity.* *Mature synapses*, such as the potentiated ones just described, are sufficiently stable to last years without disappearing, and thus can enable long-term memory storage. In contrast, *immature synapses* are constantly being created by dendrites, but are destroyed within days if not stabilized. These immature synapses have both fewer ion channels than mature ones and also lack particular *scaffolding proteins* required to structurally stabilize the synapse. It is the dynamism of these immature synapses that makes them useful for learning and memory formation.

When the dendrite of a postsynaptic neuron reaches out to make immature synapses with the axon of one of its presynaptic fellows, two possible fates await these new synapses. If no synchronized activation occurs in the two neurons, these young synapses will decay in a few short days with no lasting effects. However, if the presynaptic and postsynaptic neuron undergo synchronized activation, for example in a neural circuit that forms an episodic memory engram, then these immature synapses will be stabilized through the addition of scaffolding proteins and ion channels. These now mature, potentiated synapses, that persist after memory formation, are what allow long-term memory storage.†

* This is a broad simplification. If you want more detail, see the review on spine dynamics by Berry & Nedivi.[21]

† There is actually a related process, called *long-term depression*, that can depotentiate synapses and weaken the potential that a presynaptic neuron evokes in the postsynaptic neuron. Which process occurs depends on the details of the timing in pre- and postsynaptic activity. Notably, this process can also be used to encode information. It is important to keep in mind that it's not the absolute strength of the synapses that matter, it's the difference before and after memory formation.

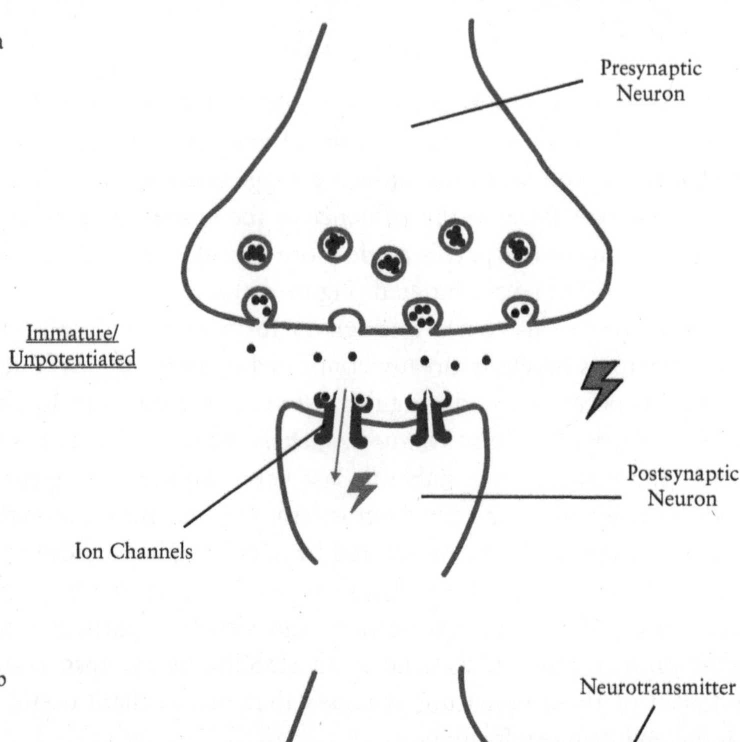

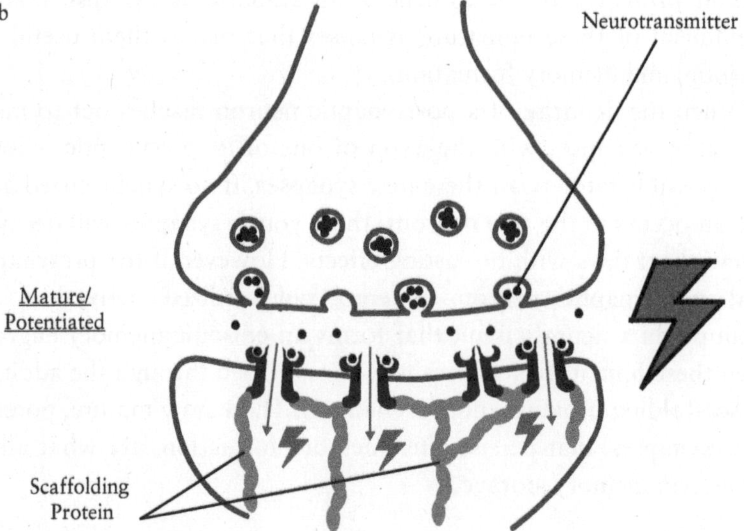

Figure 15. a) Immature and unpotentiated synapses transmit only weak signals when neurotransmitters released by the presynaptic neuron's axon are detected by the postsynaptic neuron's dendrites. b) If the presynaptic and postsynaptic neuron are often firing at the same time, this regular coactivation can lead to synapse potentiation and maturation. More ion channels are inserted into the postsynaptic dendrite and scaffolding proteins are added to ensure the long-term stability of the dendrite. As a result, neurotransmitters released by the presynaptic neuron will now elicit a larger response from the postsynaptic neuron.

Teaching mice acrobatic skills elegantly demonstrates just how this is the case. In one study from 2009, researchers trained mice to balance on a rod that gradually rotated faster and faster. As the mice struggled to avoid falling, the scientists simultaneously observed synapses in a region of their cortices used for learning these new movement skills, named the *motor cortex*. As the mice gained experience with the task, they were able to balance for longer and longer without falling off. At the same time as these improvements occurred, the researchers observed a significant increase in the number of synapses produced in the motor cortex. Most of these new synapses were subsequently eliminated, but a small fraction of them were retained indefinitely. It is these kinds of mature synapses that provide the basis for lifelong memory retention, ensuring you never forget how to ride your bike.[14]

Another group of scientists used the same acrobatic task, in combination with optogenetics, to identify and control the specific synapses that formed during learning. To clarify, this optogenetic technique was applied to the motor cortex of mice in a somewhat different fashion than that described earlier in this chapter. Instead of activating ion channels, shining light on these motor cortex neurons forced them to eliminate any synapses that they had recently potentiated. When this optogenetic method was applied to the brains of mice that had recently learnt the rotating-rod task, it erased their memory of how to balance and led them to fall off almost as quickly as mice who had never been trained on the task. Interestingly, if the mice were subsequently retrained on the same task, they would repotentiate the same set of synapses that were strengthened the first time. In contrast, if they were taught a different acrobatic skill more akin to traversing a high wire, they instead potentiated a different set of synapses.[22] Altogether, these memory-erasure experiments, along with many other recent works, strongly support the claim that long-term memories are stored in particular ensembles of synaptic connections between neurons in the cortex.

Just before finishing this section, it's worth re-emphasizing a point I have made several times throughout this book: it's not the specific physical components of the synapses that matter for storing memory, but rather the information that they represent. While mature synapses can remain stable for years, the molecules they are made of are constantly being recycled and replaced.[23] The ion channels and scaffolding proteins have a typical turnover rate of hours to days, meaning that almost none of the original components of a synapse will be left after a few months. As mentioned back in the chapter on personal identity, the continuity of a person and their memories over time cannot depend on the particular cells, molecules, and atoms they are made of, because these are continuously being changed out. Much like the information in a book doesn't depend on the particular ink used during printing, or the video files that let you watch a movie don't have to be stored on any particular hard drive, neurophysiological memory doesn't care which specific molecules make up a synapse.

MENTAL TIME-TRAVEL

Although we've been focusing on the nitty-gritty neurophysiological details of how memory works, we should be careful we don't miss the forest for the trees. Impressive as they are, the ways in which intricate nanoscale structures of synaptic connections store data are not important to us in and of themselves. Ultimately, we are only exploring neurophysiology so as to understand the physical basis of psychological connectedness between our past and future selves. With this perspective in mind, we want to know how it is that we use our engrams to remember clambering over playgrounds when we were children, to recall the sights, sounds, and smells of a foreign city we visited ten years ago, or to bring back into consciousness countless other things that happened during our lifetimes.

The capacity to put yourself back into your younger self's shoes is known in psychology as *mental time-travel.*[24] It works by virtue of a few key components. Intuitively, you need to have data on what happened at previous moments in your life. As already covered, this data is stored in the engrams that were originally created during the formative experiences. Less immediately apparent is that you also need the ability to use this data to actively reconstruct your past experience. This process is as impressive in its versatility as it is notorious for its fallibility, and thus worth examining a little more closely.

Let's begin with a finding you might find surprising: when we reconstruct past episodes from our lives, we make use of remarkably similar processes to those employed in imagining entirely hypothetical experiences. The key evidence for this claim is that problems with memory and imagination often go together. For example, try to visualize 'the sun rising above the horizon on a hazy day'. Although most people say they cannot do so as vividly as if they were actually viewing a sunrise, the majority claim to experience at least a 'moderately clear and lively' version of the scene. In contrast, around 1 per cent of people state that they have essentially no visual experience at all when prompted in this way. This phenomenon, where people lack visual imagination, is labelled *aphantasia*.[*,25]

Aphantasia is relevant to our discussion because the condition is associated with deficits of episodic memory. People categorized as aphantasic typically describe themselves as having difficulty vividly recalling their past experiences, even in the absence of visual impairments and while still reporting normal visual experiences during dreams.[26,27] Related evidence comes from the observation that patients who develop memory impairments due to hippocampal damage often simultaneously develop problems with visual imagination. For example, one such patient, when asked to imagine 'lying on a white sandy beach in a beautiful tropical bay' responded by saying 'The only thing I can see is blue.'[28]

Further support for the similarity of memory and imagination comes from observing how memory 'fails' even when operating normally in healthy individuals. For example, assume that I have a cherished memory of a warm summer's night from shortly after I graduated high school. On recalling that pleasant evening, I can once again hear snippets from the album *AM* by the Arctic Monkeys, feel the sway of the hammock in which I lay, and bring to mind the scenery beyond the front veranda of the house where I was staying. Were I to believe this was an accurate memory of mine, I might find it somewhat shocking to later learn that the house actually had a veranda only at the back of the property, that I did not visit until my second year of university, and that *AM* was not released until three years after I finished school. This can happen because, as impressive as human memory is in retaining information over decades, it is still notorious for altering details, filling in gaps, accidentally adding in information only learnt after the

* From the Greek *a-* ('without') and *phantasia* ('imagination').

fact, and introducing numerous other flaws.[29–31] It follows that mental time-travel is not equivalent to the passive playback of a video recording, and thus that the point of memory is presumably not to maintain high-fidelity records of the past to the exclusion of all other considerations.

Rather, the primary purpose of episodic memory is probably to improve predictions of the future.[32,33] Consider how we frequently need to imagine what might occur in times to come, so as to better ready ourselves for all sorts of eventualities. When preparing for a job interview tomorrow, and considering whether it would be better to brag about your past achievements or to let your humble professionalism speak for itself, it helps to have some memory of how similar situations have gone before. Engrams serve to enhance these mental simulations, by providing ground-truth data on past events known to have definitely happened from which to extrapolate possible futures.

But given memory recall needs only to portray the past accurately in so far as this improves predictions of the future, it can tolerate a process which fills in gaps with plausible approximations where necessary. In essence, it is only a fortuitous side effect of needing to look forwards that we are also able to look back. As such, it is unsurprising that the process of remembering often introduces errors, from erasing details that were irrelevant to your interests, to adding embellishments from information one could not have known at the time. Rather than bemoaning the inaccuracies of memory, though, it is fairer to be grateful that we can recall our earlier selves as well as we can using a method not explicitly designed for such a purpose.

There is some final evidence worth mentioning to support the supposed similarity between imagination and recall: performing either of these functions bears a distinct neurological resemblance to what is involved in perceiving an object in the present.* For example, remember the study mentioned in the previous chapter where behaviourally unresponsive patients were identified as conscious by asking them to

* Another interesting source of evidence in favour of this hypothesis is that memory and imagination develop in parallel, with children gaining the ability to answer questions about their past and imagine their futures roughly simultaneously between the ages of three to five.

remember walking from room to room in their house, or alternatively to imagine playing tennis?[34] This study relied on the fact that recalling or imagining an event requires reactivating some of the same brain regions that are active during perception in the present. Or, to provide another example, assume once again that you are looking at a bright red strawberry. When examining brain activity involved in actually seeing, imagining seeing, or remembering seeing such a delicious object, all three cases will show clear and overlapping activity in areas of the visual cortex.[35]

That is not to say that perception of the present, remembering the past, and imagining the future are all exactly the same thing, either in terms of how they feel or in terms of their underlying mechanisms within the brain. Individuals with aphantasia might have impaired memory recall, but they do not completely lack the ability to remember and identify details of their previous selves. Some people who have blindsight, including TN, can still remember or imagine visual experiences, demonstrating that not every brain region initially required for conscious experiences is later necessary for recall.[36] Patients suffering from semantic dementia, a rare neurodegenerative disorder where individuals primarily lose their knowledge of facts about the world rather than of memories from their own life, show significantly greater losses in their ability to imagine than to recall.[37] These three processes can come apart to a degree, and the fine details of how the various mechanisms are related and differentiable are yet to be fully elucidated.

But that said, it is still indubitable that perception, memory, and imagination are intimately related. In the end, all three are ultimately about knowing which states of the world did, do, or might occur, out of all the possible ways that things could be. Whether we are recalling a past episode or imagining a future event, we rely on many of the same neural functions and structures we use to experience a scene in the present. Our brains are constantly trying to construct and update our model of the world and our place within it, and will use evolutionary memories, engrams, expectations, or any other tool available to do so. From past to present to future, it is through these mechanisms that we bind ourselves together over time.

CONSOLIDATING OURSELVES

From Penfield's original experiments on artificial memory-recall in the 1950s, through to today's optogenetic demonstrations of the selective erasure of specific memories, the past century has seen incredible advances in understanding the mechanisms of memory. As a necessary consequence of the wealth of knowledge that has accumulated, I have had to restrict my scope to only the science most relevant to brain preservation. Unfortunately, this has resulted in the exclusion of a large amount of brilliant work by many talented scientists.

The most glaring omission is that while I have largely discussed long-term episodic memories, there are many other kinds of memory present in the brain. When you remember how to swing a tennis racket, ride a bicycle, or crack an egg, you are making use of *procedural memories*. Given Henry Molaison could learn to draw despite his amnesia, it is clear procedural memories work through different means to those we primarily discussed. Alternatively, when you recall that a green banana is underripe, a yellow one ready to eat, and a brown one should become banana bread, you are making use of *semantic memories*. There are further kinds still. Consider how, when you visit a friend's house and they tell you the Wi-Fi password, by constantly rehearsing it in your head you can keep it in mind long enough to type it into your computer. This is *working memory*. In fact, there is an entire taxonomy of memory that I have not discussed. While each memory system largely depends on the same underlying neurophysiological principles, there are still considerable differences in how each is implemented in the brain.

Since I am making confessions, I should also admit that, while neuroscience has made substantial progress this past century, there is still much we do not know. For example, we are still not entirely sure what exactly constitutes the lowest-level unit of memory in the brain.[38] It could be that memory is so finicky as to rely on almost the exact location of every kind of ion channel and intracellular protein in every last neuron. Or it might turn out that the neurophysiology of memory is robust enough that only broad clusters of synapses considered in aggregate are necessary to read out data. Similarly, up at the higher level of conscious recollection, we do not know the means by which people voluntarily select and recall specific memories. For example, consider how you can know you have a memory for a fact or event on the tip of your tongue, but are not quite able to bring it back to the surface. Annoying as this experience is, it is even more frustrating for the neuroscientists still struggling to understand how the phenomenon occurs. And lastly, an important caveat with everything I have discussed is that much of the work done on the basic neurophysiology of memory has come from studies involving rodents.* Although memory is an evolutionarily ancient ability, and there is no reason to suspect its fundamental neurophysiological processes would differ between mice and men, there may remain some level of undiscovered interspecies differences.

But even though there is still much for neuroscience to uncover, there is a clear and strengthening consensus consolidating around the neurophysiology of memory. This is nothing like the problem of consciousness considered in the last chapter, and there are no equivalently deep philosophical divisions in beliefs on the very nature of memory itself. Whether memory is considered in the broad sense of how any kind of data is stored in the brain, or the narrower sense of how an animal may acquire and retain information from its lived experiences, neuroscientists have a clear idea of the general processes involved. It is through the connections between neurons, and the varying sizes and strengths of these synapses, that information exists within the brain for any extended length of time.

To be clear, this consensus on how information is stored goes far beyond just episodic memory. I have focused on memory because it is one of the most complicated and dynamic processes within the brain, fully shaped by an animal's interaction with its environment and thus requiring constantly changing and updating neural circuits. But patterns of synaptic connections record more than just these memories; they provide all aspects of our minds that persist across our lifetimes. Our reflexes and instincts. Our personalities and inclinations. Our

* Ethics committees are somewhat reluctant to approve research studies that involve injecting humans with genetically modified viruses and then implanting their brains with fibre-optic cables when there isn't a justifiable medical need to do so.

desires. Our moral compasses. Our beliefs about the world. Everything. Whether or not a facet of our minds is genetically determined, environmentally created, or some combination of the two, all constancy within ourselves is ultimately due to the stability of our synapses.

Neuroscientists have a name for this specific pattern of synaptic connections that provides you your unique way of being. In a homage to the term *genome*, which describes the unique set of genetic memories carried within each person's cells, the full set of a specific person's synapses is referred to as their *connectome.** And in the words of eminent neuroscientists, such as the Head of Samsung Research and Princeton University professor Sebastian Seung, 'You are your connectome.'[39] In containing and specifying all of your mental attributes, in maintaining your memories across time, and in uniquely defining you out of all the other people who could be, your connectome is the physical manifestation of your personal identity.

With our journey through the philosophical and neuroscientific background now complete, it is time to finally come out and say what we've been building towards these past four chapters. *As long as your connectome continues to exist, you exist.*

As we'll very shortly see, the implications of this realization are profound. Medicine does not know how to cure all cancers, reverse organ failure, or turn back aging. We cannot yet prevent decay in a biologically active body. But even as the flesh fails, there are ways to keep a connectome intact. We already have the means to capture a person through their connectome, place them in stasis away from the ravages of time, and keep them safe until they can be restored to health. And as we just concluded, while their connectome still exists, so do they. At long last, we can now turn to the practical methods by which, should someone want it, we can save them from death.

* This isn't just the connections alone, but also the kinds of neurotransmitters released and other biomolecules present at each particular synapse.

PART THREE

How

If we are to abolish death, we need to put the knowledge gained in Part II to work.

I'll start by finally explaining the neurobiological, chemical, and surgical details of how a brain preservation procedure can actually stop a person from dying, before turning to cautious speculation on the technological advances that will be required to later bring them back into the world.

From there we'll go on to consider what it would take for healthcare systems across the globe to provide universal access to the procedure, and set these costs in the context of what we already spend on end-of-life care. Through comparison with the health economics analyses used to calculate whether novel therapies are worth their expensive price tags, we'll come to see that brain preservation is already affordable enough to be provided to essentially everyone.

7
How We Can Save Someone

No-one's dead until they're warm and dead.

Medical adage

As Anik attempted to tighten the curve of his glide into a spin, his left skate juddered, causing him to trip. While the early winter ice had previously been strong enough to support his eight-year-old weight, it cracked under the impact of his tumbling body. Anik plunged into the frigid water below, pushed under by his momentum and dragged down further by the weight of his winter clothes. Terrified, shocked, and disoriented, he quickly ran out of strength to struggle. While his older sister screamed and frantically called emergency services, Anik quickly passed into unconsciousness beneath the ice.

—

Forty-five minutes passed before the firefighters managed to pull Anik from the water. The deathly pallor of his body, with its blue lips and bloodless skin, was the first indicator that his core temperature had dropped to 22°C. While a body normally keeps itself at 37°C, and uncontrollable shivering begins around 34°C, at dramatically low temperatures like this, heart and brain activity can completely cease.[1] For all appearances, the small body the firefighters handed to the paramedics was a corpse.

But with knowledge enough to look beyond appearances, and with ambulance sirens blaring, the paramedics immediately began resuscitation efforts. These became increasingly sophisticated upon arrival at the hospital, where doctors connected his major blood vessels to an extracorporeal membrane oxygenation machine, allowing Anik's blood to be rewarmed externally at around 0.5°C a minute. Meanwhile, nurses administered him myriad drugs to prevent inflammation and infection, maintain his blood sugar and acidity levels, and otherwise reignite the many vital bodily functions that the freezing waters had doused.

About half an hour after arriving at the hospital, Anik's heart started to shudder back to life, a clear sign that the treatment was working. Four days later, Anik came off the artificial circulation machine, his heart and lungs once more capable of keeping him alive on their own. Miraculously, by four weeks, Anik had been discharged and was safely back at home. For someone who had been dead for almost an hour, he was recovering remarkably well.*

***

Even more remarkable than case reports of individuals surviving prolonged periods of cold-water drowning is the fact that modern medicine can make use of this phenomenon to perform what would otherwise be impossible surgeries. People sometimes require operations during which blood circulation must be completely stopped – even cardiopulmonary bypass machines cannot be used.† As outlined in Chapter Three, under normal conditions this would ensure the patient's death if prolonged for more than a few minutes. However, if a patient is cooled to below 20°C, surgeons can operate on them for about forty-five minutes while still keeping the survival rate at around 90 per cent. During this time, most patients have absolutely no cardiovascular or brain activity, which is why the advanced medical procedure is called *deep hypothermic circulatory arrest.*[3,4] First developed in the 1970s, the technique provides proof-of-principle that patients can recover from prolonged periods of complete neural inactivity and still survive with their memories and identity intact, so long as their brains are kept under the right conditions.

* While this particular story is fictional, it's based on many similar true accounts. As a warning, the real cases are often considerably more harrowing than the simplified story I've provided.[2]

† Aortic-arch repair or surgery for some aneurysms, for example.

What exactly are the 'right conditions', and how long can a person be kept in them? This chapter will outline precisely what these are, and how if medicine properly establishes them, a person should survive neural inactivity of not just forty-five minutes, but of indefinite length.

SAVING SOMEONE'S STRUCTURE

Before explaining the strange conditions under which a dying person's life can be extended, it'll help to briefly recap what exactly a person even is. People are entities with the capacity for consciousness and self-awareness, and with some degree of continuity over time. A specific person has a unique self, which consists of all the attributes that make them distinct from other individuals. Of these attributes, their particular ways of thinking and feeling are usually considered the most important, which makes psychological connectedness the key aspect of someone's continuity over time.

The physical basis of this psychological connectedness is the stability of synapses, with the aggregate of someone's unique, person-defining synaptic patterns termed their connectome.[5] The differences between two people are reflected in differences in their connectomes, while the relative constancy of an individual's connectome across their lifespan is ultimately what makes them the same person over time.

To account for all the possible differences between individuals, connectomes are enormously complex structures. There are roughly 1 quadrillion (a million billion) synapses that make up the connectome of an adult human. To do this number justice, we need to zoom out from microscopic brain structures and compare it to the vastness of space. The galaxy in which our solar system resides, the Milky Way, comprises around 100 billion stars. But, even though this number is already unfathomably big, we would need the stars of 10,000 galaxies to equal the number of synapses that make up a connectome.[6] What this enormous complexity means is that the information storage capacity of connectomes is immense. Or, to put it another way, there are essentially innumerable ways one person's connectome can differ from another's.

To reiterate the critical point that the previous chapters had been building towards:

a person is not truly dead so long as their connectome survives in some form.

Maintaining personal identity through the persistence of psychological connectedness is equivalent to the continued existence of someone's specific connectome over time. A generic wiring map of a typical human brain, averaged over many people, is not a good enough description. My survival ultimately depends not on saving my skin, but on conserving my connectome.

To capture a person's connectome in high fidelity, we need at least three crucial things. Firstly, we need to know which neurons were connected to which other neurons, by which I mean we need a map of as many of a person's synapses as possible. Secondly, we need to know the shape and size of these synapses, as this is indicative of their strength. Small, thin, immature synapses indicate weak connections, while big, protuberous, mature synapses indicate strong connections. Thirdly, we need to know what kind of neurotransmitters and ion channels are present at each synaptic cell membrane. There are many different neurotransmitters that can be released, including glutamate, GABA, serotonin, dopamine, and others, with different combinations of these encoding different information. While we probably don't need to know the position and count of every single neurotransmitter and ion channel present at every last synapse, we do need at least a representative sample. Altogether, if we can capture these three things, we should know enough to save someone.

Obviously, saving someone's connectome while also allowing them to maintain their daily activities is ideal. That's the goal of standard medicine, where doctors aim to manage a patient's ever-increasing list of ailments as best they can so as to maximize their quality of life. Yet inevitably, over time, damage accumulation outpaces the capacity of medicine to forestall a patient's imminent death and decomposition. Historically this has been the point where doctors shift from curative medicine to palliative care, maximizing the quality of remaining life while lessening the focus on alleviating decay. Palliative patients are then cared for until the point of legal death, after which their terminal decline is seen as complete. From then on, the patient is considered beyond help.

But with our improved understanding of what a person is and what constitutes their death, we can see this is not true. There is still more that can be done even after what currently constitutes legal death. If no interventions are taken, a cessation of breathing will naturally be followed by starving neurons, decaying synapses, and before too long the irreversible loss of a person's connectome. But if, rather than passively letting nature take its course after legal death, we instead preserve the identity-defining structures of a person's brain, we can prevent their actual, information-theoretic death. As the examples of cold-water drowning and deep hypothermic circulatory arrest demonstrate, it's not an unbroken chain of neural activity that we have to ensure, but instead someone's structure that we have to save. To update the medical adage that was used as this chapter's epigraph, 'No-one's dead until their connectome is dead.'

The key consideration in keeping a person's connectome intact after their legal death is time. As brains have no energy reserves, they start decaying almost as soon as the heart stops beating. More specifically, within about three minutes neurons run out of energy, and then things get very bad, very quickly. Acidity levels rise, biomolecules start being oxidized or denatured, cellular organelles stop functioning, and neurons start generally falling apart.[7] Preserving a person's connectome requires stopping these decay processes before they have time to wipe out the information stored in synapses.

But, while time is of the essence, connectome breakdown does not happen immediately. We don't need to keep every molecule exactly in place, as these change constantly even during normal life. We likely don't even need every neuron, let alone every synapse. There are plenty of examples of people suffering mild brain injuries, destroying millions of neurons and billions of synapses, without any perceptible change in a person's identity. It takes a while for synaptic damage to accumulate to the point of erasing a person's identity, which gives us a window in which to act. Although the window is small, if we move fast we can capture a person's connectome while it's still there.

To be more precise, if someone who was otherwise previously neurologically healthy suffers a sudden cardiac arrest, my best guess as to how long it takes them to die, in an absolute information-theoretic sense, is somewhere between twenty minutes and thirty-six hours.*

* For the record, this is my 90 per cent confidence interval for the mean time to information-theoretic death for an otherwise neurologically healthy person who

The lower bound of my estimate is based on the fact that, while synapses examined at twenty minutes after blood flow cessation look almost completely normal, some visible alterations can start to occur from this point onwards.[8–10] These changes, which include minor swelling of axons and dendrites, probably don't cause problems when trying to map out someone's connectome, as synaptic contacts are still clearly visible. On the other side, my upper bound comes from the observation that extensive damage to synapses becomes clearly visible in decaying rodent brains at thirty-six hours, while evidence of total decomposition of neural structures in humans also becomes increasingly apparent from around this point.[10,11] This time window is just my best guess, though, and more research focused specifically on this topic could easily provide a clearer answer.

Obviously, the better we can preserve a dying person's brain – the more information about their connectome we can retain – the greater the chance we can save them from information-theoretic death. Indeed, there will be no complaints from future medical professionals if we end up safeguarding much more neural information than we need to, as it'll only make their jobs easier. In the absence of a clear answer to when information-theoretic death occurs, it's better to act as quickly as feasible and save as much as possible. Luckily, we already have a technique to preserve everything down to the molecular level, which is probably a level of detail beyond what is actually required. The trick is just to stop time.

STOPPING TIME

All change requires movement, and all movements require time.* If movement is arrested, no change can occur and it is as if time itself cannot pass. Biological decay is a kind of change through inappropriate

enters global ischaemia and whose body is kept at room temperature. The estimate will change dramatically based on the pre-existing health status of the individual and the environmental conditions in which their body is left.

* You can probably just trust me on this one, but if you'd like an authoritative source, see Zeno's paradox of motion.

movement: molecules move to places they shouldn't be, or react with things they shouldn't touch. If we can stop molecules from moving, we can stop decay, and by doing so we can effectively remove something from time.

Chemistry has two well-developed techniques for rendering molecules motionless. One is to sap their energy by cooling them down and removing their motive power. The other is to lock them in place, so that despite their wriggling and struggling they cannot move. To save someone we need to use both, so let's go through each in turn.

How quickly and forcefully a collection of molecules bounce off one another, otherwise known as the *average kinetic energy* of a collection of particles, turns out to be the same as what we normally think of as *temperature*. To make a fluid hotter is to force the particles that make it up to move faster, while to make it colder is to do the opposite and remove some of their kinetic energy. Cool a fluid down sufficiently and its constituents cannot move at all, instead becoming stuck in place. This is what it means for something to solidify or freeze: molecules that once moved freely around a container are now trapped.

Chemical reactions depend on molecules being able to move into contact with each other. As a substance is cooled down, the chemicals within it collide at lower frequencies, accompanied by a corresponding slowdown in reaction rates. Refrigerators make use of this principle to keep food fresh. Food going bad requires chemical reactions to occur, so cooling down food extends its shelf life. The same principle applies to humans, as demonstrated by the cases of cold-water drowning and deep hypothermic circulatory arrest. Even though people may only be cooled down to 20°C, still much warmer than a fridge, that decrease is sufficient to reduce the pace of damage progression long enough for life-saving medical procedures to take place.

But these temperatures are still too warm for a patient to be kept at for long. Sufficient biochemical reactions still occur to ensure that hypothermic surgery cannot exceed forty-five minutes without patients suffering clear neurological damage. As such, it would be great if we could go colder still. Reaction rates decrease exponentially with temperature, meaning that reactions that take place in one second at normal body temperature can take years at those of liquid nitrogen.* This implies that if we could cool someone's brain to a sufficiently low temperature, we should be able to slow connectome decay to a negligible rate.

Unfortunately, there are complications that mean saving someone is more difficult than just putting a dying person in a freezer. The main problem is due to the behaviour of water as it cools.[12] At body temperature water is a liquid, meaning its molecules move and flow in a disorganized jumble. This chaos is actually convenient, as it allows biomolecules to insert themselves freely into the watery soup that makes up the inside of cells. Yet if we cool a person's body down to below water's freezing temperature, issues start to occur with this unhindered dance of cellular components. Water molecules, stripped of their kinetic energy, cease their chaotic collisions and instead organize themselves into ordered crystals. This molecular arrangement causes problems through both taking up more space than the formerly liquid jumble, as well as by forcing other molecules out from where they are supposed to be.

To be more specific, ice formation unleashes damage through at least two different mechanisms, depending on whether the ice is forming inside or outside of cells. Ice that forms on the inside damages cells as its crystals grow, presumably by causing mechanical damage to organelles and puncturing the integrity of the cell. Alternatively, ice forming in the spaces between cells dehydrates them, causing the cells to shrink considerably.† Together, these processes can cause considerable deterioration of synapses, cells, and everything up to whole organs, doing enough damage to mean that straight freezing is a questionable method of connectome preservation.

Thankfully, with preparation, there are alternate ways to cool things down without causing ice formation. Adding an antifreeze compound, more formally known as a *cryoprotectant*, will prevent ice from forming as a liquid cools. Cryoprotectant molecules achieve this by sticking weakly to water molecules and interfering with their

* This is based on a straightforward interpretation of the Arrhenius equation, which, while directly applicable to fluids, does not apply neatly to solids. In reality, reaction rates in solid materials can essentially stop entirely when sufficiently cold.

† This process bears some resemblance to freezer burn, where moisture is lost from frozen foods.

attempts to arrange themselves into organized crystals. If you add a sufficient concentration of cryoprotectant to water, it will remain a liquid far below its normal freezing temperature.

That said, should you continue cooling the water with cryoprotectant added, it will still eventually become cold enough to solidify. However, instead of the water molecules arranging themselves into an organized crystal, at some point they will simply stop where they are and stay still within their disorganized jumble. Rather than freezing into ordered ice, the water has now *vitrified* into a disordered glass. The name is from the Latin *vitrum*, meaning 'glass', because the molecules in everyday glass are also arranged in this solid yet non-crystalline mishmash.

Vitrification has been widely employed for decades to store egg cells, embryos, and other small biological tissues indefinitely without having to worry about them decaying.[13] The procedure is particularly well suited to these cases, as vitrification is easy to use on small, thin, or diffuse collections of cells. This is because it works best in situations where the cryoprotectant can easily diffuse into the cells and the tissues can be cooled rapidly. For this reason, its use is particularly prominent in assisted reproductive technologies, where vitrification storage has led to considerably better outcomes compared to earlier egg-freezing techniques.[14]

Unfortunately, getting vitrification to work with larger segments of biological material has proven difficult. Due to their high viscosity, cryoprotectant solutions can take a long time to diffuse into and fully penetrate organs. This issue is even worse when it comes to the nervous system, as the blood–brain barrier further impedes the diffusion of cryoprotectants. Inadequate diffusion is problematic for two reasons: not only does it fail to prevent ice formation within neurons, but the higher concentration of cryoprotectant outside the brain cells also pulls water from their interiors, leading to shrinkage. As a result of this dehydration, vitrifying human brains using cryoprotectants alone causes them to shrivel down to half their usual size.[15]

I mentioned the current practice of cryonics in the Introduction. Although several existing cryonics organizations have already been offering clients this kind of vitrification procedure, severely shrinking a brain is not ideal for a treatment that is supposed to ensure the maintenance of connectomic integrity. Given that the synapses of brains vitrified in this manner are compressed and difficult to distinguish under a microscope, it is currently impossible for these organizations to say with confidence that they can capture a person's connectome.[16] Standard vitrification is thus decidedly non-ideal for a medical procedure that aims to guarantee it can preserve someone.

What we need is a method of vitrifying brains without causing shrinkage-associated damage. Specifically, we need some method of initially stabilizing neurons, synapses, and complex molecules to prevent them from shrinking or breaking prior to and during the vitrification process. Fortunately, in addition to cooling, there is another, completely different way to chemically stop time: we can also lock all the complex biomolecules in place.

Rather than stopping molecules by removing their kinetic energy, we can also bind them together using molecular chains and glue. Chemicals used for this purpose are called *fixatives*, as when they infiltrate organelles, cells, and tissues, they essentially bind, or 'fix', them at that particular moment in time. These bound molecules are still warm, and retain their kinetic energy, but now wriggle in place instead of moving about. The lack of motion prevents molecules from undergoing chemical reactions with each other or altering their spatial relationships in any way, and thus prevents biological decay. For these reasons, fixation is routinely used in biology whenever tissue preservation is required for research purposes.

The most commonly used fixatives are *aldehydes*, specifically *formaldehyde* and *glutaraldehyde*. While formaldehyde is better known, I will focus on glutaraldehyde as it is better able to rapidly fix neural tissue.[17] A single molecule of glutaraldehyde consists of a chain of five carbon atoms with an oxygen-atom cap at either end. These oxygen caps will readily bond to many of the other molecules present inside cells, particularly proteins. Because glutaraldehyde can fuse to other molecules from either end of its chain, it readily forms crosslinks that bind molecules to each other. As a consequence, within seconds of introduction into cells, glutaraldehyde forms a meshwork jail that locks proteins, nucleic acids, and other complex molecules in place.

Glutaraldehyde fixation is currently standard when preparing neural tissue for study with extremely precise microscopes.[18] For example, take electron microscopes, routinely used in neuroscience research to image tissues at resolutions below 10 nanometres. For reference, synapses occur on portions of dendrites that are around 100 nanometres wide, while a red blood cell is about 8,000 nanometres in diameter.[19] Electron microscopes are fully capable of taking pictures of neurons at or below the synaptic level, almost approaching the molecular level. When examined through an electron microscope, synapses in glutaraldehyde-fixed neural tissue look close to perfectly preserved.* As a result, we can be fairly confident that aldehyde fixation can preserve someone's connectome.

One issue with glutaraldehyde fixation though is that it alone cannot perfectly preserve a person's connectome forever. The meshwork formed by glutaraldehyde crosslinking is a maximum-security prison, but not quite a completely inescapable one. At room temperature the molecules continue to wriggle even when imprisoned in this fashion, enabling some to slowly move around the crosslinks over time, with fatty or oily molecules being particularly slippery.[20,24] This means that, while fixation by itself is great for temporary use, it is insufficient for the indefinite storage of a person's brain.

Luckily, combining fixation with cryopreservation nullifies each of their respective disadvantages while maintaining both of their unique benefits. To combine them, first aldehyde-fix the neural tissue to lock the brain's biomolecules in place. This sets the tissue up for cryopreservation, as fixation prevents the shrinkage that would otherwise occur

* The strength of this claim comes from comparing tissue examined after glutaraldehyde fixation to that prepared through high-pressure freezing. Although it can't be done on large amounts of tissue, biological samples of around 200-micrometre thickness can be flash-frozen at high pressures, which preserves them in essentially their exact native state. When comparing these flash-frozen samples to those treated by glutaraldehyde, it is apparent that aldehyde fixation provides high quality preservation that allows for synaptic and connectomic tracing. That is not to say it is completely perfect, as glutaraldehyde-fixed tissue shows some signs of a reduction in extracellular space compared to flash-frozen tissue.[20] However, as reductions in extracellular space occur within seconds after cessation of blood flow to the brain, yet temporary ischemia is already survivable with modern medicine, the loss of this extracellular space is unlikely to constitute destruction of the connectome.[21] Even so, there are ongoing efforts to develop improved techniques that can also preserve extracellular space and approach the gold standard of high-pressure freezing.[22,23]

through cryoprotectant-induced dehydration.* Next, gradually introduce cryoprotectants while also slowly cooling down the neural tissue until it vitrifies. Under these conditions, no detectable dehydration or brain shrinkage will occur, and one can be assured that the connectome within the vitrified tissue has been successfully preserved. Once complete, congratulations, you have performed *aldehyde-stabilized cryopreservation* and removed the neural tissue from the ravages of time.[25] At this point feel free to leave the brain in the freezer for a year, ten years, a thousand years, however long you need – no changes will occur and no information will be lost.

In honour of their publication of this new technique in 2015, along with subsequent demonstrations of its general applicability, Aurelia Song and Greg Fahy won the Brain Preservation Foundation's Large Mammal Prize in 2018.[26] This prize required evidence of the successful preservation of a pig brain in a manner compatible with high-quality, centuries-long storage. When provided with pig brain samples prepared through this technique, the prize judges determined that the brain tissue was well preserved, with synapses sufficiently intact to enable clear connectome tracing. As a result, aldehyde-stabilized cryopreservation, also referred to by its shorter name *vitrifixation*, was verified as a connectome-preserving technique suitable for indefinite storage.

Vitrifixation has subsequently been performed on humans shortly after their legal death, with the results likely constituting some of the highest quality human brains ever preserved.† These findings suggest that vitrifixation works just as well for human brains as it does for pig ones. However, analysis of the results under different clinical conditions has shown that prompt commencement of the procedure after a declaration of clinical death is critical to ensuring a high-quality preservation.[27] Determining just how long this window of viability exists is still a matter of ongoing research, as is ascertaining whether there

* When used in combination with small amounts of a detergent to permeabilize the blood–brain barrier.

† Much of this recent human work has been performed by the company Nectome, founded by Aurelia Song (formerly known as Robert McIntyre) to develop vitrifixation into a routine end-of-life medical procedure. At the time of writing (late 2023) they were in the process of preparing this data for publication.

are any ways of extending the window's duration. Because these investigations are still incomplete, and additionally because the vitrifixation protocol is still undergoing optimization for integration into routine medical practice, the procedure has not yet been made available outside of research settings. Nonetheless, vitrifixation has already been developed into a mostly validated brain preservation procedure for humans, at least under ideal conditions. Given this success, the time has finally come to describe the explicit, procedural details of just how we can save someone.

TIME TRAVEL THROUGH VITRIFIXATION

Remember Keiko Tanaka from Chapter Two, the eighty-four-year-old woman with terminal cancer whose daughter placed her in a time machine in the hopes that it would save her life? Unfortunately, time travel doesn't seem likely to become possible, while metastatic breast cancer is sadly already very real. As a result, we're going to have to revise the original scenario.

***

To begin, Keiko is back in 2054, stuck with a prognosis of only a few months to live. She is not in a good way. Tumours have spread to her bones, liver, and lungs, causing her considerable pain and shortness of breath. Her symptoms are becoming harder and harder to manage at home, and Keiko's quality of life is declining quickly.

As a result, and in consultation with her doctors, Keiko decides to move to a hospice, a facility halfway between a nursing home and a hospital that specializes in palliative care. The staff there are experienced at providing sophisticated pain management, and shortly after entering their care Keiko starts to feel considerably less sick. With the easing of her symptoms, she is better able to enjoy the visits she receives every day from her daughter, Ai, her grandchildren, and her friends. Although her energy levels are nothing like her pre-illness self, she can normally manage to chat for an hour or two in the late morning before she becomes too tired. While Keiko's not feeling well by any stretch of the imagination, she's still grateful to be spending what little time she has left with those she loves.

One day, in the middle of asking Ai how her grandson's first year at university is progressing, Keiko starts to violently cough. One of the tumours in her lungs has invaded an artery, causing it to burst open, and blood is now flooding into her already compromised lungs. Keiko can no longer breathe, and quickly passes out. Ai shouts for a nurse, who upon arrival quickly summons a doctor. By the time they rush into the room Keiko's heart has already stopped, and the doctor promptly pronounces her legally dead.

As her health had deteriorated, Keiko had made clear she did not wish to be resuscitated in a circumstance such as this. However, she and her doctor had previously discussed vitrifixation, including its potential complications and benefits. While Keiko was firmly of the opinion that she did not wish to be stuck in a body that could no longer function, she also wanted to take whatever chance there was to one day see her daughter and grandchildren again. If that required waiting an undetermined period of time, then so be it. While Keiko had completed a 'Do not resuscitate' order when she moved into the hospice, she had also signed the consent paperwork for having herself preserved.

Upon the doctor's pronouncement of legal death, an accompanying orderly immediately springs into action and starts wheeling Keiko's bed down to the preservation theatre. With Keiko's starving neurons beginning to destroy themselves, time is of the essence. Fortunately, the hospice is designed to handle exactly this situation. Within minutes of Ai first calling for the nurse, Keiko arrives at the preservation theatre, ready for vitrifixation to commence.

—

The next section is somewhat graphic. While the technical details are important, skip this part if surgery makes you squeamish.

The moment Keiko makes it onto the operating table, the preservation technician on standby is ready to go. A few quick scalpel cuts down the middle of her chest begins the procedure. Next, a saw is used to cut through her sternum, and a rib spreader is inserted to open up her chest cavity. A tissue sac nestled between her lungs becomes visible, which, once opened, reveals Keiko's now-unmoving heart. Carefully, the technician cuts off the tip of the bottom of the heart, allowing access to the interior chambers. They are then able to insert a large plastic tube all the way through the left ventricle and secure it snugly in place inside the aorta, the main vessel carrying blood from the heart to the rest of the body. After a final nick is cut into the right atrium, the initial setup is complete.

It has been less than fifteen minutes since Keiko's heart stopped when the preservation technician recommences the flow of fluid through her cardiovascular system. But instead of restoring the circulation of Keiko's blood, the technician is replacing it with a chilled fluid containing oxygen, anticoagulants, and acidity regulators. A pump pushes this *washout solution* through the input tube in her left ventricle, from which it makes its way throughout Keiko's body. By both cooling and delivering oxygen to her breathless cells, this wash-out solution dramatically slows decay processes throughout her brain and body. Meanwhile, the nick made into the right atrium allows blood and excess washout solution to drain from Keiko's body into a collection vessel below the operating table. Since blood stuck in Keiko's circulatory system could cause clots and blockages if not removed prior to fixation, the pump is left running for some time to ensure even her smallest capillaries are completely cleared.

With the washout solution flowing, the preservation technician can relax a bit. It will take a few minutes to fully purge Keiko's blood vessels, during which time the technician can check for any issues that might be arising. Their first glance is at the pump's pressure gauge. Too high a reading would indicate a blockage in one of Keiko's blood vessels, necessitating quick surgical work to get it cleared. Too low, and a leak would be suspected. In Keiko's case, the reading is thankfully in the low end of the target range, meaning the technician can proceed to fixation once the washout is complete.

After around ten minutes the output fluid is completely clear, indicating Keiko's circulatory system is clean of blood. Accordingly, the technician switches the pump input fluid across to the fixation solution. Glutaraldehyde begins to course through Keiko's body. Within seconds, every biomolecule, every synapse, every engram is bound in place. Keiko's body becomes a still-life snapshot of itself, frozen in biological time. Her connectome is now safe from almost all decay processes, her personal identity preserved. Keiko is now no longer dying; she is instead on pause.

To be safe, the fixative is kept pumping through Keiko's body for the next thirty minutes, ensuring glutaraldehyde reaches every last cell and organelle. During this time, Keiko's skin becomes firm and hard, providing external proof that fixation is indeed taking place. Meanwhile, the technician drills a few small holes into Keiko's skull to visually confirm that successful brain fixation is occurring. A comforting colour change from pink to a yellowy-grey provides satisfaction that there is no need to escalate the case.

Now that Keiko is out of immediate danger, she needs to be prepared for cryopreservation. The fluid streaming into her body is switched over once again, this time to a combined fixative and cryoprotectant solution. Once this fluid starts to flow, the technician hands over control of the pump to a monitoring computer. Over five hours, the computer gradually increases the concentration of the cryoprotectant while reducing that of the fixative, doing so very slowly so as to prevent dehydration damage due to osmotic pressure. By the end, once much of the water in Keiko's body has been replaced with cryoprotectant, she is ready for long-term storage.

No more surgical details; it is safe to start reading again from here.

After a short wait in the preservation-theatre holding area, where she is also changed out of her hospital gown and into a white kimono, Keiko is picked up for transportation to one of Tokyo's preservation storage facilities. As Keiko's consent documentation specified that she has no particular religious affiliation, she is taken to the closest available location to her next-of-kin's residence. She arrives two hours later at an enormous, white-painted building in Kawajima, on the outskirts of the city. The van transporting her and several other preserved people docks in the loading bay, and a door rolls open to expose the intake area of the facility. Although she doesn't know it, Keiko is about to enter her new home for the indefinite future.

From here, Keiko needs to pass through quality control before she can be moved to her final resting place. First, she receives a CT scan of her entire body. This provides a reference dataset on her current overall state, and also serves as a substitute in many cases when autopsy information might otherwise be needed. Secondly, several tiny-needle biopsies are made to extract small tissue samples from various brain locations.* These samples will later be examined under a microscope to confirm whether the preservation procedure was indeed successful down to the synaptic level.

These checks complete, Keiko next moves to the cooling room. Here, along with her fellow recent arrivals, Keiko's body temperature is slowly lowered to around −130°C.† As her body approaches the bottom of this range, after many hours, it solidifies into a glass. Any molecules within Keiko that had escaped fixation and maintained some small degree of movement or reactivity come to a complete halt, forced by the cold to wriggle weakly in place. Neither years nor centuries can harm Keiko now.

Cooldown complete, Keiko can be moved to her long-term resting place. A series of robotic conveyors, capable of operating safely at these frigid temperatures, gently transport her from the cooling room to her designated slot. While this location is mostly determined by what maximizes storage efficiency for the facility, the allocation software is required to take into account one request listed on Keiko's vitrifixation consent form. Although Keiko specified no religious requirements, she still wished to follow a common cultural practice. As a result, after a sedate journey, Keiko is eventually deposited in the slot next to Tetsuya Tanaka, her husband of forty-six years. Here, the two will wait side-by-side for as long as it takes until they can live together once more.

—

Three days later, shortly after the last guests leave the wake, Ai finds herself holding her mother's ceremonial preservation-certificate tablet. She swipes through the screens – biopsy and CT scan results, resting slot ID number, current vault temperature – and arrives at a

* These are taken through the holes previously drilled by the preservation technician.

† This is about halfway between the temperature of inland Antarctica on a cold winter's night and liquid nitrogen.

photograph of her mother from twenty years ago. Keiko is gently smiling, her silver hair framing a face full of self-possessed strength. The picture had been taken not long after Ai had given birth to her first child, and with a stabbing nostalgia she remembered how comforting it had been to have her mother around to help her manage. Keiko has only been gone three days, but Ai already misses her so badly she can't even make tea without wishing her mother was there to share it with her.

'I love you, Mama,' Ai whispers to herself. 'I'll see you later.'

HOW WE MIGHT REVIVE SOMEONE

On 13 December 1972, Eugene Cernan stood on the edge of a lunar crater with a steel tube in one hand and a hammer in the other.* Though it had required a marvel of engineering to propel him there, his current task was strikingly rudimentary. Right now, scientific progress depended on Eugene pounding lunar soil into a tube, much as a child may pack a plastic mould with beach sand.

It had been fifteen years since the dawn of the Space Age, and, with each passing year, humanity's ambition had deciphered more mysteries of the heavens. On this day, Gene was standing on the edge of this crater because scientists back on Earth wanted to know which gases, if any, were present in lunar dirt. This could not only tell them about the history of the Moon's geological formation, but also how feasible it might be for future astronauts to locally produce the water they needed to drink, the oxygen to breathe, and the fuel to power their rockets home. Were this to become possible, humanity's expansion into the cosmos could be made that much easier.†

Sample collected, Gene placed the tube inside a specially made receptacle and sealed it away with a twist of the cap. Safely ensconced, lunar soil sample 73001 accompanied him back to his spacecraft, and from there made the journey to Earth, before ultimately finding itself in the Lunar Sample Laboratory Facility at Johnson Space Centre.[28]

While many of its fellows were eagerly opened and analysed not long after their arrival, this special sample underwent a different fate. As much as contemporary scientists wanted to know which gases were present in lunar soil, they knew the analytical tools of the 1970s were incapable of detecting and discriminating such faint chemical signatures. While they could imagine how researchers might one day

* Actually, it might have been anywhere between 11 and 14 December. I couldn't find the exact date.

† This would be quite the improvement from the historical practice. In the absence of being able to resupply during their journey, the Apollo 17 mission had been forced to bring everything they needed with them on their voyage. This meant that, out of the 3 million kilograms of material present on their rocket at lift-off, only 5,000 kilograms, or 0.16 per cent of its total mass, remained unconsumed by the time they left the surface of the Moon.

craft machines that could achieve such feats, this possibility was still a distant dream. So, with admirable self-restraint, they preserved this particular lunar specimen in a stainless-steel vault, awaiting the day when scientists' tools had caught up to their aspirations.

It wasn't until fifty years later, in 2022, that sample 73001 was eventually unsealed.[29] In the meantime, the unrefined palates of 1970s analytical apparatuses had slowly transformed into the skilled sommeliers that are modern mass-spectrometry devices. With the development of equipment finally capable of detecting and examining the faintest wisps of gas, the delayed gratification of a previous era's scientists was at last achieved. Although humans have not been back to the moon since Eugene Cernan's visit, through foresight and intergenerational cooperation, a decades-long research programme could still reach its fruition.

***

Much as the NASA scientists of the 1970s could not have described the engineering that allows modern mass-spectrometers to analyse trace gases present in sample 73001, present doctors and scientists cannot currently explain the exact means by which a person who has undergone brain preservation might be revived. But, just as those earlier researchers looked at their analytical tools and foresaw how they could be made more capable and precise, we too can speculate on what might eventually be possible. As a result, we often know, today, when we should go to the effort of preserving materials for future generations if they are to have any hope of success in achieving what we could not. Just because we of the 2020s do not know precisely how a person might be revived, it does not mean it is futile to contemplate how it might be done.

And, as cautious as we should be in such an exercise, there are other precedents that show it is not always as impossible a task as it may initially seem. Among his many achievements, Gottfried Wilhelm Leibniz, one of the co-discoverers of calculus along with Isaac Newton, figured out the basics of computer science centuries before the first computer was built. All the way back in 1679, Leibniz theorized about how a machine could perform calculations. Instead of electricity moving across transistors, he imagined marbles moving through mechanical gates, with an open gate corresponding to a binary 'one' and a closed gate being a 'zero'.[30] He envisioned this 154 years before the first mechanical computer was conceived, and 266 years before the first electronic version was actually constructed.* Leibniz had no notion of semiconductors, let alone the nanometre-sized transistors used today, but his understanding of fundamental principles enabled him to anticipate technologies centuries before they were actually feasible. Following in Leibniz's footsteps, I'm going to do my best to cautiously speculate on the most likely means by which brain-preserved people will be revived. We'll start with the methods I think are most probable, before considering proposals increasingly more distant from our current capabilities.

Digitizing a connectome

Imagine it's 2124, and somehow humanity is still around. The worst effects of climate change were avoided through steep emissions reductions, and cheap energy provided by renewables and nuclear fusion is now being used to pull carbon dioxide back out of the atmosphere. Superhuman artificial intelligence turned out to be easier than expected to deploy safely, with researchers successfully working out how to align machine motivations to human values. Through a combination of luck and hard work humanity has persisted, despite the ever-present risks of deadly pandemics, nuclear wars, and other global catastrophic risks.

In fact, not only has humanity survived, but it is flourishing. Economic reforms of the late twenty-first century ensured that the enormous dividends provided by cheap energy and labour automation were shared population-wide, allowing global living standards to rise dramatically. The average Bangladeshi is now far wealthier than essentially all Americans were a century prior. While there are still social conflicts, scarcity is as distant a memory as smallpox was to those of the 2020s.

There is even enough surplus wealth available to allow government and private budgets to fund increasingly ambitious projects. The

* Charles Babbage first conceived of his analytical engine in roughly 1833, and arguably the first electronic computer was created in 1945 with the construction of ENIAC.

Diverse Futures Consortium has already achieved 47 per cent of its goal of returning Earth's biological, cultural, and linguistic diversity to its pre-agricultural levels. Mars colonization efforts have begun in earnest, with the red planet now boasting a permanent population of 1 million settlers. And, amidst these flourishing ventures, motivated by goodwill for those past generations who ushered in this era of peace and prosperity, the Ancestor Revival Project has just transitioned from its pilot phase to full operations.

One at a time, we're going to explore the various techniques that an Ancestor Revival Project could potentially use to revive someone.

The first method we'll examine is *whole-brain emulation*, one way to achieve what is colloquially referred to as *mind uploading*.[31] The aim here is to take the personal identity information stored in someone's connectome and use it to recreate a brain for the person that runs on synthetic rather than biological hardware. To do this, you'd initially want to collect their personal-identity-specifying information by digitizing their connectome. Next, you'd have to breathe life back into the person by allowing this static snapshot of their identity to become dynamic and conscious once again. Step by step, let's walk through how this might be done.

In order to digitize someone's connectome, you'd need to scan their brain at almost molecular resolution.[32,33] As of 2023, electron microscopy provides the most well-developed method for achieving this outcome, although other alternatives are becoming increasingly promising.* These microscopes function by shooting a beam of electrons at their targets and measuring the subsequent reflections to create a

* Specifically, I'm referring to a technique called *expansion microscopy*, which offers a method to visualize synaptic ultrastructure at a nanometre resolution while using light microscopy.[34] Normally, light microscopy cannot be used to visualize sub-synaptic details directly in brain tissue, because the ion channels and other structures present at this scale are much smaller than the wavelengths of visible light. To get around this issue, expansion microscopy involves a series of chemical steps that cause the biological tissue to uniformly swell in size. By making synapses much larger, they can then be visualized by traditional light microscopes. This has multiple benefits compared to using electron microscopes, such as faster speeds and the ability to more easily make use of chemical labelling methods. This technique has only been developed in the last few years so it is still quite new, but if I were writing this book five years from now there's a good chance I would be focusing on this tool rather than electron microscopy.

visualization.[18] Perform this technique across an entire brain, and you can capture a digitized image of someone's connectome.

However, examining untreated biological material with an electron microscope is a bit like taking photos of a foggy landscape during twilight – everything in view looks pretty much the same. To improve the contrast, it helps to add chemical stains that allow electron microscopes to more clearly differentiate between the various kinds of biomolecular structures present inside and around neurons. For this to be done on a preserved person's brain, you'd first need to slowly rewarm their body from the cold storage where it had been safely resting in the intervening years. Next, you would once again connect their blood vessels to a fluid pump system, and wash out the now-redundant cryoprotectants. Once complete, a set of stains could be introduced into the solution that would give each key type of biomolecule a unique tag. This would prevent the components of synapses becoming confused when they are later viewed under the microscope.

Another issue to surmount is that, while electron microscopy has excellent resolution, it can only image the surface of whatever it is analysing, and is unable to peer deep inside an object. Thus, scanning someone's connectome requires repeated cycles of imaging the surface of their brain, removing a small layer from the surface, and then imaging again. This can be achieved through a technique that's existed since the 2010s known as *ion-beam scanning electron microscopy*, which scans the top layer of a tissue surface and then mills it off with an ion beam.* Repeated cycles of this process can enable the capture of someone's connectome at 10-nanometre resolution.

With current technology, however, this process would require thousands of years to image a single human brain, which is a bit slower than ideal. There is a fairly simple solution to this problem, although it is somewhat unpalatable to imagine: just cut the brain into several thousand layers and image each of these slices in parallel.[35]

The next objective, then, after chemically staining a preserved

* This process is similar to laser cutting, but instead of burning or vaporizing the material off the surface with a laser, ion-beam milling gently mechanically knocks off atoms and molecules from the surface by throwing high-velocity ions at it. This produces a smooth surface with no heat-damaged areas.

person's brain is to prepare it for slicing. The first step is to remove any remaining water from their body and replace it with a plastic resin that will ensure its stability through slicing and subsequent scanning. In order to accomplish this, you'd need to once again pump a series of solutions through the circulatory system of the preserved person, ending with the resin.* After a few days, and without affecting any of the microscopic details within the person's body, this resin cures solid, after which the person's brain and spinal cord can be surgically extracted from their skull and spine, with the rest of their body kept safe for later. The person's central nervous system, now contained in a plastic block, can then be progressively sliced into thousands of sections, each 20 micrometres thick. Once the last sections are cut into shape and mounted onto their dedicated imaging wafers, the preparation process is complete.

The collection of brain slices is now ready for simultaneous electron-microscope imaging. Each slice is placed into a machine which cycles between scanning the surface with hundreds of electron beams before milling off the top ten nanometres with a stream of ions. It takes 2,000 iterations to scan one slice, and, excluding the spinal cord, there will be around 9,000 slices. The resulting raw image of the total brain consists of approximately 1.2×10^{21} volumetric pixels, or *voxels*. In other words, even though the ion beams blew away the atoms that were the previous physical constituents of the person's connectome, their personal identity is now captured in over 1 billion trillion voxels on the imaging facility's storage system.

This unimaginable amount of raw data needs to be converted into a more useful format before it can come back to life. A critical first step is to turn the thousands of individual image slices back into a single three-dimensional connectome. Key to this are neuron-tracing algorithms, which pore over the stacks of two-dimensional images to trace out every last neuron's dendrites and axon branches while taking note of the synaptic connections between them. Another step is to identify which particular ion channels are present at each synapse and identify

* It might actually be easier to do the resin embedding after slicing. Keep in mind that, though it is based on current protocols, my account is still speculative, and a lot of these procedures require further optimization.

whether they are sensitive to glutamate, serotonin, dopamine, or any other neurotransmitter. Once these and a few other secondary steps are complete, this tracing and labelling results in a *molecularly annotated structural connectome*, the digital snapshot of a person at the time of their preservation.*

Emulating success

At this point, the person comprised by this digitized connectome exists in a state akin to heavy anaesthesia or deep hypothermia. In a sufficiently hypothermic brain, neurons are electrically silent, cooled into unconsciousness. But, if you carefully warm a person's body up, biological neurons can transform a static brain back into a dynamic, conscious person. With emergence from deep hypothermia as a precedent, how could we achieve an analogous rewarming process for a digitized brain?

Assuming functionalism is correct, restoring consciousness to a preserved person would require ensuring their new digital neurons function analogously to their previous biological ones. To achieve this, we can take the ongoing evolution of neural prostheses to its logical endpoint, and consider how individual digital replacements of biological neurons would operate.

One method might be to allocate each virtual neuron of the digitized connectome its own space in computer memory.[36] The information specifying the shape, connections, and subtype of each formerly biological neuron would then be used to tune a corresponding set of parameters for their digital counterpart, including how sensitive they are to neurotransmitter inputs and how easily their synaptic connections

* The steps described here – neuronal tracing and molecular annotation – are definitely required, but they are not necessarily sufficient. It is moderately likely that some of the cells that support neurons, such as astrocytes, will also need to be traced in order to fully capture someone's connectome. Less clearly necessary, but possibly still important, are things like extracellular space volumes and intracellular protein phosphorylation states. On the other hand, a lot of this information may turn out to be obtainable without the need for molecular annotation at all. It is already possible to sometimes use morphological information alone to determine the molecular class of a synapse, without needing to chemically stain it.[34]

can be potentiated or weakened. This tuning would ensure that the diversity of neuron types would still be represented in a digital version of someone's brain. Once each of the person's billions of neurons have been individually defined in this way, one could then begin the process of waking them up.

Much in the way that there is effectively no passage of time for biological neurons without allowing their constituent biomolecules to move around, waking up digital neurons requires allowing their memory states to vary. For a biological neuron, its moment-to-moment activity depends on the voltage across its membrane, which in turn is determined by the neuron's shape, subtype, and its recently received signals. A digital neuron could achieve the same by taking its current parameters and updating them as new information comes in. For example, if the voltage at its cell body is set at −70 millivolts at a certain time point, but the neuron is receiving a lot of positive current due to signals from its upstream neighbours, then at the next time step its voltage might be updated to −65 millivolts. As this digital neuron's output provides inputs for each of its connected neurons at the next time step, the entire network can coordinate its activity.

If all this neural activity and plasticity is implemented properly, a digital brain could be set up to perfectly replicate the activity of its biological predecessor. For now, ignore the fact that, in order to function, this digital brain will still need some way to receive external sensory inputs and perform motor outputs, as we'll return to these embodiment concerns shortly. Instead, let's focus on how, according to many functionalist views, this return of a person's neural activity necessarily entails the restoration of their intrinsic, first-person perspective.

Because this method of revival recreates the same activity as the person's original biological brain, but using different hardware, it is called *whole brain emulation*. The aim here is not mere *simulation*, which imperfectly mimics a system's behaviour without precisely modelling its internal components. This is instead *emulation*, a much more rigorous process which faithfully recreates a system's internal components at sufficiently high fidelity to precisely restore its behaviour.*

* Consider the simulations that produce detailed weather predictions. These are often only accurate up to about a week out because they operate at a more abstract and

Provide this emulation with the appropriate sensory inputs and grant it control of a biological, robotic, or virtual body, and the process should return a person to their original state of being. As we established in previous chapters, if certain psychological views of personal identity and functionalist theories of consciousness are correct, then, despite now being made of very different materials, this emulation is the same person as the one who was preserved all that time ago.

We can get an estimate of the kind of hardware that will be needed to store a whole brain emulation by examining the complexity of biological brains.[6,37,38] An adult human brain has around 86 billion neurons and a quadrillion synapses. Each neuron is itself an intricate, finely branching structure that requires maybe 10,000 connected segments to model accurately.* This primarily involves keeping track of the electrical activity in each neuronal segment, but also potentially monitoring changes in their internal chemical composition. It is unlikely that this needs to be recorded all the way down to the individual biomolecule level, but it may well require keeping note of around 1,000 variables or so per segment. Altogether, if we assume each electrical or chemical variable can be accurately represented by 1 byte of data, i.e. by taking one of 256 possible values, then a whole-brain emulation requires 1 million terabytes of storage space, or 1 exabyte. For reference, that's an

---

coarse-grained level than the actual atmospheric processes that determine winds and temperatures. Forecasts are created by simulations that take the current weather as data and use it as input to a model which calculates the weather at the next time step. A perfect model would need to track every air molecule, but this is completely beyond our computational abilities. As a result, the approximation diverges from reality over time until it is no better than chance.

In contrast, I can run an emulation of the 1998 Nintendo 64 game Banjo-Kazooie on my laptop from 2020 without the game ever failing to behave exactly as it would were I playing it on its original console. This is because my current computer only needs to model the old console down to the level of its logic gates and memory states, rather than all the way to the atomic level, to run the game exactly as it did on my Nintendo 64 indefinitely into the future. This situation, where the desired behaviour can be achieved despite entirely doing away with the original mechanisms below some particular boundary, is known as *scale separation*.

* The number of compartments required to accurately model the behaviour of neurons is a matter of considerable dispute, so this number may well be off in either direction by a few orders of magnitude. To see an example of how these estimations can be done, see here.[39]

equivalent size to around three hours of global internet traffic in 2021.[40] That is very large, but not unimaginably so – it is already within the storage capacity of early 2020s online cloud storage.

But that only tells us how much memory space we need to hold a static snapshot of the brain at any given time point. In order for the person to be conscious, the emulation needs to be able to dynamically update themself, so we'll also want an estimate of the processing demands required for that. For this digital connectome to think and feel in real time, we need to update the state of each neuronal segment approximately 10,000 times per second. In turn, each of these segments takes about 1,000 discrete calculations to ready itself for the next time point.* Multiplying these together suggests an emulation would need around 10^{25} calculations per second, or 10 yottaFLOPS, to run in real time.† That is around 10 million times faster than the world's most advanced supercomputers in 2023, meaning we're not going to be able to run a whole-brain emulation anytime soon. Yet, given computing speeds for supercomputers have already increased by a factor of about 100 million since the 1990s, if historical trends in computing-performance improvements continue, this should be achievable sometime in the early 2040s.

That takes care of the brain, but the person is going to want to have a body too. At best, running a whole-brain emulation without providing it a body would simply not work. A brain fully disconnected from sensory inputs and motor outputs may partially or entirely fail to function, at least according to the philosophical field of *embodied cognition*.[42] At

* By *calculations* I mean 'floating-point operations', where floating-point operations per second (FLOPS) is a typical measure of computer performance.

† As a side note, the computational requirements needed to perform a whole-brain emulation are likely much higher than the actual computational power of the brain itself. We do not yet know all the ways in which biological brains perform computations, but there is likely a large degree of redundancy in neuronal processing. This means that while it might take almost a giga FLOPs to emulate a neuron, the actual neuron itself may only perform a small fraction of that many calculations based on its synaptic inputs. One estimate puts the computational power of the human brain at 10^{17} FLOPS, which would mean that a brain has 100 million times less computational power than is required to emulate it.[41] One implication of this is emulations are likely to get a lot cheaper once we figure out what level of emulation fidelity is actually required, and what is unnecessary.

worst, an unincarnated emulation would experience something nightmarishly akin to locked-in syndrome. Either way, neglecting to provide a body would significantly detract from the quality of a person's revival. This will not do, particularly as there are several plausible options available for granting one to our temporal refugee.

One method would be to provide them with a descendant of cochlear implants, bionic limbs, and other early twenty-first century neural prostheses, by which I mean a robotic body.* It's not hard to imagine that the technology of future decades will make today's prostheses seem as archaic as nineteenth-century mechanical calculators are in comparison to modern laptops. Already in the 2020s, prosthetic limbs can be controlled via neurally implanted sensors and provide limited tactile information to their user.[44] Future developments in this field could lead to synthetic bodies, custom-built to mimic a preserved person's original frame. If done right, this would allow an emulation's digital neurons to see through bionic eyes and move using artificial muscles in a way that felt indistinguishable from their original biological flesh.

In pursuit of this goal, there is thankfully some evidence that embodiment is unlikely to take anywhere near the storage or processing demands that running a brain emulation requires. For example, consider how much data flows through the optic nerves connecting your eyes to your brain. Your two optic nerves combined have a transmission bandwidth of approximately 20 megabits per second, or about as fast as an average internet download speed was in 2010.[45] What this relatively small transmission capacity indicates is that the brain is aware of only a fraction of the true complexity of the body in which it resides. In turn, this means that there is no requirement for a perfect cell-by-cell emulation to provide a revived person with something that feels just like their original body.

Okay, let's take stock. Imagine you are working for the Ancestor Revival Project, and, at the end of a long process of preserving, staining, scanning, emulating, and embodying someone, you have arrived

* Another approach would be to embody the emulation in a virtual body in a virtual environment and dispense with the difficulties of building sophisticated hardware. David Chalmers, of the 'hard problem' fame, argues that virtual worlds can be just as real and meaningful as the physical one, making this a potentially viable alternative.[43]

at the last stage: switching them on and ensuring that everything is working properly. A good first step would be to boot up the emulation into a state of dreamless sleep and verify that the activity of their digital neurons is as expected. For example, if you were to take recordings from a sleeping biological human brain you would observe characteristic slow brainwaves, so these should also be seen in a functioning emulation. More sophisticated tools could also check for reflexive responsiveness to stimuli presented to their robotic body, appropriate connectivity between regions inside their digital brain, and the expected reconfiguration of synapses that typically occurs during sleep. If all this is occurring as it should, it would be time to wake the person up.

Rehomed inside their new robotic body, our temporal refugee lies asleep on a bed in the revival clinic. As they are restored to consciousness, a doctor at their bedside begins to ask them questions, verifying that their memories are intact and that their cognition has returned. At the same time, the doctor assesses their newly awakened patient for signs of any possible discomfort, as any infidelities in how their new robotic body mimics their old biological one may cause distress, at least until they adapt to their new anatomy. Still, as all is looking good, it is time to welcome the person back into the world. The doctor hands over responsibility to the social worker team, who will bring the patient up to speed on how to adapt to all the changes that have occurred while they've been in stasis. At this point, just as Elizabeth emerged from the limbo of Dr Allen's starvation clinic in 1922 after the transformative effects of her insulin treatments, so too should our successfully revived person be now ready to get started with the rest of their life.

Sufficiently advanced technology is indistinguishable from magic

Should it be shown to be a philosophically acceptable method of survival, whole-brain emulation using standard computer hardware presents the simplest proposal for revival. This is because it only requires equipment that either already exists or whose development would largely be a straightforward extrapolation from modern technology. Certainly, those who hold a functionalist theory of consciousness and a psychological view of personal identity should be confident that this revival method is viable. Yet even if everything appears to be functioning well in this scenario, there are still academics who would dispute the feasibility of this style of revival. If their objections are not invalidated in the decades between now and when an Ancestor Revival Project can be commenced, there would be reason to consider alternative revival methods.

For example, no matter how closely the emulation's behaviour matched its biological predecessor, proponents of the integrated information theory of consciousness claim it would feel nothing like the biological brain on which it was based.[46] Traditional computing hardware has a very different architecture to biological neurons, which in turn produces a very different pattern of integrated information. Typical computers physically separate their processing units, which perform calculations, from their memory units, which store data. In contrast, a biological neuron integrates both logic processing and memory in the same cell. These differences in architecture mean that there will be differences in the integrated information present in each system, even though functionally equivalent circuits can be built out of both silicon and biology. In turn, this means that a computer running an emulation might have close to zero integrated information, rendering it akin to an unfeeling philosophical zombie. Alternatively, some parts of the machine might have some degree of integrated information, meaning parts of the emulation would have some degree of consciousness but in a manner very different from that of biological humans. Either way, these theorists claim that as long as the patterns of integrated information differ between the emulation and the biological brain on which they are based, revival attempts would fail.

That being said, integrated information theory doesn't imply that revival is a forever unachievable goal. While it looks unfavourably upon traditional computer architectures, which isolate processing from memory in a non-biological fashion, it has no such disapproval for *neuromorphic* computer designs, which more closely imitate neurobiology.[47] Instead of being built primarily out of transistors, some neuromorphic computers incorporate *memristors*, synthetic analogues of biological neurons. Remember how when one neuron's activity frequently coincides with that of its downstream target, their synaptic connection will strengthen? Memristor physics mimics this history-dependent sensitivity to inputs, enabling synthetic circuits to be built that resemble neurophysiology. In principle, it should be possible to construct neuromorphic hardware that structures integrated information in an equivalent manner to a human brain. Once built, at least according to integrated information theory, any emulation run on such a device should feel conscious in the same way they did back when they were flesh and blood.*

But, to make matters worse, a small number of philosophers go even further than the integrated information theorists, suggesting that not even neuromorphic computers would suffice for restoration of consciousness. Some claim that a human-like first-person perspective is probably only achievable with biological brains, or at least that being biological strongly influences what it feels like to be conscious.[48,49] Synthetic neurons will not do, as they lack the multitude of internal biological processes that are supposedly critical for consciousness, from maintaining homeostasis to excreting waste products. From this viewpoint, an emulation built out of silicon rather than cells will not feel like their old self, and thus revival will fail.

Yet even if this minority perspective on consciousness turns out to be accurate, we needn't give up hope. In the chapter on death, we discussed how both stem cells and neural prostheses provide a means to replace dead neurons and restore functions to individuals with brain damage. While artificial neurons are advancing at a faster rate, and seem to me to be a more feasible option for revival in the long run, there is still evidence to suggest that, should we need to, we could one day build a biological brain out of stem cells capable of running an emulation.

* Unfortunately, running an emulation using neuromorphic hardware is a much more distant prospect than proposals to use traditional architectures. Current circuit designs using anything more than a trivial number of memristors are still very bulky and inefficient, reminiscent of the early days of electronic computers. There is no consensus on the best materials to use for building memristors, as all approaches have issues with precision, reliability, or energy efficiency. To compound these problems, improvements in neuromorphic computer performance are progressing slower than for their conventional counterparts due to considerably less investment. Now, all of these challenges are likely surmountable, and the potential utility of these devices for artificial intelligence applications is already spurring further developments. Nonetheless, if integrated information theory is correct, then any Ancestor Revival Project will have a tougher time getting started.

In 2022, a group of neuroscientists and engineers reported successful construction of a cyborg system made of stem cells that could play the arcade game Pong.[50] In Pong, the aim of the game is to move a paddle so as to prevent a continuously bouncing ball from falling through a gap. In order for the cyborg to play, its stem cells were first induced to develop into neurons, and were then placed on top of an array of electrodes. Next, these freshly grown neurons were provided with electrical stimulation that indicated the current position of the paddle and the ball. At the same time, the cyborg system's neuronal firing was recorded and used to move the paddle left or right. Over several play sessions, the neurons were programmed via a feedback system to produce better and better Pong performance by playing longer and longer rallies.

This kind of biological system is incredibly crude by the standards of modern computers, let alone human brains. Even so, it suffices to suggest that we can build arbitrary, programmable devices out of living neurons. Given enough time and investment, it is plausible that one could devise a more sophisticated system that could run a whole-brain emulation. If this were ever shown to be the case, it would allay the concern that revivals are only possible if the emulations run on biology.

Even so, all this talk of futuristic synthetic or biological hardware is irrelevant to the most common objection to the possibility of revival via whole-brain emulation. Most people are not concerned about whether an emulation would function by using digital or biological neurons. Instead, they are worried that an emulation wouldn't revive *them*, but just a copy of them. In the chapter on personal identity, I discussed why I and many others think this viewpoint is wrong, and that the psychological connectedness provided through preservation and emulation is sufficient to ensure someone's survival. Even so, it would be disingenuous to ignore the fact that some philosophers and members of the general public still object to this position for a variety of reasons. A few believe survival can only occur through continuity of the physical material of one's body.[48,51] Others accept the psychological view, but assert that uploading fails to ensure survival for a variety of technical reasons.[52–54] If it turns out that I am wrong, and they are right in asserting that emulation would never produce anything but an unsatisfying copy of the person we were hoping to save, does that mean brain preservation is pointless and we should abandon hope?

No. Losing emulation as an option doesn't make revival theoretically impossible, it just makes it a lot harder. In this circumstance, preserving a person's body still allows their personal identity, and thus them, to survive. It's just that, instead of being free to pick any possible medium with which to restore the person to consciousness, we're limited to somehow reversing the preservation process and returning their diseased and vitrifixed body back to health. Now, no current technology under development is even close to being able to reverse the vitrifixation process, let alone do so while simultaneously curing whatever was causing someone to be dying in the first place. But a person under preservation has infinite patience, and with enough time and effort anything that is not physically impossible is in principle feasible.

In 1959, the Nobel Prize-winning physicist Richard Feynman presented a lecture entitled 'There's Plenty of Room at the Bottom', in which he hypothesized that one day it would be possible to swallow a microscopic medical robot that could perform surgery from within a patient's body.[55] This was the first recorded articulation of the concept of *nanotechnology*. Almost thirty years later, and without modern knowledge of vitrifixation and connectomes, the nanotechnologist Eric Drexler imagined how nanoscale robots might one day be used to revive a preserved person.[56] He imagined introducing these robots into a person's blood vessels, from which they would roam around the body, cutting the cross-linked bonds that occurred during fixation and repairing damaged cells. Once the initial repairs are complete, the person would be slowly rewarmed and have their cryoprotectant removed. With careful monitoring, and possibly several rounds of nanobot medical attention, the person would be revived into a state similar to just before they entered vitrifixation, albeit in much greater health. It is through the potential for this kind of nanomedicine that those who believe in the necessity of bodily continuity for survival can maintain hope.[57]

By the standards of today's primitive technology, this vision of nanomedicine is so far beyond current medical capabilities that it borders on magical thinking. Correspondingly, it would be easy to mock and dismiss dreams of nanomedicine, if not for the fact that we are already surrounded by alien technology that appears fantastical to our simple human science. For cells, the building blocks out of which all the majesty of biological life is built, are nothing but microscopic bags of nanomachinery designed through billions of years of evolutionary processes. No human device can pass through blood vessels to perform repairs on microtears, but platelets can. Humans cannot build an invisibility cloak, but octopuses can deploy pigments in their skin cells to perfectly mimic their environment in a fraction of a second. Life on Earth is 4 billion years old, while human science has had barely more than four centuries to develop. Imagine what we might be capable of once we've had even a fraction as much time.

LIMINAL, BUT NOT ELIMINATED

As late as 1839, the esteemed surgeon Alfred Velpeau said, 'The abolishment of pain in surgery is a chimera. It is absurd to go on seeking it [. . .] "knife" and "pain" are two words in surgery that must forever be associated in the consciousness of the patient.'* A mere seven years later, William Morton gave the first public demonstration of anaesthesia and ushered in a new era of medicine.[58] One should be very wary of making claims that certain medical advances will never be achieved.

Letting the brains of dying people decay because modern computing power cannot yet emulate the human nervous system, or because nanomedicine is incapable of vitrifixation reversal, is equivalent to 1970s scientists throwing away moon rock samples for a lack of sufficiently advanced analytical equipment. Even though we are currently unable to revive a preserved person, it does not follow that they must be dead. As long as a person's connectome is intact, there is still a chance for their revival, just as Elizabeth's years in limbo enabled her recovery once insulin arrived. The means by which a preserved person could be restored to consciousness, however complicated they may turn out to be, are just a matter of details.

That is not to say that details don't matter, or that people considering such a treatment should not be educated as to how it might work. A key part of making any medical decision is providing informed

* I discovered this quote while reading Eric Drexler's book on nanotechnology, *Engines of Creation*.

consent, and, given the stakes involved in preservation, it is imperative that patients be able to specify their beliefs and requirements. If a patient holds a particular view of personal identity, or on the physical basis of consciousness, they should be able to specify that they do not wish to be revived until a method is available that is compatible with their beliefs. Preservation empowers people to turn fate into choice, and these decisions should be theirs to make.

That being said, I would personally tick the box on the consent form labelled 'default to whatever the scientific and philosophical consensus is at the time revival technology becomes available'. Leibniz might have been able to guess at the broad strokes of how a computer could be built 400 years before they were first constructed, but he certainly didn't get many of the details right. I am sure that researchers 400 years from now will have a much better idea of how to revive people than anyone today, so long as we provide them with the necessary connectomes.

What I am not so sure of is whether this discussion of technological feasibility and philosophical beliefs is even the most important part of a preservation consent form. I suspect that, for many people, the technical details of how their revival will be performed concerns them less than whether their friends and family will also be there when they wake up. For – while we are first and foremost our connectomes – our spouses, siblings, and other social connections are almost as important for defining our identities.[59] Many would likely have no desire to be revived unless their partner would be there beside them, while others would be pained to return to a world that their children had forever departed. A discussion of these social concerns should be a critical part of any preservation consent form.

The best way to ensure these social requirements for revival are satisfied is to make certain that every single dying person who wishes to undergo preservation has access to the procedure. Saving an additional person does not just help them, it enriches the lives of everyone else who cares about them. This chapter has looked at the technical feasibility of preserving someone, and speculated on how we might bring them back. But, as admirable as it is to save any individual life, our real aspirations should be to save *everyone*. Up next: what it would cost to abolish death entirely.

8
How We Can Save Everyone

In the long run we are all dead.
John Maynard Keynes, *A Tract on Monetary Reform*

Even for a child misfortunate enough to develop cancer, five-year-old Emily was unlucky.[1] Eighty per cent of all children with acute lymphoblastic leukaemia are cured of the disease with a single course of chemotherapy, yet Emily suffered two relapses within a five-month period.[2] Given the low efficacy of the remaining treatments available in 2011, she was likely to die within a few years. Emily's medical team recommended that she be placed in palliative care, spending what little time she had left with those who loved her.

I suspect that, by this point in the book, you know that is not how this story is going to go. Emily's parents were unwilling to accept her terminal diagnosis, just as Elizabeth's had been back in 1919. They searched desperately for a treatment that would provide another option, hoping that some recent medical breakthrough could save their daughter. They found one at the Children's Hospital of Philadelphia.

In cancer, a population of rebellious cells stop playing their part as components of a greater whole, instead replicating with no regard for the broader needs of the body. Now, if these cells were foreign invaders such as bacteria, the immune system would have no difficulty recognizing the intruders and trying to destroy them. But with cancer, the immune system is incapable of distinguishing the rebels from still-obedient cells. Unable to tell friend from foe, it sits idly by even as the multiplying mutineers cause greater and greater destruction. If only the immune cells could be given some way to identify the traitors in their midst, they could wipe the cancer from the body.

Emily became the first paediatric patient enrolled in a clinical trial to do exactly that. This new treatment, called CAR T-cell therapy, involved extracting some of Emily's own immune cells from her blood and genetically re-engineering them to recognize the insurgents within her. Once reintroduced into her body, her newly unblinded immune system could now discern the traitorous cancer cells and proceed to quash their rebellion.

A week after her seventh birthday, a bone marrow biopsy showed she was in complete remission. As of 2023, over ten years later, a now eighteen-year-old Emily remains alive and cancer-free. Every breath Emily takes is a testament to our age of miracles and wonders. This was no less the case for Elizabeth, Trent, or Anik before her, nor for anyone else who would be dead if not for modern medicine.

This far into the book, it's possible the magic of medical discoveries may be starting to feel somewhat mundane. My apologies, if so, as that sentiment is only going to intensify from here. Now in the home stretch, we have mostly finished with the miraculous and must increasingly turn to the prosaic and administrative. As such, the point I need to focus on is not the relief of Emily's parents, nor the brilliance of the researchers and healthcare workers who made it possible, but the vulgar financial details of her treatment. Putting together her CAR T-cell therapy, hospital stays, medication for side-effects, and other attendant expenses, Emily's treatment costs may well have exceeded $1 million.* Human lives might be priceless, but they still need to be accounted for.†

***

As we must now focus on the unromantic aspects of reality, I should start by recounting a case with a much less satisfying ending than Emily's story that is sadly still relevant to our discussion. On an overcast morning in April 2018, the parents of Jordan, a six-month-old

* If not otherwise specified, all monetary figures in this chapter have been converted into US dollars at their historical conversion rate and inflation-adjusted to 2022 dollars.

† I first came across Emily's story in the excellent health-economics textbook *The Right Price* by Daniel Ollendorf, Joshua Cohen, and Peter Neumann.

boy from South Australia, awoke to discover him uncharacteristically listless and quiet in his cot.[3] They rushed him to hospital, where upon examination he was found to have a purple rash spreading across his small body. His doctors, recognizing this as an extremely grave sign of an infection in his blood, frantically endeavoured to administer him antibiotics and rush him to an intensive care centre. Despite their best efforts, though, Jordan died within a few hours of his parents having first noticed any symptoms.

The tragic part of this story is not only Jordan's untimely death, but also that a readily available course of vaccines costing roughly $200 might have let him live. As of 2018, a vaccine for meningococcal B, the disease that claimed Jordan's life, had already been available in Australia for five years. Given a three-dose course of the vaccine can begin at two months of age, with the second dose occurring as early as four months, Jordan could potentially have had some protection from the disease by the time he contracted it at six months old.

Nor was his failure to be vaccinated a result of negligence on the part of his parents. Australia has a national childhood immunization programme, and Jordan's parents had diligently taken him to receive all of his routinely scheduled vaccinations. The problem was, despite being available, the meningococcal B vaccine was not part of this schedule. What could possibly have prevented the inclusion of this life-saving medicine into the routine childhood vaccination programme? The Australian government's reasoning was that, despite the vaccine's modest price tag, saving the life of Jordan and other children in his position just wasn't worth the cost.

What makes this story all the more confusing is that Australia's socialized healthcare system will provide expensive CAR T-cell therapy to children like Emily for free, but won't pay for $200 vaccines to save children like Jordan. To understand how this could possibly be justified, we must consult the reasoning of the Pharmaceutical Benefits Advisory Committee, the body that determines which medicines will be publicly funded in Australia.

When the meningococcal B vaccine first became available in Australia in 2013, the committee issued a ruling on why it would not be added to the public registry.[4] They did not dispute that the vaccine was likely clinically efficacious in providing some protection against the disease. Instead, their sticking point was the cost it would take to provide the vaccine to all children, relative to how many of them would ever contract the illness.

It turns out that Jordan was actually even more unlucky than Emily. Before CAR T-cell therapy was introduced, about one in 17,000 people were killed by acute lymphoblastic leukaemia. In contrast, only around one in a million people died from a meningococcal B infection. The rarity of the disease meant that hundreds of thousands of children would have to be vaccinated for a single life to be saved. The committee calculated that an initial rollout would require $525 million to vaccinate 4 million children. They estimated this would prevent approximately nine deaths, meaning each life saved would cost around $58 million. For context, if each of the 160,000 Australians who died in 2020 could have been saved for $60 million, it would have cost $9.6 trillion, over six times the Australian economy's GDP. Accordingly, the committee rejected publicly subsidizing the vaccine, concluding it did not provide value for money. The Australian population's health would be overall improved by using the funds elsewhere.

***

I am aware that this calculus may appear abhorrent. A child's worth is immeasurable to their parents, just as a life of any age may be for its possessor. In principle, we should be spending whatever it takes to save each and every one. In practice, though, our resources are limited, even if our desire to save lives is unbounded. For whether it is a government or household budget, healthcare already comprises a huge percentage of all spending. In 2020, spending on healthcare already represented 19 per cent of GDP in the US, 11 per cent in Japan, 10 per cent in Australia, and 11 per cent globally.[5] This proportion has been growing, too.[6] As countries develop and grow richer, more and more of their resources are spent on improving the quantity and quality of their citizens' lives. The UK government spent under 1 per cent of GDP on healthcare in 1900, 2.9 per cent in 1960, 4.5 per cent in 1980, 5.5 per cent in 2000, and 9.9 per cent in 2019. This looks less like a callous world leaving people to die in misery, and more like a caring one striving to provide ever-more medicine while juggling multiple priorities.

As always in life, we must make tradeoffs. Evolution through natural selection is eager to throw away decades of our lives if it will marginally improve our reproductive fitness. Humans are much more compassionate, but we are still bound by the limits of reality. We are willing to spend huge amounts of money to improve our health, but we need to save some of it for the other things that make life possible and enjoyable. At the very least, some money needs to be reserved for agriculture, lest we starve, critical infrastructure, lest our cities collapse, and education, so as to sustain our civilization. Even beyond these absolute necessities, we want to have some money left to spend on art, food, entertainment, and all the other luxuries that make life worth living. In the absence of infinite budgets, this implies a finite limit to our healthcare spending. In turn, that means there must ultimately be a maximum price we are willing to pay to save lives.

The contention of this book is that we should abolish involuntary death entirely by providing universal access to brain preservation. But, for this to be possible, it is not enough to show that it is technically feasible. We must also know at what cost. If preservation requires millions of dollars per procedure, it is of no use to anyone but billionaires. The ancient Egyptians may have been willing to spend a significant fraction of their economic output building pyramids to ensure comfortable afterlives for their Pharaohs, but modern democratic governments have no such interest in funding expensive projects that benefit so few of their citizens. Unless it can be made cheap and ubiquitous, brain preservation has no hope of helping the typical individual, their family, their community, or humanity at large.

Given this, there are two key questions we need answered to determine if preservation is going to work at scale.

The first: how much are we willing to pay to keep people alive? Considering the stories of Emily and Jordan, the Australian government clearly values its citizens at more than $1 million but less than $60 million. When economists and bureaucrats perform these macabre calculations, what is the threshold value they determine we can afford to spend?

The second: how much does brain preservation actually cost? Are its expenses more like CAR T-cell therapy, available only to the rich citizens of wealthy nations? Or might it be more like insulin in the modern day: not trivially cheap, but at least affordable for most in all but the poorest countries?

It might be taboo to put a price on lives, but it has to be done. There is no way to run a public healthcare system or a private insurance company without an evaluation of the tradeoffs people are willing or unwilling to make to extend lifespans. Failing to perform this kind of analysis does nothing to address the scarcity of healthcare resources. Instead, it merely leads to their misallocation, and consequently more sickness and death than need otherwise occur. I understand that there is a painful loss of innocence in learning that necessity demands placing base monetary values on the sanctity of human lives. My consolation to you is that once your disillusionment is complete, at least you will see that the price of saving everyone is a cost our societies can comfortably bear.

THE VALUE OF A LIFE

As with all goods, how much we're willing to pay to 'save lives' depends on how much life we're buying. For example, imagine there are two different treatments for advanced cancer, each costing $100,000. The first treatment extends the lives of patients by only three months, while the second is sufficiently effective to ensure 95 per cent of patients will still be alive after five years. It is uncontroversial to assert that public healthcare systems, insurance companies, and private individuals are all going to be far more willing to pay for the second treatment than the first. What this demonstrates is that people don't just care about saving lives per se, they also care about the number of years of life that they have saved. One of the reasons we are generally willing to pay more to save children's lives than adults' is that, since they still have their whole life ahead of them, healing a five-year-old saves much more life than treating someone in their eighties. As such, when considering how effective a treatment is, economists calculate its benefit in terms of increased *life years* rather than simply 'lives saved'.

That said, people do not necessarily consider all of their life years to be of equal value. Consider Camila, a forty-five-year-old resident of Mexico City, who has suffered a painful arm fracture courtesy of a careless driver as she cycled to work. Over the following year she experiences considerable pain and distress, from both the original injury itself and a series of corrective surgeries. She misses out on participating in her community baseball team, and has to forego leisure time to attend frequent rehabilitation sessions. When, after twelve months, her arm feels almost completely back to full function, Camila is certain the new year to come will be better than the painful one she has just completed. Her experience indicates how people care not just about the number of years they live, but also about the quality of those years. As a result, economists typically use *quality-adjusted life years* as the fundamental unit of concern in healthcare.

Given this perspective, considering whether a novel therapy is worth funding first depends on assessing the quantity and quality of life it can provide to patients relative to the status quo. Determining the new treatment's supposed benefits requires two pieces of information. The first is the currently expected lifespan for prospective patients who might use it, and the quality of that lifespan. The second is the degree to which the new medicine will extend and improve the lives of these patients. Both of these things need to be established before even considering the treatment's cost.

Lifespan is easy to quantify objectively, but measuring quality of life requires some sophistication. The most direct method is to just query people on how much they prefer being in one health state compared to another. In the *time tradeoff* paradigm, researchers first ask people to imagine suffering from a certain health-limiting condition for a period of time, such as having diabetes for ten years. Next, the researchers ask them to imagine they are in perfect health for some shorter period of time, such as three or seven years. Finally, people are asked to decide exactly how much lifespan of lower health quality they would be willing to sacrifice in order to live for a shorter period in perfect health instead. For example, one individual might report that ten years with chronic lower back pain would be equal to eight years in perfect health. This time tradeoff indicates the participant believes back pain reduces someone's health status by 20 per cent compared to full health, providing a quantitative measure of quality of life.

To make these calculations more broadly applicable and practical, instead of exhaustively collecting time tradeoff information for every possible comparison of health conditions, economists frequently make use of more convenient classification systems. One such scale is the EQ-5D, which assigns any person's health status a score between 1 (perfect health) and 0 (dead).* It does so by again asking people to consider a particular disease, but this time to assign it a value on each of five dimensions: Pain, Self-Care, Usual Activities, Anxiety/Depression, and Mobility. Specifically, EQ-5D requires individuals to select a level for each dimension, where level 1 is 'completely unaffected' and level 5 is 'most severely affected'.

To make this concrete, consider how Camila might score herself while suffering from her badly broken arm. She might assign herself a level 3/5 on the Pain dimension, given her arm is quite sore; a level 2/5 on Self-Care and Usual Activities, given she cannot properly use her arm for her activities of daily living; a level 2/5 on Anxiety/Depression, given she's missing out on her treasured baseball games with friends; and a level 1/5 on Mobility, as she doesn't generally need her arm to walk or move around. Running these values through a classification algorithm calibrated on a 2019 survey of the general Mexican population would mean Camila's overall health status would be scored at 0.76, or a 24 per cent reduction compared to perfect health.[†,7]

This information provides the baseline against which to assess

* It's also possible to designate certain health statuses 'worse than dead' by providing them negative scores, or 'better than perfect health' by scoring them greater than 1.

† Under ideal conditions, these classification systems allow for relatively easy assignment of quality-adjustments for years spent in any possible health status. Yet, as with all tools, it's important to be mindful of assumptions and implicit choices in the way these scoring systems are designed and implemented. One of the biggest issues is deciding who sets the score for the severity of any particular health condition. Should it be the general public? This is the easiest group to survey, but there's reason to question the accuracy of their responses. People often overestimate the badness of visually salient impairments, such as reduced mobility due to leg amputations, while underestimating the suffering of those with less visible conditions, such as depression or anxiety. Maybe instead it should be the patients with a particular condition? Perhaps, but surveying patient populations can have its own difficulties. Possibly healthcare workers, with their broad overview of a diversity of patient experiences, would be a useful group to ask? Whichever way researchers decide, the results should be interpreted with the choice kept in mind. That's not to say there's no agreement between the scores assigned by different groups, but merely to point out that inclusiveness and

improvements from proposed novel therapies. And assess we must: thanks to the ongoing efforts of medical researchers and pharmaceutical companies, there is an ever-expanding list of therapeutics that could be funded. For example, in the November 2022 edition of the monthly meeting of the Australian Pharmaceutical Benefits Advisory Committee, the body considered such treatments as asciminib, for a particular kind of leukaemia, empaglifozin, for chronic heart failure, and etanercept, for various autoimmune conditions including rheumatoid arthritis.[8] Which of these should be added to the public subsidies list, and which rejected, depends on just how many extra quality-adjusted life years they can provide and for what cost.

Examined in isolation, there is no answer to which treatments should be funded, as it depends on the size of the available budget. For an organization with very few resources available, such as a relief agency providing healthcare in a developing country, the number of quality-adjusted life years is maximized by using the limited funds on cheap and effective treatments such as vaccines and antibiotics. On the other hand, in wealthy countries like the UK, rather than just purchasing the most cost-effective treatments until a fixed budget is consumed, it is more common to fund all treatments that fall below a certain cost-to-benefit threshold. That is to say, if a new treatment for a certain condition is cheaper than an otherwise equivalent pre-existing therapy, or more expensive but also proportionally more effective, it will typically be funded.

SO, HOW MUCH?

The price an organization is willing to pay for a treatment providing an additional quality-adjusted life year compared to existing therapies can be described as their *threshold*. A few countries list these thresholds explicitly.[9] For example, take the National Institute for Health and Care Excellence (NICE), which determines which new healthcare

---

careful consideration is required when evaluating the subjective health status of human lives.

interventions will be publicly funded in England and Wales. In 2004 the institute endorsed a threshold of £20,000–30,000 per quality-adjusted life year, although they maintained that factors of equity and wider social circumstances could lead to certain exceptions.[10] An independent 2015 analysis of decisions made by the Institute showed that 75 per cent of treatments costing under £27,000 per quality-adjusted life year were accepted, while 75 per cent of those costing over £52,000 were rejected. Overall, this implies an actual threshold of around £40,000 per quality-adjusted life year.[11] An equivalent body in Thailand considers a new treatment good value for money if it provides an additional quality-adjusted life year for less than the Thai GDP per capita, equivalent to about $7,000 in 2021.[12]

While most other countries are less explicit about their threshold, they still use one behind the scenes. The Pharmaceutical Benefits Advisory Committee is coy about their specific cut-off, but the pattern of pharmaceutical company applications in Australia and a history of the Committee's decisions suggests an implicit threshold of around $60,000 (US dollars, not Australian).[13] They and other health bodies typically decline to provide an explicit threshold on the grounds that additional concerns also influence their decisions. For example, given a disease currently lacking any viable treatment, many organizations are willing to pay extra on the grounds of ensuring equity and meeting unmet clinical needs. Even so, this only smears the threshold across a blurry range, rather than removing it entirely. The threshold of acceptable cost per quality-adjusted life year remains the major determinant of which new treatments will or won't be added to public healthcare systems.[9]

The story is more complicated for countries like the United States, which lack a single major public payer for healthcare. Costs and payments in the US are set by multiple actors across the federal government, individual states, and private insurance companies. None of these bodies is capable of setting a standard threshold for all the other players, whose willingness to pay for specific treatments is influenced by the particular populations they serve and the political pressures they experience. To complicate things further, organizations in the US have an aversion to explicitly calculating thresholds, as the idea of a willingness-to-pay for a quality-adjusted life year evokes a cultural fear of healthcare rationing. As an example, although the Affordable Care Act legislation passed in 2010 created an institute that advises Medicare about what treatments it should provide, it explicitly prohibited the body from performing analyses that could provide a threshold for cost-effective treatments.[14]

Yet a lack of an explicit threshold doesn't mean that American organizations will fund any beneficial healthcare treatment, no matter how small the benefit nor how high the cost. Instead, a threshold is set implicitly by each organization through murky decision-making based on precedent, pharmaceutical company lobbying, and political pressure from patient groups. Doctors are aware that, even in the richest country on Earth, resource limitations mean a threshold must be considered when deciding which treatments are cost-effective. Accordingly, researchers often reference a value of $50,000–100,000 when publishing cost-effectiveness analyses for new treatments.[15] In the end, both private and government healthcare agencies end up deciding which treatments to fund by liaising with non-governmental groups willing to perform independent cost-effectiveness analyses, such as the US Department of Veterans Affairs coordinating with the Institute for Clinical and Economic Review.[16]

Overall, instead of benefiting from transparent and consistent decision-making about which treatments will and will not be funded, the US populace ends up beholden to a system where funding decisions are made by policy makers with unclear incentives. This is somewhat shocking for a country that spends around 18 per cent of its GDP on healthcare, or around $4 trillion per year, with some arguing that up to 25 per cent of this is wasted on low-quality care.[17] One cannot help but wonder how many lives could be saved with a more coherent allocation of this money.

Ironically, even as Medicare is effectively prohibited from calculating a pragmatic price to pay for a year of healthy life, other branches of the US government routinely put an explicit value on human lives.[18] If adding crash barriers to a highway is expected to save one person's life over the course of the highway's lifespan, but the barriers would cost more than $10.4 million to install, the Department of Transportation wouldn't deem the project worthwhile. In the same way, the Environmental Protection Agency doesn't recommend river clean-ups or toxic waste site decontaminations unless they cost less than $9.4 million per life saved as a result. In general, when creating regulations on safety, transportation, and environmental standards in the US, these and other agencies have decided that imposing a cost of less than $10 million dollars per life saved provides good value for money.*

They are able to do this this because, rather than determining the cost of medicine they are willing to pay to extend a person's life, these government departments are instead calculating the value of a safety-standard improvement that would statistically ensure a person will be saved who would otherwise have died. While both amount to the same thing in the end, the more indirect nature of saving lives through installing road upgrades rather than administering drugs means these agencies elude the ire of those who campaign against perceived rationing in healthcare.

Indeed, the very abstractness of the term *value of a statistical life*, belies the impact it has on the decisions of policy makers and subsequently the lives of real, ordinary people.[19] Whenever a government agency in the US or any other country decides whether speed bumps should be installed on certain roads, or how much pollution a power plant can emit into the atmosphere, the value of a statistical life determines the threshold at which the costs of increased safety regulations exceed the benefits of averting deaths.[20] But even if statistical lives are less sympathetic than patients explicitly visible in hospital beds, the threshold still determines whether real people will live or die. For Camila, who would not have lost a year of her life had the road she cycled on had a dedicated bike lane, this number is far from abstract.

To be fair to governments, their decisions on how to set the value of a statistical life are ultimately determined by how much their citizens are willing to pay to protect their own lives. Agencies read and commission research on the spending behaviours of individuals that reveal how they tradeoff between shelling out for increased safety and saving money for other purposes.[18] For example, someone purchasing a car might be informed that their risk of death from driving is 1 in 10,000 per year, but if they bought a vehicle with upgraded safety

* These figures are from 2016 and will increase over time.

features this would be halved. If the maximum this person would be willing to pay for this improvement is $500, this would imply they value their life at $10 million.* Analysis of this sort quickly makes clear that individuals are unwilling to spend their entire budgets on safety and healthcare. Even if they were, with their limited savings they would still have to decide how they rank necessities like surgeries and shelter against the more marginal health improvements of dentistry and bike helmets. People may say that you can't put a price on human lives, but their own spending habits will reveal otherwise.

Unpleasant as it is, there is no way to avoid putting a value on human lives in some way, shape, or form if one is going to make any sort of coherent and consistent set of healthcare or safety policies. It helps to remember that this number does not reflect the inherent moral value of each person's life, but only the practical limit of our willingness to trade off life against other important things. And thankfully, as our economies grow, and our healthcare budgets along with them, so too does our ability to pay for the ever more sophisticated and expensive interventions necessary for saving lives.

In understanding how healthcare expenditure varies with the size of economies, you should know that the World Health Organization has historically recommended countries deem cost-effective any treatments providing an extra year of healthy life for less than between one and three times their GDP per capita. As of 2023, in rich places like the US, the UK, the EU, and Australia, a year of healthy life is valued at anywhere from $40,000–100,000, or $3–10 million per life saved. In contrast, the same threshold in the poorest places in the world is around 1,000 times less.

This is evident when examining possibly the most cost-effective health intervention anywhere in the world that is incompletely funded: the provision of insecticide-treated bednets to people living in sub-Saharan Africa. These bednets reduce the frequency with

* They are willing to purchase a 0.5 in 10,000 risk-reduction (halving their risk of death) for $500. With the assumption that their willingness to pay for risk-reductions in their chance of death is linear, dividing $500 by 0.5 in 10,000 equals $10 million. See the other references in this section for more examples.

which people are bitten by mosquitos, and thus prevent deaths from malaria, particularly among children and pregnant women. GiveWell, an organization dedicated to using money to save lives as effectively as possible, estimates it takes about $5,500-worth of bednets to save one life.[21] If one takes a global perspective on whether any new treatments deserve to be funded over those that could already use more money, this is the threshold to keep in mind.*

But even though our willingness to help those in need is often found wanting if they reside in foreign countries, our commitment to pay for life is clearly on display when we make funding decisions regarding treatments aimed at extending the lives of our fellow citizens who are imminently dying. Upon examination, in this circumstance we are certainly no misers. Globally, 8–11 per cent of annual healthcare expenditure is made on those who end up dying in any given year.[23] In the US, while only 5 per cent of Medicare enrollees die in any particular year, they consume 25 per cent of Medicare's budget.[24] In the UK, about $22,000 per patient is spent on those dying from cancer in the last six months of their lives.

It is not that this money is all being wasted on fruitless attempts to eke out more life for the doomed, so much as it is a commitment to provide care for all those who may benefit from continued treatment. When researchers have tried to make predictive models of patients who would die within twelve months, only 10 per cent of those who actually died had been assigned a probability of death over 50 per cent.[24] What this means is that 90 per cent of those who die in any given year appeared ahead of time to have a reasonable chance of surviving at least a little while longer. All this is to say

* Fortuitously, though, the costs of many effective healthcare interventions fall well below the thresholds of any healthcare budget. Take the treatment costs for diarrheal diseases like cholera and dysentery as examples.[22] Untreated, the mortality rates from these infections can reach 30–50 per cent, due to patients suffering fatal dehydration. A simple oral rehydration solution made of salt, sugar, and some additional electrolytes can bring the death rate down to almost zero. The costs amount to a few cents per patient, well below the cost-effectiveness threshold of essentially everywhere in the world. Cheap and efficacious treatments like these are a boon for society, posing no difficult tradeoffs nor requiring painful sacrifices in order to preserve lives.

that, at least in some circumstances, our expenditures indicate we are willing to pay a lot of money to try and give people as much life as we can.

***

When assessing the economic feasibility of saving everyone from death using brain preservation, these are the figures to take note of. Globally, we spend about 10 per cent of economic activity on healthcare, or approximately $10 trillion in 2022. In wealthy countries, we are willing to pay about $50,000 for a year of healthy living, or $10 million to save an entire life. Even for those in their last few months of life, we will spend tens of thousands of dollars to maybe give them a bit more time. For our poorer fellow humans in developing countries, the threshold is sadly less, but it is at least increasing over time as economic development pulls more and more nations out of poverty. However, even in rich countries, $60 million for a life is a higher cost than we are able to bear, as shown by the case of Jordan's death from meningococcal B. The naive view that we will spend whatever it takes to save lives is clearly not true. Even so, we sure are willing to spend an awful lot.

THE PRICE OF PRESERVATION

The key takeaway from all that background is that the more life a treatment can provide, the more we're willing to pay. Correspondingly, if we're to know whether brain preservation is worth the cost, we need to have some idea of how many years of healthy life it can provide to someone who would otherwise die.

During the initial rollout of any new medical technology, the answer is always going to be highly uncertain. Even well-established medical procedures can retain a considerable degree of unpredictability. For example, heart transplantation has a 10 per cent mortality rate at one year post surgery, and 30 per cent at five.[25] In Australia, the initial surgery costs $190,000, and the total comes to $250,000 when considering the first twelve months of ancillary costs.[26] This is a lot of money to be spending on patients where one in three of them will be dead within five years. Despite the risks, we provide these treatments because their probability of success multiplied by the benefits they provide, also known as their *expected value*, is still worth the cost.

So, how much benefit do we expect brain preservation to provide? Evaluating this consists of answering two sub-questions. Firstly, what is the probability someone will be successfully revived after brain preservation and subsequent storage? Secondly, how long, and with what quality of life, will people live post-revival?

Assuming someone is maintained under adequate storage conditions, I think the potential for a properly preserved person to be eventually restored to consciousness is extremely high. For revival to turn out to be entirely impossible would require neuroscience to discover new ways that the brain stores information which turn out to be impossible to capture with a vitrifixation procedure. There are still many mysteries about the brain, but it still seems unlikely that neuroscientists will uncover entirely novel domains of human neurophysiology at this stage. I am not so confident as to assign the chance of revival as fully 100 per cent, but given a well-preserved brain and sufficiently advanced science I expect the probability to be pretty close.

However, I am by no means certain that successful long-term storage can be guaranteed. This is not because I anticipate there being any problems with the technical aspects of running preservation facilities for indefinite periods of time. That should be a relatively easy engineering challenge, should society have the will to meet it. Rather, my concern is that a global nuclear war, a devastating pandemic, or some other global catastrophic risk will damage civilization to the point that there will be no-one willing or able to perform revivals in the future. As mentioned back in Chapter Two, the expert on apocalyptic scenarios Toby Ord assigns some variant of global catastrophic risk a one-in-six chance of occurring in the next hundred years. Should that come to pass, nothing else we can do to improve preservation quality will matter. Still, even if we accept this pessimistic perspective, the optimistic take is that doomsday is less likely to arrive than not, and, if it doesn't, I think revival is highly plausible.

Assuming a person is successfully revived, the next question is what their post-revival quality of life will be. As ridiculous as it feels to speculate on the living conditions of a century from now, extrapolating past trends forwards suggests that, if we don't destroy ourselves, our prospects look rather good. One hundred years ago, even in a rich city like London, many women could not vote, there were no antibiotics for people suffering from infections, and the air was filled with toxic smog. Worried as we should be about issues like climate change and wealth inequality, a historical perspective suggests that our circumstances are still mostly improving. In fact, there has never been a better time in history for the average person to be alive than today, and current trends indicate that is still likely to be true in most possible futures. I do not know how people will spend their time a century hence, but it will probably be in better health and happiness than our own time.

What about the lifespan of someone revived and freed from the vicissitudes of biological aging? Forever is an awfully long time, but certainly their expected number of years to live would now be essentially indefinite. Rather than condemned by nature to a handful of decades, someone revived could take their life into their own hands for as long or as little time as they desired. Another century? A millennium? Until the heat death of the universe? Who knows how long a person would wish to live for if actually allowed to make choices about their own fate.

If this were a traditional healthcare cost–benefit estimation, we would multiply the chance of revival success by the number of quality-adjusted life years it would provide, and arrive at the expected value of the brain preservation procedure. But if we try that in this circumstance, the estimates we end up with are absurd. Assigning revival any chance of success greater than zero, and then multiplying that by an indefinitely large number of life years, leaves one with an arbitrarily large number. This answer of 'Lots!' to the question of how many quality-adjusted life years preservation could provide might be satisfying to some, but many others will conclude the exercise with a feeling that the result is frustrating and the reasoning untrustworthy. If we finish this calculation with a sense of unease rather than satisfaction, then this method has not really helped at all.

So, instead, let's approach the question from the opposite direction. Given a credible estimate of the costs involved with preservation and long-term storage, would these seem like a reasonable price to pay for a chance of saving someone's life? What comes next is an attempt to try and calculate exactly that.

At the outset, though, I must note the caveat that the numbers which follow are a rough guide rather than a detailed analysis. Formal cost estimates for vitrifixation and storage when deployed at a widespread scale have yet to be performed, and I am a neuroscientist rather than an accountant. Having said that, enough information exists to provide a ballpark estimate of what the costs are likely to be. Let's work through it all and find out.

Cold and calculating

When embarking on a cost calculation for any product, one crucial variable to ascertain is the potential market size. The larger the consumer base, the greater the justification for expensive production methods. For example, constructing a semiconductor foundry to manufacture modern computing chips rings up a bill on the order of $5 billion, beyond the financial reach of essentially any individual. However, because there are a multitude of eager purchasers willing to pay a few hundred dollars per chip, these production costs can be spread out over millions of consumers.

Assuming widespread adoption of preservation as a practice, the demand for the procedure would be similarly large. Globally, 2021 saw approximately 69 million deaths, or about 0.8 per cent of the world's population.*[27] To give some examples broken down by country, that was 13 million people in India, 3 million in the US, 1.6 million in Japan, 650,000 in the UK, and 166,000 in Australia. The only upside of these horrifyingly large numbers is that, be it through private payments or government funding, the costs of providing preservation can be distributed over an enormous number of potential users.

For any commodity with a sufficiently large market, the initial research and development expenses quickly become spread out over

* You might be confused as to how the death rate can only be 0.8 per cent even though mean life expectancy is seventy-three, which would imply a rate of 1.25 per cent. The reason is that the world is disproportionately young. The human population is still growing, which means there are more young than old people, which in turn means the death rate is lower than the world's average life expectancy. If the global human population stabilizes around 2100, as expected, the two numbers will reach equilibrium then.

so many consumers that they become negligible in determining the product's ongoing cost. In our situation, this means we can ignore the substantial outlay it will take to finish optimizing vitrifixation into a routine medical procedure and integrating it into the healthcare system. Instead, the long-term cost of providing preservation is dominated by the labour, consumables, and storage space required for each new person to undergo the procedure. Given that, let's run through last chapter's description of Keiko undergoing vitrifixation once more, this time keeping track of the costs that accumulate along the way. If you want to see these listed in spreadsheet form, along with the corresponding sources, see the website companion to this book.*

* * *

We'll commence shortly after the pronouncement of Keiko's legal death, just as she is being wheeled into the preservation procedure room attached to the hospice. Even before the surgery commences, there are some immediate costs to tally.

First, there is the required rental of the procedure room itself. While it need not be as sophisticated as a hospital operating theatre, a standard medical procedure room still comes in at around $100 per hour. Keiko will need it for approximately eight hours, totalling $800.

The room is of no use without qualified professionals to perform the procedure, so their wages need to be included too. Each procedure will require a specialized preservation technician, talented at performing vitrifixation and troubleshooting when things go wrong. No such job currently exists, but the skill and training level is roughly comparable to a physician's assistant or perfusionist, each of whom cost about $50 an hour. To be maximally efficient, they will likely also need an aide who can be trusted to handle tools, move things around, and otherwise provide general assistance, costing $25 an hour. If we need both these people for the full preservation procedure, that would total $600 in labour.

—

* www.arielzj.com/the-future-loves-you

Warning: the next section is again somewhat graphic. While the technical details are important, skip this part if surgery makes you squeamish.

At the beginning of the procedure, these staff move Keiko to the operating table and commence the surgery to expose her circulatory system. Most of the tools and other durable equipment in the room can be reused again and again for each procedure, so their costs can be largely factored out. Between replacing bone saw blades as they blunt over time, cleaning tools between cases, and changing out the filters for the fluid pumps, depreciation of the equipment may cost around $75 per procedure.

After a cannula is surgically inserted into Keiko's aorta, the washout solution used to clear the blood from her vasculature becomes the first major consumable aside from labour. A human body contains only 5 litres of blood, but it takes a flow-through of ten times as much solution to ensure all of it is removed. The washout solution itself is mostly just cheap saline, but there is some cost in the drugs and anticoagulants mixed in to help slow decay and prevent blockages. For 50 litres of it, at $15 per litre, the total comes to $750.

Once complete, the technicians will start pumping through the fixative. This consists of glutaraldehyde dissolved in saline, plus a tiny bit of detergent to better penetrate the blood–brain barrier. The fixation solution costs about $12 per litre, entirely dominated by the cost of the glutaraldehyde. Its affordability is due to it already being produced in large quantities for other medical and industrial purposes. However, to make absolutely sure every part of Keiko's body is permeated with fixative, 340 litres – around two oil barrels' worth – needs to flow through her blood vessels. With an improved protocol it may be possible to reduce waste by capturing and recirculating some of this fluid. However, using the open flow cycles that have currently been trialled, this will total around $4,000-worth of fixative.

After thirty minutes of pure fixation solution, the perfusion-pump computer starts to gradually ramp up the concentration of cryoprotectant included in the mix. Over the next five hours, more and more of the saline is switched out for the antifreeze chemical ethylene glycol, replacing the water in Keiko's body so that she can later be cooled without damaging ice crystals forming. Ethylene glycol is already produced at an industrial scale, so adding it to the fixation solution only increases its cost by around $10 per litre. As with the fixative alone, though, we still need a lot of cryoprotectant to ensure full saturation of Keiko's body. At around 180 litres, or one oil barrel's worth, this adds another $4000 in expenses.

No more surgical details; it is safe to start reading again from here.

Tallying up the costs at the end of the initial eight-hour procedure, including placing her now chemically-fixed body into a protective container, preserving Keiko has come to about $10,000. Eighty per cent of that is due to the expense of the large volumes of chemical solutions required, with the rest largely from room rental and labour costs. A more sophisticated method of fluid recapture, filtration, and reuse could likely bring this down considerably. Yet, even at its current cost, the procedure is fairly inexpensive as far as surgeries go.

Initial preservation done, there needs to be somewhere safe and cold to leave Keiko's body for however long it takes until she can be revived. There's no need for this to be in the centre of a bustling metropolis, as a long commute is not likely to trouble Keiko for quite some time. At the same time, a city of 5 million people suffers around one hundred deaths per day on average, so putting the storage location far out in the countryside would result in excessive transportation costs. The most economical place is likely to be a very large warehouse just outside a city, close enough for easy access but far out enough for the land to be affordable.* Assuming it takes a van a 50-kilometre round trip to drive Keiko's body to such a facility, then $60

* That said, if we're willing to spend a bit more money, I'd recommend creating a space more similar to a traditional cemetery, enabling people to visit their preserved relatives and providing them with a sense of connection. If we want to express our gratitude towards earlier generations and remind society why we should work towards reviving them, it'd be nice to have a more spiritually and aesthetically satisfying place for them than a drab industrial estate.

for three hours of the driver's time and $20 in refrigerated-van hire would come to about $80 in transportation costs.

Upon arrival at the warehouse, intake of Keiko's body starts with several quality-control steps. A CT scan providing reference images of the state of her body costs about $75. Slightly more expensive are the needle biopsies that sample a tiny amount of tissue across several of Keiko's brain regions. If three biopsies are required to confirm successful preservation of her connectome, capture and analysis of these samples may come to around $300. Once these checks are complete, the induction can conclude, and Keiko's body is ready for long-term storage.

***

Although many of the figures involved when costing a novel medical procedure are highly uncertain, the expenditure required to maintain long-term storage of preserved bodies is the one I am most uncertain about. Storage costs would be lowest if keeping people at room temperature were sufficient to maintain a fixation-preserved body without decay. If that were the case, the rent for the required warehouse space would only cost around $50 per year. However, if it is critical for high-fidelity preservation that bodies be kept at cryogenic temperatures, this will be considerably more expensive. Exactly how much more is unclear, as no organization has – or is currently trying to – develop warehouse-sized freezers that could store material at around −130°C.*

Still, there are some relevant comparators. For reference, the costs of long-term storage of small amounts of human biological material are already well established. Sperm, eggs, and embryos are routinely vitrified and stored submerged in liquid nitrogen at −196°C. This is economically feasible because liquid nitrogen is cheap, costing as little as 50 cents per litre when bought in bulk.

It would be convenient if entire human bodies could be stored in this

* The closest extant facility that I know of is a −80°C, 2,500-square-foot walk-in freezer built by BioFisher for an undisclosed client.[28] I've been assuming that a human-body container requires 2 metres x 1 metre x 1 metre of space and that three can be stacked on top of each other in a warehouse setting. As only thirty-five bodies could be stored in the BioFisher facility, we're going to need something a lot bigger.

way, but naively pursuing this approach is far from ideal. Submersion of large volumes of tissue, like entire bodies, into fluid at 60°C below the temperature at which vitrification occurs will cause fracturing of organs due to uneven thermal contractions. To avoid breaking people's brains, we should instead be aiming to keep preserved patients only a few degrees below their vitrification point.

Despite these problems, the traditional cryonics organization Alcor is currently holding around 200 bodies in their care submerged in liquid nitrogen. Alcor's hope is that the dehydrative and fracturing damage these bodies will have suffered as a result is not so bad as to destroy these people's connectomes. In 2011 they claimed this was costing them $2,200 a year per body. This figure serves as a probable upper bound for storage costs, as any organization operating at a larger scale and storing bodies at warmer temperatures should be experiencing lower costs.[*,29]

A precise estimate of the cost of keeping bodies cool at −130°C would require a detailed engineering analysis considering all the relevant variables, which include the size and capacity of the facility, the degree of feasible insulation of the warehouse walls, the frequency of intake of bodies, the local cost of electricity, and the lifespan and replacement cost of refrigeration compressors, among many other variables. In the absence of this analysis, my best-informed guess, after consulting with colleagues and perusing the relevant comparators, is that keeping bodies cool at −130°C in a warehouse setting would cost $1,000 per body per year if done at a large scale.

These cost estimates are by no means definitive, but they serve as a rough guide to the expenses that would be necessary should society embrace brain preservation as the standard means of treating people otherwise dying. After tacking on an additional 25 per cent for

* Specifically, this is because the smaller the difference between the ambient air temperature outside the storage facility and the temperature at which bodies need to be stored, the less energy it takes to keep the facility refrigerated. This relationship is not linear: as the temperature difference drops, the corresponding cost falls even faster. While Alcor is demonstrating $2,200 a year for −196°C storage, the equivalent space in a cold-storage warehouse used to keep frozen goods at −20°C comes to about $140.

administrative expenses, the total comes to around $13,000 for the initial procedure and $1,300 a year in ongoing storage costs.*

***

To finally return to the original question, then: do these costs seem like a reasonable price to pay for a chance of saving someone's life? We're now ready to compare the price of preservation to healthcare fees that our societies already deem reasonable. If someone like Keiko has to be kept in storage for one hundred years before revival is feasible, the total costs, including the initial procedure and long-term storage, come to around $150,000, or less than the cost of a heart transplantation surgery.†

If we compare this to the pre-existing threshold of $50,000 that rich countries are willing to pay for a quality-adjusted life year, preservation would be good value for money as long as we expect there's a decent chance Keiko will live at least another three years. If the neuroscience and philosophy presented in the previous chapters has convinced you that someone who has undergone brain preservation has any chance of revival at all, it's hard to avoid the conclusion that this procedure is worth the cost.

Preservation is not actually a particularly complicated or expensive procedure compared to many medical and surgical practices already in place. The costs could be substantially greater than my estimates and the expected benefit presented by an indefinite extension to lifespan would still make this a worthwhile project. Developing and deploying the physical infrastructure and human capital required to provide preservation on a universal scale would certainly be a

* This isn't to say that would be the approximate cost of every single procedure. Some patients will have medical complications, such as a haemorrhagic stroke, that will cause the initial procedure to be much more involved and correspondingly more expensive. In contrast, scientific and engineering advances into recapturing fixative and cryoprotective fluids, allowing vitrification at higher temperatures or reducing the electricity costs of refrigeration, could all notably decrease the cost of routine procedures.

† Readers with some economics training might be annoyed that I have avoided applying a discount rate to both the future storage costs and the eventual benefits from revival. My apologies, but doing so properly would both overcomplicate this preliminary analysis and exceed my accounting skills.

substantial addition to healthcare budgets, but it is an expense that wealthy countries could reasonably absorb. The major remaining developments necessary to start saving everyone are not fundamental scientific breakthroughs, or engineering insights that massively reduce costs, but simply for people to realize that this is something that they want for themselves and those they love, and to act accordingly.

COSTS WORTH BEARING

Hundreds of millions of lives have been lost and tens of billions of dollars spent fighting the War on Cancer since it was declared by the US President Richard Nixon in 1971. While humanity has made some progress in the intervening years, the enemy still holds the higher ground. Cancer continues to be the second leading cause of death globally, accounting for one in six deaths worldwide.[30] Metastases remain inescapably fatal foes against which we have extremely limited armour. That is not to say our efforts to fight back have been entirely in vain, as Emily's story demonstrates. Nonetheless, the world spends billions of dollars annually on cancer research with great uncertainty as to what the outcome of this expenditure will be. Most clinical trials of novel therapies fail. We have no overall strategy for curing cancer entirely. Maybe one day a collection of breakthroughs similar to CAR T-therapy will score a definitive victory. In the meantime, society pursues its hugely ambitious and expensive goal of researching how to defeat cancer, because life is worth fighting for.

We believe this even in the face of prospects much bleaker than that posed by cancer. Doctors at least know what traitorous cells make up metastatic cancers, even if they often can't treat them, but scientists have not yet even managed to work out what causes Alzheimer's disease. Spending on Alzheimer's research was at least $1.4 billion globally in 2016 and exceeded $3.4 billion in the US in 2023 alone, yet medicine has very little in therapeutics to show for it.[31,32] Despite occasional media hype about new and exciting discoveries in recent years, every single trial of a therapy to slow Alzheimer's tested so far has yielded clinically insignificant results, let alone found something that could reverse the damage. Be that as it may, we spend enormous sums trying to treat a disease that almost exclusively affects the elderly because, even in what currently passes for old age, we still think human lives are valuable. Despite the absence of any promising treatments on the horizon, and with all the uncertainty and financial sacrifice that research spending entails, we are willing to bear these costs in the hope of increasing the quantity and quality of even our eldest's lives.

We do so in part because a history of previous medical breakthroughs gives us the courage needed to tolerate the unpredictability of medical research and its concomitant costs. In fact, a historical view makes it clear that we are at least ready, if not eager, to accept the expense of developing novel medical technologies and integrating them into the healthcare system. To pick one country as an example, the change in the UK's healthcare spending from under 1 per cent of GDP in 1900 to 10 per cent in 2019 is likely eminently acceptable to British citizens when they consider the host of ways their medical care has improved over the last century.

For an often overlooked yet important example of what this increased spending has bought for Britons, look to radiology. Up until the late nineteenth century, there was no way to examine the interior of a patient's body except through incisions made by a surgeon's scalpel. The era of non-invasive imaging opened in 1895 when Wilhelm Röntgen, who had serendipitously discovered X-rays six weeks earlier, used them to take a photograph of the bones of his wife's hand. By the First World War, the two-time Nobel Prize winner Marie Curie had developed mobile X-ray machines that could be deployed to French field hospitals.[33] Demonstration of a medically useful ultrasound imaging device began in the 1950s, with investigations showing ultrasound could distinguish some cancers from benign growths.[34] Their use was widespread by the 1970s, by which point the digital ultrasound scanner had become a routine tool in medical diagnostics. Developing at the same time was computed tomography, the practice of combining a series of two-dimensional X-ray images to construct a three-dimensional model. The initial CT scans enabled by these hardware and software improvements were performed in the early 1970s, while by 1980 the new devices had already enabled millions of examinations.[35] Lastly, the combined use of strong magnetic fields and radio waves to produce clear images of soft biological tissues enabled the first MRI of a human in 1977.[36] Clinical scanners started to be installed in hospitals from the 1980s. The culmination of this century of improvements in imaging techniques was achieved in 1992, when functional MRI first visualized the real-time changes of blood flow in the brain that correspond to the very act of thinking itself.

These astonishing improvements to the physician's toolkit have come with a correspondingly stupefying price tag. An MRI machine, which requires coils of superconducting magnets cooled with liquid helium to −269°C, can easily cost over $1 million to purchase and install. Subsequently using the machine, perhaps to check whether a patient has a torn a ligament in their knee, could not happen without an entire ecosystem of expensive and specialized professionals, including the engineers who first developed and installed the device, the technicians who performed the scan, the radiologists who interpret the images, and all the secondary suppliers who provide the liquid helium and perform the necessary maintenance. The enormous capital required and ongoing expenses mean that a single diagnostic scan typically costs at least several hundred dollars.

Yet all this time, money, and effort is worth it because it enables people to live longer and healthier lives than they otherwise would. That is what people have always wanted, and that is what people will continue to want more of. As long as people still die from heart disease, cancer, and dementia, and while they still suffer due to chronic illnesses like depression and arthritis, there will never be a point where people think the healthcare system is sufficiently mature and there is no further need to develop new medical treatments. As shown by anaesthesiology in the nineteenth century, and radiology in the twentieth, our societies have continued to add more healthcare whenever they have been able to afford it. Whatever we end up calling the nascent field of brain preservation, I am hopeful this expansion will continue into the twenty-first.*

* 'Preservology'? 'Preservistry'? 'Preserviatry'? If we wanted to keep a Greek etymology, perhaps '*diatir*ology'? I'm open to suggestions.

Intergenerational credit

A glaring omission from this chapter is that, while I have shown the costs of the initial procedure and subsequent storage to be relatively affordable, I have provided no details on the resources it would take to eventually revive someone. For this I can only apologize: by whatever means revival one day becomes possible – be it through emulation, nanotechnology, or any other method – its cost to a society capable of performing such feats is beyond my capacity to estimate. An aviation engineer from the 1920s might have been able to guess at the principles governing the interplanetary rockets that would exist fifty years later, but they would have been hard pressed to give any indication of their price.

That said, my intuition is that, as with all new inventions, revivals are likely to start off incredibly expensive and then come down in price as the technology matures. The first microwave oven, introduced in 1954, cost $2,500 at the time, or $28,000 in 2023 dollars.[37] A contemporary microwave is better, safer, and can be obtained for under $100.* And, as a side note, no matter how long it takes for the costs of revival to fall in a similar manner, the great strength of preservation is that no patients need die waiting for revival to become affordable.

Even so, there is still a financial problem with revivals: those who would benefit from the procedure have no way to pay for its cost. When we place the dying of our time into storage, with a desperate request to future generations to please revive them, we owe a debt to any descendants who may choose to heed the call. As such, the question arises: how can we possibly pay them back?

We cannot contract with revival companies that do not yet exist. Even if we could, any material goods we may try to sequester for future payments would likely be of trivial value to a society with the resources capable of reviving a person. Moreover, regardless of if we somehow had something of value to offer in exchange, there is no way we could hold them to their end of the bargain when the time comes. Hoping that future generations will perform revivals out of a

* For a more biomedically relevant example, it cost at least $100 million to produce the first human genome sequence, while today it can be done for under $1,000.

pure generosity of spirit is thus an uncomfortably precarious position to be in.

Yet, just as it is precarious to place our lives in the hands of our descendants, their own existence is contingent on the choices that we make today. It is not at all guaranteed that we will be responsible enough to ensure future generations are given the same opportunity to live that all you reading these words have had. In our anger, madness, and inability to compromise, we may destroy the world in nuclear fire. Through carelessness and greed, we run the risk of letting loose artificial intelligences whose destructive powers we cannot control. If we continue to show the same contempt for our environment that has historically caused a string of ecological disasters, including climate change, ozone layer depletion, deforestation, and the shrinking of the Aral Sea, there may be no Earth upon which our grandchildren can live. Herein lies the method for paying the first instalment of our debt to our descendants: pushing the probability of global catastrophic risks as close to zero as we can, and thus ensuring that there is even a world for them to live in.

Even so, securing their existence alone is a rather miserly price to pay to our descendants for the bother of reviving their ancestors. If we are asking them to bring us back to life, we should first be giving them a world prosperous enough to justify the request.

Beyond the basics of safety and security, we must strive to improve our systems of governance to allow the benefits of social and technological progress to accumulate to all across every generation. Through democratic reforms, legal codes, and institution building, we have already made progress in removing power from the jewelled fists of chiefs and kings and placing it into the hands of common people. Yet there is still work to be done in eliminating corruption, aligning the incentives of policy makers with those whose decisions they affect, and ensuring power is used to serve people rather than people serving those with power.

Aside from developing brain preservation, we must continue fighting to eliminate diseases. Whenever the burden of a chronic illness can be ameliorated by a new medicine, it makes the lives of all current and future sufferers that much more worth living. Every time a child's life is saved from a disease that would have historically been a death sentence, we gain an adult grateful for the efforts of their elders. It is hard to look upon the drug that stands between oneself and death – to know the hundreds of careers, thousands of experiments, and billions of dollars that went into developing it – and not feel attachment to the creators who made one's own life possible.

And from our vantage point, standing at the cusp of a new age of economic productivity enabled by artificial intelligence, we must endeavour to use that wealth, and all the other technology we have built, to usher in an era of leisure, freedom, and plenty. Not only should we be continuing to grow our industries and improve our productivity, but our aim should also be to ensure the fruits of these achievements are distributed equitably so that all may thrive rather than merely survive.

Our own lives today are as dependent on the choices of our ancestors as those of our descendants will be upon our current decisions. We owe our forebears a great debt for their efforts to nurture us, to work to provide for us, and to solve the challenges of their time so that our own existence need not be as harsh as theirs was. Their struggles to improve the lives of their children and build the civilization that we have today were done without any expectation of repayment, but instead out of a desire to leave the world better than they found it. It has been said since at least Roman times that 'A society grows great when the old plant trees in whose shade they shall never sit.' As the beneficiaries of hundreds of thousands of years of culture, and over 5,000 years of civilization, the forest in which we live is ancient.

If we're going to ask our descendants for more than our ancestors have asked of us, for a chance to sit once more beneath the sun, then we should be working hard to leave them even greater gifts than our own forebears provided us. After all, the only enforcement mechanisms for ensuring intergenerational credit is repaid are gratitude and love. If we build a world of peace and prosperity for our children, where people are empowered to pursue their agendas at their leisure, then the only limits to their projects will be their own imaginations.

Think of a loved child, safe and happy in their home, bringing a freshly drawn picture to their grandparents to see them beam with pride. Should we succeed in providing our descendants with a similarly nurturing world, perhaps some of them will want to bring us back, if only to show us the wonders they can make.

Conclusion

One evening in April 1902, a journalist approached the physicist Lord Kelvin with a question: would it ever be possible for an aircraft to soar over the vast Atlantic Ocean? The dawn of the twentieth century had been marked by unprecedented technological advancements, and who better to ask about the possibility of humanity one day taking to the skies than the pre-eminent scientist of the age. After all, Lord Kelvin had helped uncover the fundamental rules of the universe described by the first and second laws of thermodynamics, identified the absolute coldest temperature theoretically conceivable, and aided in designing and deploying the submarine cables that now enabled instantaneous communication between London and New York. If anyone was equipped to gaze into the future, surely it would be this visionary who had sculpted so much of its foundation.

Kelvin considered the question seriously and carefully, as he did all important matters. Balloons had floated aloft for over a century, but their trajectories were determined by the whims of the wind. Otto Lilienthal had demonstrated the possibility of unpowered heavier-than-air flight a few years prior, yet the would-be pilot had plummeted to his death after losing control of his glider. Kelvin pondered all the problems that would have to be solved for human flight to ever become practical: developing a robust yet lightweight engine, stabilizing an aircraft despite constantly changing atmospheric conditions, crafting wings that could generate sufficient lift without being fragile or unwieldy . . . the list was endless. As he deliberated, he recalled the ancient Greek myth of Icarus, and its timeless message of the dangers that befall those whose hubris leads them to fly too close to the sun. No human had ever made a controlled, powered flight in all the aeons of human history, and, despite the recent progress that science and technology had made, it seemed likely that no-one ever would.

'No; I think it cannot be done. No [. . .] aeroplane will ever be practically successful.'[1]

—

A year and a half later, the Wright Brothers made the first powered human flight above the sand dunes of North Carolina. Fifteen years after that, Lord Kelvin was proven definitively wrong when the first transatlantic flight took off from Newfoundland, Canada, and touched down in Galway, Ireland. Most remarkable of all, if there had been any children present that evening to hear Kelvin's sceptical words, they might well have lived long enough to see Neil Armstrong first set foot upon the Moon.

***

As humanity's history makes patently clear, we are an ever-changing, ambitious, and often arrogant species. Almost a century ago, when my grandparents joined the other 2 billion humans on the Earth at the time, horses were still more common than cars, and a computer was a person who was fast at arithmetic. Fifty years ago, when my mother entered university, the world population had doubled to 4 billion, humans had landed on the Moon six times, and a computer was an extravagantly expensive device that could store a few kilobytes of memory. As I am writing these words in 2023, humanity has again doubled its numbers to 8 billion people, and there are serious discussions as to whether our machines have already achieved some degree of human-level intelligence. Ours is an exponential age. Only through the narrowest view of history could one see the current time as normal.

One thing that has always been consistent across history, though, is fear of new ideas and changing circumstances. When books first began to proliferate following the spread of the printing press in the fifteenth century, many worried they would 'make the following centuries fall into a state as barbarous as that of the centuries that followed the fall of the Roman Empire'.[2] As childhood education became widespread in the late nineteenth century, one doctor worried that schools would 'exhaust the children's brains and nervous systems with complex and multiple studies'.[3] In 1908, as women clamoured to become equal participants in democracies, a leader of the Women's Anti-Suffrage League wrote that allowing women to vote would be 'the prelude to a social revolution which must set back progress' and would 'cut into the peace and well-being of families'.[4] The changes posed by technological innovation have always felt scary, and worrying that social disruption will lead to society's unravelling is a similarly timeless tradition.

Even so, for as long as humans have been tinkering, there have been those who saw the potential benefits of new technology as alluring enough to overcome their fears of change. Over a million years ago, some brave person, undeterred by burning heat and choking smoke, first learned to tame fire. Their reward for turning this elemental, forest-destroying force into a human tool was the ability to make the inedible into the palatable, and keep the cold at bay. At another moment in the distant past, some courageous soul gazed out over the vast alien ocean and, instead of running back to the comfort of the forest, took the forest with them into the unknown by hollowing out a log to make a boat. Even more remarkable is that these discoveries have happened again and again, at different times and in different places, as the ingenuity of the human spirit meets the challenges of material reality.

In the more recent past, we begin to have records of those courageous enough to risk the stabilizing doctrines of tradition and dogma in pursuit of truth and the discomforting power it provides. In the sixteenth and seventeenth centuries, the observations and theorizing of Copernicus and Galileo demoted our planet from the centre of the universe to a small, remote rock in the endless void. Yet, in exchange for our world's diminishment, we ironically gained new powers, granting humans everything from improved nautical navigation in the eighteenth century through to the pinpoint accuracy of global positioning systems today. Similarly, in the nineteenth century, Darwin proved that we humans are not a standalone species but instead just another kind of ape, subject to the same evolutionary pressures as all our fellow animals. Painful as this loss of status was for humanity, from its acceptance comes much of modern biomedical insight and understanding. Again and again over time, we have lost our naivety by straying beyond our comfort zones and seeing the world for what it truly is. In turn, each daunting step into the unknown has been commensurately rewarded with increased mastery over the once-totalizing forces of nature and concomitant improvements in our standards of living.

To assume things must be as they have always been is to be blind to how much has changed for humanity over the millennia. Approximately 120 billion *Homo sapiens* – modern humans – have already lived and died before our time. A sizeable fraction of those people lived as hunter-gatherers, with foraging instead of fridges, huddling instead of heating, and walking instead of wheels. But in the 7,500 generations since modern humans first evolved, many made incremental progress at leaving their children a better world than the one they entered into.

That is not to say each generation has always had it easier than the one before it. Human history has not been like an elevator, ascending blissfully towards a technological paradise with each level better than the last. Indeed, there have been setbacks along the path to developing even the most fundamental aspects of modern life. The change from foraging to agriculture increased the availability of food, but rendered premodern farmers susceptible to crop failures, malnutrition, and famines. Houses give much better protection from the weather than simpler dwellings, but, until chimneys became common in the sixteenth century, and plumbing in the nineteenth, most were smoky, smelly places that could kill their inhabitants through pollution and disease. Readily available food and dry shelter are such basic conveniences of modernity that it is easy to forget that their development often involved initially dangerous steps. We reap the benefits of sacrifices made by our ancestors, who risked change and suffered stumbling blocks to craft a world where their descendants could live longer, healthier, happier lives than they did.

Despite this, there is still much work to be done. The proposal to abolish the inevitability of death is only one effort among many to liberate individuals from the shackles of seemingly immutable circumstance, and help them find the agency to live life on their own terms. Consider how the quality of a person's life is often evaluated in terms of the freedoms they are afforded. Freedom to pursue their own dreams rather than be chained to the desires of others; freedom to practise their faith or beliefs without restriction or persecution; freedom to express who they are without fear of retribution. Freedom from death is just one further ideal that should be registered within the public consciousness.

That is not to deny that it is a scary and disquieting proposition. Taking it seriously requires us to gaze steadfastly upon our own mortality, a deeply unpleasant task. It forces us to make active decisions, where before there was no option but to acquiesce to fate. It demands the acknowledgement that our bodies are made of decaying flesh, in turn composed of base and breaking physical components. And it necessitates re-examining the traditions and rituals in which our approach to death is normally ensconced, leading us to potentially set aside the psychologically protective barriers our ancestors developed to shield us. But, as disturbing as it is to challenge death, the alternative is worse.

Seen clearly and put simply, my argument is straightforward: involuntary death is bad. It is bad because it disempowers people. It is bad because almost all people want to live longer than they are able. It is bad because it prevents people from pursuing all of their dreams and ambitions, witnessing the growth and achievements of their loved ones, and experiencing the beauty and wonder of the world. It is bad because death is the ultimate thief, robbing people of their futures and stealing away their family and friends. It is bad because it ends our journeys, thwarts our plans, extinguishes our joys, and deprives us of our abilities to make a difference to the world. For every reason that life is good, and for every joy and laugh and love that it deprives from the world, death is bad.

WHAT YOU CAN DO

If I have convinced you that abolishing death is a worthy cause, or if you were already on board from the get-go, at this stage you may be wondering what you can do to help. The first thing I would ask of you – after thanking you for having been open-minded enough to stick with me this far – is to reflect on the strong will to live remaining in many terminally ill patients, and remember the surveys showing that people want more years than they are typically able to enjoy. I ask this because, if we are going to act on our desires to extend the quantity and quality of our lives, I would appreciate your help in removing the taboos on talking about death and dying, and enabling frank discussions about exactly what we want and how it can be achieved. Public discussion of our shared wish to extend life, and awareness of the technological means by which this may be done, are crucial for establishing public mandates for pursuing such goals. So, then, here is the primary thing that anyone can do to help achieve the goal of saving everyone: just talk about these aspirations with your friends, or family, or colleagues, or neighbours, or acquaintances at a party, or strangers on the internet, or anyone at all.

***

But if you happen to be a neuroscientist, philosopher, or any other related researcher, your opinion on death abolition is particularly important for your community to hear. Even if you use your voice to speak up against mine, it is important that we hear it at all. Now is the time to establish an academic consensus on the current and near-term feasibility of extending lives through brain preservation, and collectively determine whether the proposal has sufficient merit to pursue.

If you would like to contribute more than just your voice, there is also plenty of direct work that still needs to be done. Even if health-care systems everywhere commenced universal rollout of vitrifixation immediately, our work would not be complete. Although we currently have enough knowledge to hit the ground running, there are still unknowns obscuring the ultimate finishing line of a fully optimized medical procedure. Exactly how long, for example, is the window between when an individual suffers loss of blood flow to the brain and when sufficient damage has occurred to constitute their information-theoretic death? Are there better or cheaper brain preservation protocols that could be developed than vitrifixation?

Even if those challenges are overcome, there are further obstacles on the path to bringing people back into the world, rather than just saving them from death: can we give greater precision to the constraints and methods by which revival may eventually be possible? As a proof of principle, how long until we can demonstrate whole-brain emulation of a small animal? None of these important questions have yet been systematically investigated.

***

If you are a healthcare worker, there is similarly much you will be able to do to help directly, in addition to vocalizing your support. Best-practice guidelines for performing vitrifixation in different medical settings need to be developed and tested. From technical procedural details through to patient consent forms, we need to establish specific schemes for how brain preservation can be integrated into end-of-life care. To give some examples of the necessary details that are currently absent: how might a particular patient's medical history affect administration of the procedure, such as how stroke victims may require a more invasive protocol for ensuring complete brain fixation? Are there any interactions between patient medications and some of the necessary vitrifixation chemicals? What should the framework be to regulate which staff perform the procedures? How will they be trained? Should these professionals form their own medical speciality, or be incorporated into a pre-existing one? Widespread rollout and implementation of the procedure would also no doubt uncover issues of concern as of yet unknown. The sooner these problems can be identified through the collaborative efforts of all relevant medical professionals, the more efficiently we can refine this new technique for saving lives.

***

Should you be a policy maker, you already know that rendering brain preservation universally accessible will be virtually impossible without your efforts. We need only look to progress on combating climate change for a clear example of the inertia of scientific knowledge until it is incorporated into public policy. Scientists first suggested that carbon dioxide emissions could cause global warming as early as the end of the nineteenth century. Beyond theoretical concerns, the earliest evidence the phenomenon was actually occurring was reported in the 1950s. An initial meeting of concerned experts was convened in 1963, and the first US government investigations of the issue started in the 1970s and 1980s. However, it wasn't until the Intergovernmental Panel on Climate Change was established in 1988, and particularly the pledges and policies made by governments as part of the Kyoto Protocol in 1997 and Paris Agreement in 2015, that large-scale and effective efforts to mitigate climate change have actually started happening. The concerns of scientists are entirely impotent unless shared by those who wield power, and the suggestions of researchers completely irrelevant unless developed and implemented by policy makers. To avoid another fifty-year-plus lag between identifying the problem and implementing a solution, brain preservation could use quick action from leaders experienced at motivating and mustering all relevant stakeholders and strategists.

Apart from planning the procedure's logistical implementation, politicians and policy makers can also help by allocating the budgetary resources required to save everyone. Assuming my costing model of $13,000 per procedure and $1,300 in storage costs per person per year is remotely plausible, the financial commitment required to provide universal access already falls comfortably within the bounds of economic and political viability for affluent nations. As an example, the required ongoing yearly budget in the UK would be under $10 billion, representing an additional 4 per cent of the current healthcare budget of around $300 billion. For reference, Britons already collectively spend more than that on the National Lottery every year.[5] Compared to playing the lottery, brain preservation has better odds, higher stakes, and a much grander payoff. Efforts by politicians and policy makers to procure the necessary funds sooner rather than later would be among the most impactful actions anyone could take to aid this cause.

***

If you are a philanthropist, entrepreneur, or investor, now is a unique time when your agile approach can particularly complement public-sector efforts. Governments often act only long after shifts in public opinion have become clearly apparent, while academic institutions are typically constrained by funding bodies and entrenched in their current programmes. There is therefore plenty of scope for private investment in the research and implementation of brain preservation, particularly during the pilot and transitional phases preceding widespread usage. Individuals creating companies to develop and improve the protocols and procedures stand not only to benefit from helping ensure their own survival, but also to profit from already having products in place as mass-market demand develops. The few extremely small organizations already working in this space could certainly be joined by many more. Even if and when governments start to enter the field and purchase preservations for their own citizens en masse, there will still be scope for philanthropists to subsidize the procedure in developing countries with fewer resources. Because brain preservation is limited by funding constraints, rather than still-needed scientific breakthroughs, a huge amount of progress can be made by simply investing in solutions to the problem.

***

Yet, once more, I should note that no matter what profession you have or what influence you wield, you can still aid in saving everyone. For all of us, the primary and most important way to help is simply to think seriously about what we want the future of the world to look like, and to talk openly about how we can make those aspirations happen.

THE FUTURE LOVES YOU

This book has argued that brain preservation provides a viable method of abolishing death's enduring cruelty. But even if the procedure were to become universally accessible, the overall project is still far from guaranteed, as eventual revival relies on a future which is by no means certain.

It would be comforting to assume a safe and steady march of progress will ensure a bright tomorrow for all, but casting our eyes back on the past reveals that our ancestors' attempts to improve their lot sometimes had devastatingly counterproductive effects. The European quest for a faster route to India, while a testament to rapidly improving seafaring technologies, caused the deaths of tens of millions of Indigenous Americans.[6] This duality was seen again when the Scientific and Industrial Revolutions, which should have heralded unadulterated progress, paradoxically became enablers of the brutalities of slavery and colonization. Even in the last century, we have observed how the utopian ideals of Russian revolutionaries set their nation on a path to gulags, corruption, and eventual disintegration. While overall we live longer and healthier lives than our ancestors, that is cold comfort to those who suffered from the mistakes made and the crimes committed along the way. The arc of the moral universe might eventually bend towards justice, but from the perspective of those living in the middle, it's more a jagged, chaotic smear whose upward trend is apparent only from a distance.

Even worse, as our capabilities have increased, so too has the risk that we accidentally destroy the world in our attempts to improve it. While humanity has some precedent for slowly learning from its mistakes, there is no second chance from a failure that kills you. In powering our way out of poverty since the Industrial Revolution, we risk cooking the Earth on which we live. Through our quest to understand the fundamental forces of nature, we enabled the possibility of nuclear annihilation. By building artificial intelligences to take over the burden of our labours, we hazard summoning forces we do not understand and whose goals we cannot control. And as the powers of our governments and corporations grow, so does their ability to drift into self-interested authoritarianism if not held carefully in check. Unlike the tools of yesteryear, failing to handle these new technologies correctly risks not only our own generation's lives, but could destroy the entirety of our children's inheritance.

Yet, as dangerous as the flame of innovation can be, it is crucial to remember that it is kindled out of a hope for a brighter future. While it's more than fair to question whether social progress is really the inevitable outcome of technological advances, there is no doubt that breakthroughs have been a prerequisite for many of our modern achievements. In turn, rejecting further technological developments means resigning those with currently incurable ailments to their fates, and forsaking countless others to the clutches of perpetual poverty. Even if these were sacrifices we were willing to make to ensure our perpetuity, the lesson of the dinosaurs' meteoric demise is that eschewing technology's gifts offers no guarantees of long-term safety. We must press on, but, by treading carefully and remembering the mistakes of the past, we can aim to sidestep the potential pitfalls on the path towards a brighter tomorrow.

For while humanity's strides beyond the natural order are as risky as they are ambitious, we have much to look forward to if we make it across the precipice. Tragic as the missteps of history have been, the only time better to be alive than now is likely sometime in the future. Ninety per cent of all people alive in 1820 lived in extreme poverty; this was under 10 per cent as of 2020.[7] A typical worker in a Western country laboured for fifty-eight hours per week in 1870; this was down to thirty-one hours in 2017.[8] In inflation-adjusted 2011 dollars, global GDP per capita was around $1,100 in 1820; in 2018 it was up to $15,000.[9] Assuming developmental trajectories like these ones hold, economic and technological progress is on track to produce sufficient surplus to release people everywhere from resource constraints and place them entirely at liberty to pursue their own goals and dreams.

Should this hardly imaginable future actually arrive, what might people choose to do? In a world freed from mandatory employment, no doubt there will be those who choose to continue working to eliminate whatever injustices still remain on Earth, be they pockets of poverty, burdens of disease, or vestiges of corruption. Others may seize the opportunity provided by this newfound freedom, combining leisure with advancing technology to create new worlds of games, art, and culture. Some would likely just want to relax, spend time with those they love, and enjoy the fruits of civilizational success.

And a dedicated few might find themselves new, voluntary challenges to replace the existential ones of old. With all the time and resources of a world of peace and prosperity, there would still be plenty left to do. Determining the limits of free will. Uncovering a unified theory of physics. Watching a sunset on Mars. Be it any individual, or humanity as a whole, there is little risk of boredom no matter how much time we get. Should we secure our future, what we know of the human spirit tells us that we will not be going gently into that good night, but all engines blazing towards the stars.*

* Some examples of excellent science fiction that bucks the dystopian trend and provides a positive vision of what the future of humanity could be like are the *Culture* series by Iain M. Banks and the *Terra Ignota* tetralogy by Ada Palmer.

It is certainly the case that some of those who worked so hard in earlier times to give us today's world wished that they could have seen the fruits their efforts would bear. In 1773, the American polymath and founding father Benjamin Franklin wrote

> I wish it were possible [...] to invent a method of embalming [...] persons, in such a manner that they might be recalled to life at any period, however distant; [I have] an ardent desire to see and observe the state of America a hundred years hence [...] to be recalled to life by the solar warmth of my dear country![10]

I am sure that many Americans would agree that his struggles to develop democracy, advance science, and promote social goods have more than earned him some extra time under the sun, if only it were possible to provide.

In exactly the same way, if we of the present can succeed in delivering a bright and prosperous future to our children, I cannot help but think there would be some among our descendants who would consider it a noble goal and an exciting challenge to bring back those ancestors who made their own lives possible. If future generations come to believe we did a good job of building them a better world, they may well feel it is only right that we should be allowed to share it with them.

Appendices

APPENDIX 1. PERSONAL IDENTITY PROBLEMS

Psyching oneself out

A common attack levelled at the psychological view of personal identity is that it doesn't seem to deal well with failures in the transitivity of mental properties across a person's lifespan. To clarify what that actually means, let's again consider the case of Shruthi from Chapter Four, at different stages of her life. Suppose that, as a young girl, Shruthi enjoyed a magical summer's day at the beach. Later on, in middle age, Shruthi is working hard as a farmer harvesting rice. While daydreaming on her lunch break, she fondly recalls the one sunny beach day she experienced in her youth. Finally, in her old age, Shruthi remembers her long days in the fields, but can no longer recall that distant summer's day of hermit crabs and sandcastles. Overall, the beach memory connects the young to the middle-aged Shruthi, while the farming memory links the elderly to the middle-aged, but the young and elderly Shruthi are at least partially disconnected. How could young and elderly Shruthi be the same person if their memories are not consistent?*

One possible response is to claim that the persistence of personal identity relies not upon perfect accumulation and maintenance of memory across the lifespan, but instead merely on a chain of overlapping memories and personality that provides a kind of psychological

* This is a modified version of Thomas Reid's criticisms of a Lockean theory of personal identity, which he published in 1785. People have been arguing about these ideas for a long time.

continuity.[1] Even though the elderly Shruthi is missing some of her younger self's memories, a continuous chain of intermediate Shruthis ensures the two remain connected.

This response might appear to do the trick, but there are theoretically circumstances where it produces counterintuitive results. Remember the hypothetical procedure mentioned in Chapter Three, where a person's neurons are randomly reconnected to each other in a way that erases their original memories and personality, resulting in a person with a new set of psychological characteristics? This time, imagine a scenario where, instead of that happening to someone suddenly, it progresses gradually over an extended period of time. In this case, while the person at the end is completely psychologically different from the person at the start, there is still a continuous chain of similar states to bridge the intermediate steps.

This imaginary case might seem irrelevant in practice, but there are real and tragic medical conditions to which it bears a partial resemblance. In frontotemporal dementia, patients can undergo gradual but profound changes in their personality. For example, one case history records a man who progressively changed from a devoted, sensitive, and supportive husband into a sarcastic, dishevelled, and selfish individual, to the extent that his wife stated 'it is as if a different person has crawled into [his] skin'.[2] Accordingly, it would be better to develop our working theory of personal identity with an argument that does not rely on psychological continuity alone.

APPENDIX 2. MORE ON CONSCIOUSNESS
Once more, with feeling

In Chapter Five, we examined global workspace theory as an explanation of consciousness. While the theory sits well with current neuroscientific experiments, deeper philosophical issues become apparent when trying to generalize the theory to creatures different from ourselves.* What would our response be if we came across an intelligent

* There are also more technical issues with the theory as it applies to humans, but a route to resolving these is easier to see. Examples include: how many brain areas must

animal whose brain structure seemed to preclude ignition and broadcast within a global workspace? For example, if the neuroanatomy of an octopus did not allow for information to be shared in ways that would constitute a workspace, should we conclude that the animal is not conscious or that global workspace theory is wrong?* Similarly, newer artificial intelligences are capable of increasingly sophisticated behaviours, but their software and hardware does not typically resemble a system capable of containing a global workspace.[4] If a future artificial intelligence becomes capable of performing all recognized consciousness-associated behaviours, even while lacking a global workspace, would we still feel confident in denying its claims of consciousness? Or what if the opposite occurred – were we to find a workspace within a system that seemed otherwise unintelligent and alien, would that be grounds enough to deem it conscious?

This questioning of the necessity and sufficiency of a global workspace reveals a problem not just with this particular theory, but with functionalism more broadly. Theorists can choose to be more or less inclusive about which functions they believe are required for consciousness, but both options will attract criticism. If a proposal is restrictive, such as choosing to ascribe consciousness only to creatures that possess at least every function of a healthy adult human, its critics will label it as needlessly anthropocentric and discriminatory. If instead a theory is inclusionary, allowing any number of functions and behavioural traits to count as evidence of a creature's consciousness, then it risks assigning subjectivity to creatures on insufficiently strong grounds.[5] Unfortunately for functionalism, at least at the moment, there seems no obvious way to draw a principled threshold.

But there is perhaps an even larger issue for functionalism still. A dissatisfying deficiency of all functionalist theories, global workspace included, is that they do little to explain the fundamental question of why our experiences feel the particular way they do. Sure, seeing a

---

be disconnected for the global workspace to cease to function? Does loss of consciousness through partial workspace disconnection happen in a graded fashion, or is it lost all-or-nothing?

* There have been suggestions octopuses do in fact have a global workspace. See Mather's *Cephalopod Consciousness* for more details.[3]

strawberry might induce ignition of strawberry-conveying information into a global workspace, but why should this be accompanied by an experience of 'redness'? Why doesn't this same information feel like 'blueness', or 'coldness', or 'hunger'? Functionalism does not have an easy answer to whether my 'red' is your 'green', or why any qualia should accompany functions at all.[6] In failing to provide an explanation here, functionalism seems to sidestep, rather than solve, the hard problem of why subjective experiences should accompany brain functions.

Some philosophers argue this characterization is not entirely fair, and that facts about the nature of our experiences can support an answer to the hard problem within a functionalist framework. Take, for example, the observation that an experience of 'red' is never found in isolation, but is always seemingly attached to some object in the world: a red strawberry, a red ball, red lips, and so on. In this sense, qualia appear to *represent* features of our external environments, in that our sensations bear some trace resemblance to properties of the real world. These representations are also useful once compartmentalized into classes and subclasses, as the features our experiences represent are generally structural regularities in the world that can be exploited to our advantage. Red fruits are likely to be ripe, while green fruits are possibly inedible. Shiny things are likely to be metals, which also means they might conduct electricity. Given that our experiences are understood only in relation to a conceptual dictionary of possible meanings, and those meanings were gleaned originally from representations of the physical world – either as sensations of the world beyond our bodies or as feelings of the goings-on inside ourselves – then perhaps an explanation of why 'red' feels the way it does can ultimately be grounded in the ways a subjective experience corresponds to the objective state of the world. To the best of my knowledge, this *representationalist* idea is yet to be fully fleshed out in a way that can systematically explain why the cognitive functions we have are necessarily accompanied by the kinds of experiences we enjoy, but perhaps this will one day be achieved.[7–9]

Other philosophers instead embrace the accusation that functionalism cannot answer the hard problem of why physical processes could ever be accompanied by the seemingly immaterial companions of colours, pains, and other subjective experiences. In place of believing there is a mystery of why it feels like anything to be us waiting to be solved, *illusionism* is a variant of functionalism that claims we are instead mistaken in thinking there is anything to consciousness beyond our cognitive functions.

Take the issue of whether what you see as 'red' might be what your friend sees as 'green', known formally as the problem of *qualia inversion.** Assume for the moment that your friend truly does have inverted qualia compared to you – where you see red, they see green. Further, let's assume that this happens without changing any of their reactions to the stimuli that they observe, so that you and your friend both still report a strawberry and a cherry as looking similar, and a banana and a blueberry as looking different, even though you have completely different colour experiences when looking at these objects.† Assume further that all the links between colour experiences and other aspects of the mind like emotions and evaluative judgements are inverted too, such that not only does a flame elicit a green-blue experience in your friend but that this colour also feels warm and comforting to them. In this case, even though your friend's colour experience is different from your own, it could never alter their behaviour, nor make a functional impact on the world in any other way.

Illusionism takes this causal irrelevance of qualia as strong evidence against their existence. While a dualist theory of consciousness can accept entities without causal effects on the world, illusionists argue this should sit very uneasily with the widespread physicalist leanings of most modern consciousness researchers. If our intuition is that qualia exist, but that seems incompatible with physics, then illusionists would have us discard the intuition rather than search vainly for an explanation. They would also point to historical precedent for support. Just as nineteenth-century biologists once thought that biochemistry required a 'vital spark' to enable life before they were

* Also known as the problem of *inverted spectrum*. The problem gets worse the more you think about it, too – see the related issues of *dancing qualia*, *fading qualia*, and *qualia compression*.

† If we don't make this assumption, then the experiences can readily be detected as different from a third-person perspective through structural analysis.[10]

disillusioned, illusionists believe that qualia are an unnecessary supposition that will be proved non-existent in time.

Through this line of argument, illusionists insist that a great deal of what we believe we know about our own experiences, such as our certainty that there is something that it is like to experience the colour red, is in fact wrong when viewed as anything more than our functional ability to categorize the visual similarity of apples and raspberries. They instead argue that the only real mystery to be solved is why we have such muddled beliefs about consciousness in the first place. Though this position of denying our first-person experiences has seen its proponents labelled as 'crazy, in a distinctively philosophical way', it has found prominent defenders in the philosophers Keith Frankish and Daniel Dennett, and is intimately related to a neuroscientific theory developed by the scientist Michael Graziano.[11–15] Even David Chalmers, the inventor of the hard problem, has said 'if I were to be a materialist, I would be an illusionist'.[16] Perhaps, if its supporters can clarify exactly how and why the rest of us are so confused, illusionism will succeed in showing there is no mystery of consciousness at all.

Measuring integrated information theory

In this section, I'll go into a little more detail on the experimental methods alluded to in Chapter Five that are relevant to integrated information theory. To test integrated information theory's applicability to consciousness, it would be ideal to take recordings of activity from across multiple brain regions in humans, then use these recordings to calculate the integrated information present. There's a notable practical problem with this approach, though: integrated information is too computationally challenging to measure directly from these detailed brain recordings. To compensate for this, researchers in the study from 2013 – who wanted to measure integrated information in humans who were awake, asleep, and anaesthetized – designed a proxy measure that arguably correlates with integrated information. Their approach was to analyse the complexity of collected brain recordings, rather than integrated information directly.

Complexity has a specific meaning in this context, which is how difficult it is to compress the information present in the participants' EEG recordings. Each recording was obtained by sticking sixty electrodes to the head of a participant and measuring how the voltages at these sites changed over time. If, at a certain time point, the voltage measured at every electrode was the same, instead of recording the value for each electrode individually, one could just write down '5 microvolts everywhere'. Such a recording would be highly compressible into a short description, and hence not very complex. Conversely, if the voltage at one electrode was not very informative about the value of any other electrode, one would have to write all the electrodes' values down individually, making the recording incompressible and thus complex.

There's another interesting part to this experiment, also. Rather than just passively recording, the researchers actively perturbed the participants' brains to generate an activity signature that they could assess for compressibility. Near the start of each participant's EEG recording, they would send a harmless magnetic pulse into a certain location on the surface of their brain. In a healthy, awake patient, this pulse was expected to reverberate to other locations in the brain at complicated intervals, making a highly complex and incompressible pattern detectable by all sixty electrodes. However, if a patient's brain had low integration at the time, as was expected during anaesthesia, the pulse was not expected to travel far, with the corresponding brain recordings showing low complexity.

Integrated information theory: Strengths and weaknesses

In this section, I'll go into more detail on the theoretical evidence for and against integrated information theory that I mentioned briefly in Chapter Five.

Integrated information theorists mainly claim support for their position from experiments demonstrating how integrated information is different for individuals experiencing different levels of consciousness, but there is much more to consciousness than just being awake versus asleep. At any given moment of waking life, we are drenched by a torrent of subjective experiences, specific to our activity, psychology, and environment. These qualia can be sorted into categories like visual, auditory, emotional, proprioceptive, or interoceptive, to name but a few, and, if we consider Tononi's proposition, individual qualia in combination also create new, indivisibly unified experiences. Each of these qualia comprises a particular 'feeling', but how does this come about? As a physicalist theory of consciousness, integrated information theory needs to explain why any particular integrated information feels like 'redness' instead of 'the taste of chocolate ice-cream'. We've already seen how functionalist approaches like global workspace theory struggle with this issue. Can integrated information theory do any better?

Potentially, yes.[17] To explain how, look around wherever you are right now and pay attention to different objects in different locations, their sizes and boundaries, and the distances between them. This is the feeling of three-dimensional space mediated through vision, an often overlooked but ever-present aspect of our subjective experiences. One way of formalizing what it is like to have spatial experiences is to note that the canvas of our visual world appears to be composed of countless spots that can be grouped together in various ways to form edges and regions. Overall, this forms an extended grid-like arrangement, with each distinguishable point in our visual experience corresponding to a location in the grid. Conveniently for integrated information theory, neurons in the visual cortex are known to be connected together in a grid-like fashion. Not only that, but the integrated information that these neurons are expected to create should also have 'grid-like' properties.

To explain what this means, we need to move beyond the previous example of integrated information corresponding to an aspect of consciousness that can vary only along one dimension, such as how someone's level of alertness can range from 'none' (dreamless sleep), to 'some' (drowsy), to 'full' (awake). Instead of integrated information just coming in greater or smaller amounts – and perhaps being related to whether someone is more or less awake – the integrated information present in physical systems can also be analysed structurally. Think of how the left- and right-hand versions of gloves are made of the same amount of material, but, placed in different arrangements, that material produces two distinct gloves that are not interchangeable with one another. Similarly, two physical systems can have the same amount of integrated information, and be made of the same kind of units, but still have their integrated information exist in a different kind of abstract arrangement. By this, I mean that the integrated information present within any particular system, when visualized in a particular mathematical fashion, can form different patterns termed *complexes*.

The argument made by integrated information theorists is that each unique abstract complex of integrated information is identifiable with a particular subjective experience. The similarities and differences between these complexes correspondingly accounts for the similarities and differences between qualia themselves. By this reasoning, realizing that visuospatial experiences consist of an extended arrangement of lines and spaces created by an interconnected series of points, while also noting the existence of an equivalent abstract complex of integrated information arising from the physical structure of the visual cortex, provides grounds to identify the subjective spatial experience and the abstract complex as fundamentally the same. This logic suggests that TN's loss of spatial experience is due to the destruction of the physical structures underlying these abstract complexes, while his blindsight is enabled by other brain circuitry that lacks the appropriately structured integrated information required to consciously experience visual information.

Integrated information theorists have not yet described the complexes that should underlie non-spatial qualia, but propose that the same idea will hold for all experiences. An integrated information complex that corresponds to an experience of redness will be very similar to one that corresponds to pinkness, quite different from one of greenness, and extremely different from one corresponding to itchiness. Just as earlier scientists eventually found the DNA sequences that pass traits on from parent to child, these modern neuroscientists suggest we will eventually find abstract integrated information complexes in the brain that correspond to every qualia that we can possess.

Still, while integrated information theory claims to have solved the hard problem of how consciousness relates to the physical through this structural analysis approach, I am aware that your ability to judge its merits would require a much more detailed explanation. Its absence here is partially because integrated information theory is still somewhat light on the required details, and partly because the discussion gets especially technical from here on out. So as to avoid making this material even more confusing than it needs to be, I will leave the mathematical and philosophical minutiae to those readers interested in following up the provided references.

But if you feel you cannot make an informed evaluation of the theory with only the minimal information I have provided, here's a cheat sheet of the critiques of integrated information theory provided by experts with a detailed understanding of its ideas. Some criticize it on the grounds that its mathematical framework is insufficiently specified.[18,19] Others believe its axiomatic formulation is ill defined.[20] The most common concern is that there are many things that have integrated information even though it is questionable that they are indeed conscious, as discussed in the main text.

And, at the higher level of characterizing the structure of consciousness, there are still those who take issue with a qualia-structure approach to identifying the physical basis of subjective experiences. The general programme is grounded in the assumption that introspection can reliably reveal the nature of experiences, which is not without its detractors. Citing evidence of numerous examples where humans struggle to assess their own psychology, from failures of insight into the causes of their behaviour to overestimation of their own task performance, illusionists call into question the validity of relying on introspection. At the same time, functionalists worry about how using first-person reports of introspection alone to characterize consciousness could lead one to dismiss any requirement for a necessary relationship between consciousness and functions.[21,22] They fear this could entail the opposite of blindsight: a situation where someone claims to have a subjective experience, say of intense bliss or pain, while saying it does not affect their behaviour in any way that would allow for third-person verification. If someone claims to see a new primary colour that is neither red, green, yellow, nor blue, but indescribably different from all normal colours, should we believe them or accuse them of lying?

APPENDIX 3. MORE ON MEMORY

Pattern separation and pattern completion

Back in Chapter Six, we explored how the hippocampus is able to make memories by indexing the brain activity that was present in your cortex during particular episodes from your life. But, after learning about the indexing function of the hippocampus, two further important questions immediately present themselves.* First, how does hippocampal indexing operate without engrams becoming muddled together, so as to keep memories distinct from each other? Second, how do we actually use the index to retrieve episodic memories and bring them back into awareness? While neuroscience is still unable to give a completely comprehensive description of the necessary processes, we know enough to give a preliminary account.

Memories would be of little use if they could not be separated out from one another. Episodic memories are defined by distinct details and contexts, such as where you parked your car today rather than yesterday, that your sister was delighted when you bought her concert tickets for her birthday, or that the bakery with delicious croissants near your office was shuttered when you walked by on a Monday. Without these particularities you would lose your car, disappoint your sister with rock music she does not care for, or find yourself ravenous outside of a closed bakery.

So as to keep our memories separable, a process named *pattern separation* keeps engrams in the hippocampal index distinct from one another.[23,24] It relies on the special properties of neurons located in a subregion of the hippocampus called the *dentate gyrus* (Fig. 16).† The most important feature of these neurons is that even if they receive two separate inputs from the cortex that are very similar to each other, they still output very different activity patterns. To make this more concrete, imagine three scenarios: you are at the market buying

* I mean, actually a lot more than two, but we'll stick to these or the book will quickly turn into a neuroscience textbook.

† *Dentate* ('tooth') + *gyrus* ('ridge'). When viewing a cross-section of this portion of the hippocampus, it kind of looks like it has tooth-like projections.

apples, you are at the market buying bananas, and you are cycling in the countryside. Your subjective experience of buying apples at the market is similar to that of buying bananas, while both are quite different from going cycling. Correspondingly, the activity patterns in your cortex will have far greater overlap in the 'buying apples' and 'buying bananas' scenarios compared to a situation where you went cycling. However, the dentate gyrus will produce very different outputs regardless, the key requirement for pattern separation.*

These seemingly-random outputs from the dentate gyrus are received by another part of the hippocampus, known as the *CA3*.† What makes the CA3 different from other areas is the way its input and output connections are wired up. While CA3 neurons receive some connections from the dentate gyrus, as well as some directly from the cortex, the vast majority of their inputs and outputs are from and onto the CA3 itself. As a result, CA3 neurons are very highly connected to each other, allowing them to perform a function called *pattern completion*.

To explain how pattern completion occurs in the CA3, it's once again helpful to consider what happens before, during, and after formation of an episodic memory. To set the scene, imagine you are sitting at home with a hot drink on a cold day, scrolling on your phone, when you suddenly find out you've won the lottery. In a flash, the Earl Grey tea you were drinking, the rainy weather outside your window, and the sequence of numbers you chose for that week's lottery ticket, are all burned into your memory.

Prior to the formation of this momentous memory, each of the roughly 2 million neurons in your CA3 were already connected by synapses to thousands of their neighbours.[25] As this particular memory formed, the dentate gyrus randomly selected a small subset of CA3 neurons to activate, out of your full population of CA3 neurons. Some of these CA3 neurons had pre-existing connections to other CA3 neurons that were simultaneously activated by the dentate gyrus.

* This is somewhat analogous to the use of a hash function in computer memory systems.

† CA stands for *Cornu Ammonis*, literally meaning 'Amun's horns'. It's named after an Egyptian god sometimes depicted as having the head of a ram, as a cross-section of the hippocampus looks somewhat like a ram's horn. The different sections are labelled CA1–CA4.

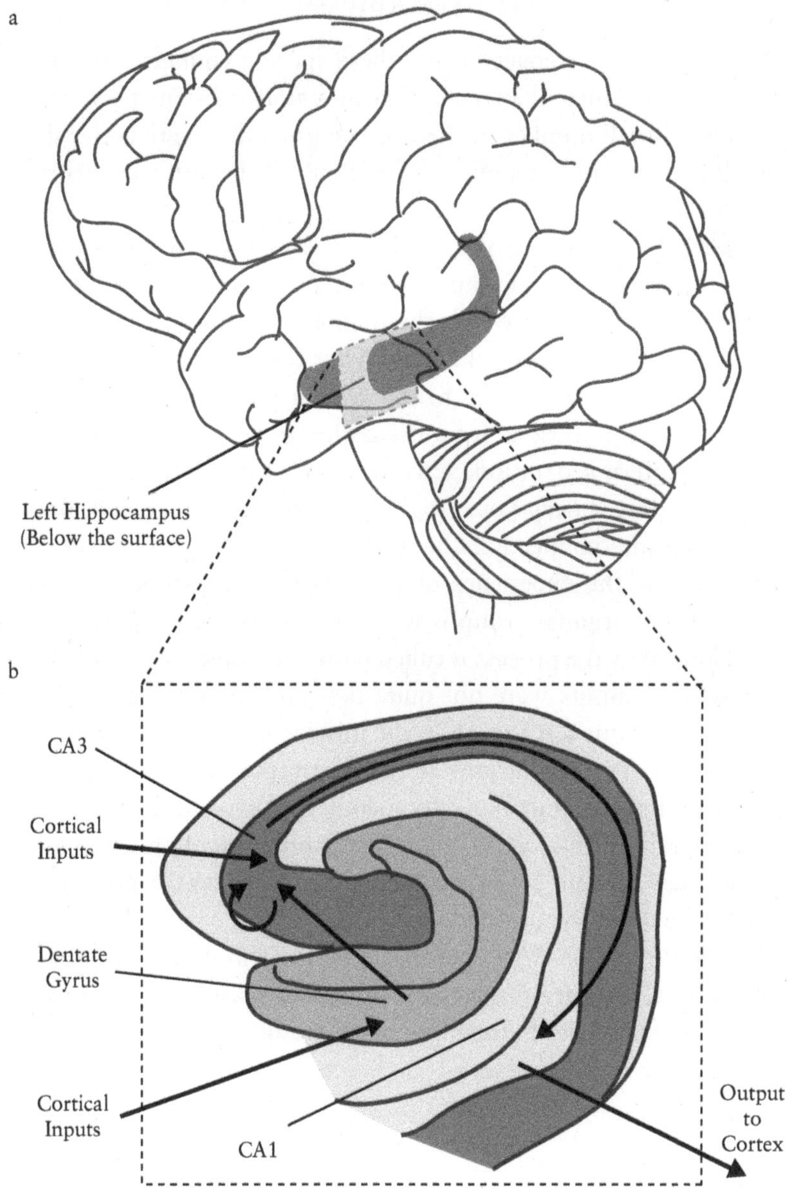

Figure 16. a) The hippocampus is a sea-horse shaped brain region located deep inside the brain, under the bulk of the cortex. b) A cross-section through the hippocampus. Most inputs to the hippocampus from the cortex enter into the dentate gyrus. The dentate gyrus transmits this information to the CA3 after performing pattern separation on the cortical inputs. While the CA3 also receives some inputs directly from the cortex, most of the connections in the CA3 are from CA3 neurons back onto other CA3 neurons. The CA3 uses these recurrent connections to perform pattern completion. Outputs from the CA3 are directed to the CA1, and ultimately back out into the cortex.

As a result of their coactivation, these specific connections are now strengthened. This enhancement ensures that subsequent activity in even just a small number of the CA3 neurons that were active during your lottery-winning memory formation will be sufficient to reactivate the entire set.

A week later, imagine you walk past a café when you smell Earl Grey tea, or see a phone number with some of the same digits that comprised your sequence of lucky numbers. Because this new experience shares some features of the old, your current cortical activity will also bear some resemblance to that which you had previously. As a result, direct connections from the cortex to the CA3, which do not undergo pattern separation, activate some of the same CA3 neurons that were firing during your original experience a week ago. Because the mutual interconnections between these CA3 neurons were reinforced during the experience of your lottery win, stimulating just a subset of this original group is now enough to trigger activity in the rest. This is why the process is called pattern completion – even though your sensory inputs were not quite the same as previously, they are sufficient for your CA3 to fill in the missing details. With the full original set of CA3 neurons now active, the output they send back out to the cortex returns your brain to a similar activity state as during the initial engram formation. In doing so, the presence of only a small part of the original event sends the memory of your recent good fortune flooding back into your mind.

It is these sets of CA3 neurons, with their mutually strengthened connections, that are thought by some neuroscientists to constitute the individual entries in the hippocampal index.*

* This presentation of hippocampal-indexing theory is admittedly a simplification. In particular, it leaves out the role of the CA1, the final, crucial part of the 'tripartite circuit' of the hippocampus. Still, I believe my description captures the essence of current theories of the hippocampus's contribution to memory formation. If you want to read an account with a higher level of detail, including some of the complications and controversies, see some of the recent reviews in the references.[26]

Acknowledgements

As per this book's dedication, first and foremost thanks must go to all those from previous generations who nurtured, worked, and innovated in earlier times so that we may live now. While it seems almost too obvious to write, it still bears remembering: were it not for the care and support of our parents (biological and spiritual) who raised us, and their parents who raised them, and their parents before them, all the way back to whenever love first evolved, none of us would exist and I would never have written this book.

Still, I must express my particular appreciation for all the scientists and scholars throughout history whose prior efforts formed the foundation that this book was built upon. Every researcher whose shoulders I stood upon, cited or not, played a part in the creation of this text.

Specific thanks are due to those who offered their guidance and expertise directly. Anders Sandberg, who provided some initial advice and pointers when I was just starting out on this writing journey. Jennifer Ross-Nazzal, who provided insights into whether NASA scientists of the 1970s really were forward-thinking when it came to saving samples for future analysis. Kevin Berryman, who clarified a query on Buddhist philosophy. Nick Bostrom, who first put me in touch with my eventual editor at Penguin. Everyone at Our World in Data, whose work provided me with an excellent and accessible database with which to easily check almost any important fact about the world and how it has changed over history. And, of course, the many who helped me in ways that I have now forgotten – please do not let my failure to record your aid in any way diminish your contribution.

In addition, I have the utmost gratitude for all of my friends, family, and colleagues who reviewed individual chapters or full drafts at any point in the book's various stages of development. Whether you were providing an expert review, or simply helping improve the text's comprehensibility, your efforts helped make the book immeasurably better than it would otherwise have been. Alexander Cochrane-Davis, Andrew Steele, Anton Jermakoff, Augustus Hebblewhite, Daisuke Shimaoka, Dylan Holmes, Florence Kant, Ivan Balbuzanov, James Cochrane-Davis, Jan Kabátek, Michael Lovell, Naotsugu Tsuchiya, Niamh Peren, Niccolo Negro, Roger Kant, Tuna Nguyen, Ville Lidberg, and Youlin Koh, your help was much appreciated.

My greatest thanks must go to the brain-preservation community, who developed much of the work that I have discussed. Andrew McKenzie, Anna LaVergne, Aurelia Song, Emil Kendziorra, John Smart, Keith Wiley, Kenneth Hayworth, Michael Cerullo, Oge Nnadi, and Randal Koene, thank you for taking the time to share your perspectives with me and to provide expert technical feedback on many and varied matters. For the record, if anyone should be credited for contributing most to the development of this new field, and thus given the privilege of choosing its name, that person is Ken.

This book would not exist without the support of Keith Mansfield, my editor, who shepherded me admirably at each step along the way. Thank you, Keith, for being uniquely sympathetic to what I was trying to achieve. My sincere thanks also to all those who helped turn my ill-formatted manuscript into an actual book, including: Alba Ziegler-Bailey, Jacob Blandy, Imogen Scott, Anna Tuck and Louisa Watson.

Even before I had professional support, I had some early and remarkably proficient editing help from my brother. David, thank you for always pushing me to be a more considerate, articulate, and empathetic writer (and brother). When I envision a glorious future full of art and wonder, it is your creations I most wish to see.

Lastly, and most importantly: my dearest Joyce, thank you for helping me with years of brainstorming, proofreading, editing, fact-checking, medical consulting, and all the other innumerable things you did to help me write this book. You have been my greatest supporter in every way. If I am lucky, this book will help me repay you, should it aid me in upholding my vow to protect all those that you hold dear. But, no matter whether I succeed or not, there is still one thing you should know: even though it is the future's love that may yet save us all from death, the love I truly cherish most is yours.

References

INTRODUCTION

1. Roser, M., Ritchie, H. & Dadonaite, B. Child and infant mortality. *Our World in Data* (2013).
2. Cox, C. Elizabeth Evans Hughes – surviving starvation therapy for diabetes. *The Lancet* 377, 1232–1233 (2011).
3. DiMeo, Nate. Elizabeth. *The Memory Palace* (2017).
4. Life Expectancy. *Our World in Data* https://ourworldindata.org/grapher/life-expectancy.
5. Obenchain, T. G. *Genius Belabored: Childbed Fever and the Tragic Life of Ignaz Semmelweis*. (University of Alabama Press, 2016).

1. WHY DON'T WE GET MORE TIME?

1. Jonathan the tortoise | Saint Helena Island Info: All about St Helena, in the South Atlantic Ocean. *Saint Helena Island Info* http://sainthelena-island.info/jonathan.htm.
2. 'Clive of India's' tortoise dies. *BBC News* (2006).
3. Bowhead Whale | NOAA Fisheries. *NOAA* https://www.fisheries.noaa.gov/species/bowhead-whale (2021).
4. Valcu, M., Dale, J., Griesser, M., Nakagawa, S. & Kempenaers, B. Global gradients of avian longevity support the classic evolutionary theory of ageing. *Ecography* 37, 930–938 (2014).
5. Austad, S. N. Retarded senescence in an insular population of Virginia opossums (*Didelphis virginiana*). *J. Zool.* **229**, 695–708 (1993).
6. Stearns, S. C., Ackermann, M., Doebeli, M. & Kaiser, M. Experimental evolution of aging, growth, and reproduction in fruitflies. *Proc. Natl. Acad. Sci.* **97**, 3309–3313 (2000).

7. Psalms 90:10. *King James Bible Online* https://www.kingjamesbible-online.org/Psalms-90-10/.
8. Cave, C. & Oxenham, M. Identification of the archaeological 'invisible elderly': An approach illustrated with an Anglo-Saxon example. *Int. J. Osteoarchaeol.* **26**, 163–175 (2016).
9. Gurven, M. & Kaplan, H. Longevity among hunter-gatherers: A cross-cultural examination. *Popul. Dev. Rev.* 33, 321–365 (2007).
10. Hill, K. *et al.* Mortality rates among wild chimpanzees. *J. Hum. Evol.* 40, 437–450 (2001).
11. Hill, K. & Hurtado, A. M. *Ache Life History: The Ecology and Demography of a Foraging People.* (Routledge, 2017).
12. Australian Bureau of Statistics. Stat Data Explorer (BETA)· Deaths, Year of registration, Age at death, Age-specific death rates, Sex, States, Territories, and Australia.
13. Finch, C. E. & Austad, S. N. Primate aging in the mammalian scheme: The puzzle of extreme variation in brain aging. *Age.* 34, 1075–1091 (2012).
14. Finch, C. E. Evolution of the human lifespan and diseases of aging: Roles of infection, inflammation, and nutrition. *Proc. Natl. Acad. Sci.* 107, 1718–1724 (2010).
15. Canudas-Romo, V. Three measures of longevity: Time trends and record values. *Demography* 47, 299–312 (2010).
16. Byars, S. G. & Voskarides, K. Antagonistic pleiotropy in human disease. *J. Mol. Evol.* 88, 12–25 (2020).
17. Wang, G. D., Lai, D. J., Burau, K. D. & Du, X. L. Potential gains in life expectancy from reducing heart disease, cancer, Alzheimer's disease, kidney disease or HIV/AIDS as major causes of death in the USA. *Public Health* 127, 348–356 (2013).
18. Coles, L. S. & Young, R. D. Supercentenarians and transthyretin amyloidosis: The next frontier of human life extension. *Prev. Med.* 54, S9–S11 (2012).
19. Pearce, D. Utopian surgery? The case against anaesthesia in surgery, dentistry, and childbirth. https://www.hedweb.com/anaesthesia/index.html.
20. Farr, A. D. Early opposition to obstetric anaesthesia. *Anaesthesia* 35, 896–907 (1980).
21. Simpson, J. Y. *Anaesthesia, Or the Employment of Chloroform and Ether in Surgery, Midwifery, Etc.* (Lindsay & Blakiston, 1849).
22. Williams, B. The Makropulos case: Reflections on the tedium of immortality. in *Problems of the Self: Philosophical Papers 1956–1972* (Cambridge University Press, 1973). doi:10.1017/CBO9780511621253.

23. Seligman, M. E. & Maier, S. F. Failure to escape traumatic shock. *J. Exp. Psychol.* **74**, 1–9 (1967).
24. Weissman, J. S. *et al.* End-of-life care intensity for physicians, lawyers, and the general population. *JAMA* **315**, 303–305 (2016).
25. NIH Professional Judgment Budget for Alzheimer's Desease and Related Dementias for Fiscal Year 2023. *National Institutes of Health* https://www.nia.nih.gov/sites/default/files/2021-07/bypass_budget_executive_summary_508.pdf.
26. Fiscal Year 2021 Budget. *National Institute on Aging* http://www.nia.nih.gov/about/budget/fiscal-year-2021-budget.
27. Fiscal Year 2021 Budget. *National Institutes of Health.* https://officeofbudget.od.nih.gov/pdfs/FY21/cy/FY%202021%20NIH%20Operating%20Plan_Web.pdf.
28. Steele, A. *Ageless: The New Science of Getting Older without Getting Old.* (Anchor, 2021).

2. WHY SAVE EVERYONE?

1. Bostrom, N. & Ord, T. The reversal test: Eliminating status quo bias in applied ethics. *Ethics* **116**, 656–679 (2006).
2. Bowen, C. E. *et al.* Living too long or dying too soon? Exploring how long young adult university students in four countries want to live. *J. Adult Dev.* **27**, 157–169 (2020).
3. Pew Research Center. *Living to 120 and Beyond: Americans' Views on Aging, Medical Advances and Radical Life Extension.* 69 https://policycommons.net/artifacts/621356/living-to-120-and-beyond/1602586/ (2013).
4. Ambrosi-Randić, N., Nekić, M. & Tucak Junaković, I. Felt age, desired, and expected lifetime in the context of health, well-being, and successful aging. *Int. J. Aging Hum. Dev.* **87**, 33–51 (2018).
5. Yokokawa, Y. *et al.* How long would you like to live? A 25-year prospective observation of the association between desired longevity and mortality. *J. Epidemiol.* JE20210493 (2022) doi:10.2188/jea.JE20210493.
6. Donner, Y. *et al.* Great desire for extended life and health amongst the American public. *Front. Genet.* **6** (2016).
7. Ord, T. *The Precipice: Existential Risk and the Future of Humanity.* (Hachette Books, 2020).
8. World GDP over the last two millennia. *Our World in Data* https://ourworldindata.org/grapher/world-gdp-over-the-last-two-millennia.

9. Gautam, R., Mawn, B. E. & Beehler, S. Bhutanese older adult refugees recently resettled in the United States: A better life with little sorrows. *J. Transcult. Nurs.* **29**, 165–171 (2018).
10. Tran, T. L. N. *et al.* The diversity of social connectedness experiences among older migrants in Australia. *Int. J. Intercult. Relat.* **89**, 208–222 (2022).
11. Haslam, C. *et al.* Ageing well in a foreign land: Group memberships protect older immigrants' wellbeing through enabling social support and integration. *Ageing Soc.* **42**, 1710–1732 (2022).
12. Malthus, T. An Essay on the Principle of Population. 134 (1798).
13. Raftery, A. E. & Ševčíková, H. Probabilistic population forecasting: Short to very long-term. *Int. J. Forecast.* (2021) doi:10.1016/j.ijforecast.2021.09.001.
14. Fertility rate: children per woman. *Our World in Data* https://ourworldindata.org/grapher/children-per-woman-UN.
15. Lima, M. *et al.* Ecology of the collapse of Rapa Nui society. *Proc. R. Soc. B Biol. Sci.* **287**, 20200662 (2020).
16. Lipo, C. P., DiNapoli, R. J. & Hunt, T. L. Claims and evidence in the population history of Rapa Nui (Easter Island). In *The Prehistory of Rapa Nui (Easter Island)* (eds. Rull, V. & Stevenson, C.) Vol. 22, 565–585 (Springer International Publishing, 2022).
17. Evenson, R. E. & Gollin, D. Assessing the impact of the Green Revolution, 1960 to 2000. *Science* 300, 758–762 (2003).
18. Stevenson, J. R., Villoria, N., Byerlee, D., Kelley, T. & Maredia, M. Green Revolution research saved an estimated 18 to 27 million hectares from being brought into agricultural production. *Proc. Natl. Acad. Sci.* 110, 8363–8368 (2013).
19. Wang, K. Yuan Longping (1930–2021). *Nat. Plants* **7**, 858–859 (2021).
20. Global Food Explorer. *Our World in Data* https://ourworldindata.org/explorers/global-food.
21. Pörtner, H. *et al. IPCC, 2022: Summary for Policymakers.* (2022).
22. Per capita CO_2 emissions. *Our World in Data* https://ourworldindata.org/grapher/co-emissions-per-capita.
23. Tyson, A., Kennedy, B. & Funk, C. *Gen Z, Millennials Stand Out for Climate Change Activism, Social Media Engagement with Issue.* 100 https://www.pewresearch.org/science/2021/05/26/gen-z-millennials-stand-out-for-climate-change-activism-social-media-engagement-with-issue/ (2021).
24. IPCC. FAQ 3: How will climate change affect the lives of today's children tomorrow, if no immediate action is taken? https://www.ipcc.ch/report/ar6/wg2/about/frequently-asked-questions/keyfaq3/.

25. Cost of space launches to low Earth orbit. *Our World in Data* https://ourworldindata.org/grapher/cost-space-launches-low-earth-orbit.
26. Elon Musk [@elonmusk]. @PPathole @Erdayastronaut @rweb11742 Yeah, looks like marginal cost of launch will be less than $1M for more than 100 tons to orbit, so it's mostly about fixed costs divided by launches per year. *Twitter* https://twitter.com/elonmusk/status/1328770804222468097 (2020).
27. Virginia Uber driver was Somali war criminal. *BBC News* (2019).
28. Can a huge solar flare break everything, what if dictators didn't age, & more from Oxford's Dr Anders Sandberg. (2018).
29. Costa, P. T. Personality across the life span. *Annu. Rev. Psychol.* 30 (2019) doi:https://doi.org/10.1146/annurev-psych-010418-103244.
30. Levin, S. G., Stephan, P. E. & Walker, M. B. Planck's principle revisited: A note. *Soc. Stud. Sci.* **25**, 275–283 (1995).
31. Azoulay, P., Fons-Rosen, C. & Zivin, J. S. G. Does science advance one funeral at a time? *Am. Econ. Rev.* **109**, 2889–2920 (2019).
32. Jones, B. F., Reedy, E. J. & Weinberg, B. A. Age and scientific genius. in *The Wiley Handbook of Genius* (ed. Simonton, D. K.) 422–450 (John Wiley & Sons, Ltd, 2014). doi:10.1002/9781118367377.ch20.
33. Salthouse, T. Consequences of age-related cognitive declines. *Annu. Rev. Psychol.* **63**, 201–226 (2012).
34. Salthouse, T. A. When does age-related cognitive decline begin? *Neurobiol. Aging* 30, 507–514 (2009).
35. Silver, N. Change doesn't usually come this fast. *FiveThirtyEight* https://fivethirtyeight.com/features/change-doesnt-usually-come-this-fast/ (2015).
36. Daley, J. & Woods, D. *The Wealth of Generations.* https://melbourne-institute.unimelb.edu.au/assets/documents/hilda-bibliography/other-publications/2014/Daley-etal_820-wealth-of-generations.pdf (2014).
37. Williford, M. Bentham on the rights of women. *J. Hist. Ideas* **36**, 167 (1975).
38. Schwabach, A. Thomas Jefferson, slavery, and slaves. *Thomas Jefferson Law Rev.* 33, 1–60 (2010).
39. Army – Regiments In India. *UK Parliament* https://hansard.parliament.uk//Commons/1866-04-17/debates/d4ba0459-2d9f-468f-b589-7321ecc1dfb3/Army—RegimentsInIndia (1866).
40. Plato. *Apology*. (Project Gutenberg, 1999).
41. Aurelius, M. *Meditations*. (167AD).

42. Kass, L. R. L'Chaim and its limits: Why not immortality. *First Things* 11 (2001).
43. Sallnow, L. *et al.* Report of the Lancet Commission on the Value of Death: Bringing death back into life. *The Lancet* **399**, 837–884 (2022).
44. Lucretius Carus, T. *On the Nature of Things.*
45. Minerva, F. *The Ethics of Cryonics: Is It Immoral to Be Immortal?* (Springer, 2018).
46. Bowen, C. E. & Skirbekk, V. Old age expectations are related to how long people want to live. *Ageing Soc.* **37**, 1898–1923 (2017).
47. Gawande, A. What should medicine do when it can't save you? *The New Yorker* (2010).
48. Chochinov, H. M., Tataryn, D., Clinch, J. J. & Dudgeon, D. Will to live in the terminally ill. *The Lancet* **354**, 816–819 (1999).
49. Tataryn, D. & Max Chochinov, H. Predicting the trajectory of will to live in terminally ill patients. *Psychosomatics* **43**, 370–377 (2002).
50. Shrira, A., Carmel, S., Tovel, H. & Raveis, V. H. Reciprocal relationships between the will-to-live and successful aging. *Aging Ment. Health* **23**, 1350–1357 (2019).
51. Linden, I. P. *The Case against Death.* (Massachusetts Institute of Technology Press, 2022).
52. Diener, E. & Diener, C. Most people are happy. *Psychol. Sci.* **7**, 181–185 (1996).
53. Morrison, M., Tay, L. & Diener, E. Subjective well-being and national satisfaction: Findings from a worldwide survey. *Psychol. Sci.* **22**, 166–171 (2011).
54. OECD. 8. Subjective well-being. In *How's Life? 2015: Measuring Well-being* (OECD, 2015). doi:10.1787/how_life-2015-en.
55. MacAskill, W. *What We Owe the Future.* (Basic Books, 2022).
56. Carmel, S., Shrira, A. & Shmotkin, D. The will to live and death-related decline in life satisfaction. *Psychol. Aging* **28**, 1115–1123 (2013).
57. Gerstorf, D. *et al.* Late-life decline in well-being across adulthood in Germany, the United Kingdom, and the United States: Something is seriously wrong at the end of life. *Psychol. Aging* **25**, 477–485 (2010).
58. Diegelmann, M., Schilling, O. K. & Wahl, H.-W. Feeling blue at the end of life: Trajectories of depressive symptoms from a distance-to-death perspective. *Psychol. Aging* 31, 672–686 (2016).
59. Bourget, D. & Chalmers, D. Philosophers on Philosophy: The 2020 PhilPapers Survey. 46 (2021).
60. Nussbaum, M. Chapter 1: Therapeutic arguments. In *The Therapy of Desire: Theory and Practice in Hellenistic Ethics* (Princeton University Press, 2013). doi:10.2307/j.ctt2tt8tt.

61. Cancer data in Australia, Cancer incidence by age visualisation. *Australian Institute of Health and Welfare* https://www.aihw.gov.au/reports/cancer/cancer-data-in-australia/contents/cancer-incidence-by-age-visualisation (2022).
62. Prince, M. *et al.* The global prevalence of dementia: A systematic review and metaanalysis. *Alzheimers Dement.* 9, 63 (2013).

3. WHAT IS DEATH?

1. Miraculous recovery for 13-year-old declared brain dead. *ABC News* (2018).
2. Alabama 'miracle' boy wakes before doctors pull plug. *BBC News* (2018).
3. Australian and New Zealand Intensive Care Society. The ANZICS Statement on Death and Organ Donation. (2013).
4. Canadian Blood Services. International Guidelines for the Determination of Death – Phase I. https://professionaleducation.blood.ca/sites/default/files/Determination-of-Death_Lit-Review_20121.pdf (2012).
5. National Conference of Commissioners on Uniform State Laws. UNIFORM DETERMINATION OF DEATH ACT. In 5 (1980).
6. Nair-Collins, M., Northrup, J. & Olcese, J. Hypothalamic–pituitary function in brain death: A review. *J. Intensive Care Med.* 31, 41–50 (2016).
7. Wijdicks, E. F. M. & Pfeifer, E. A. Neuropathology of brain death in the modern transplant era. *Neurology* 70, 1234–1237 (2008).
8. Delimiting death. *Nature* 461, 570–570 (2009).
9. Gardiner, D., Shemie, S., Manara, A. & Opdam, H. International perspective on the diagnosis of death. *Br. J. Anaesth.* 108, i14–i28 (2012).
10. Veatch, R. M. & Ross, L. F. *Defining Death: The Case for Choice.* (Georgetown University Press, 2016).
11. Pana, R., Hornby, L., Shemie, S. D., Dhanani, S. & Teitelbaum, J. Time to loss of brain function and activity during circulatory arrest. *J. Crit. Care* 34, 77–83 (2016).
12. Fleidervish, I. A., Gebhardt, C., Astman, N., Gutnick, M. J. & Heinemann, U. Enhanced spontaneous transmitter release is the earliest consequence of neocortical hypoxia that can explain the disruption of normal circuit function. *J. Neurosci.* 21, 4600–4608 (2001).
13. Hofmeijer, J. & van Putten, M. J. A. M. Ischemic cerebral damage: An appraisal of synaptic failure. *Stroke* 43, 607–615 (2012).
14. Xie, Y., Zacharias, E., Hoff, P. & Tegtmeier, F. Ion channel involvement in anoxic depolarization induced by cardiac arrest in rat brain. *J. Cereb. Blood Flow Metab.* 15, 587–594 (1995).

15. Chalkias, A. & Xanthos, T. Post-cardiac arrest brain injury: Pathophysiology and treatment. *J. Neurol. Sci.* 315, 1–8 (2012).
16. Kalimo, H., Garcia, J. H., Kamijyo, Y., Tanaka, J. & Trump, B. F. The ultrastructure of 'brain death'. *Virchows Arch. B Cell Path.* 14 (1977).
17. Larsen, M. P., Eisenberg, M. S., Cummins, R. O. & Hallstrom, A. P. Predicting survival from out-of-hospital cardiac arrest: A graphic model. *Ann. Emerg. Med.* 22, 1652–1658 (1993).
18. Sharma, H. S., Miclescu, A. & Wiklund, L. Cardiac arrest-induced regional blood–brain barrier breakdown, edema formation and brain pathology: A light and electron microscopic study on a new model for neurodegeneration and neuroprotection in porcine brain. *J. Neural Transm.* 118, 87–114 (2011).
19. Khot, S. & Tirschwell, D. Long-term neurological complications after hypoxic-ischemic encephalopathy. *Semin. Neurol.* 26, 422–431 (2006).
20. Tresch, D. D., Sims, F. H., Duthie, E. H. & Goldstein, M. D. Clinical characteristics of patients in the persistent vegetative state. *Arch. Intern. Med.* 3. (1991)
21. Bernat, J. L. Chronic disorders of consciousness. *The Lancet* 367, 1181–1192 (2006).
22. Owen, A. M. Disorders of consciousness. *Ann. N. Y. Acad. Sci.* 1124, 225–238 (2008).
23. Arnold, C. Jellyfish caught snoozing give clues to origin of sleep. *Nature* nature.2017.22654 (2017). doi:10.1038/nature.2017.22654.
24. Mateen, F. J. *et al.* Long-term cognitive outcomes following out-of-hospital cardiac arrest: A population-based study. *Neurology* 77, 1438–1445 (2011).
25. Moulaert, V. R. M. P., Verbunt, J. A., van Heugten, C. M. & Wade, D. T. Cognitive impairments in survivors of out-of-hospital cardiac arrest: A systematic review. *Resuscitation* 80, 297–305 (2009).
26. Krassner, M. M. *et al.* Postmortem changes in brain cell structure: A review. (2023) doi:https://doi.org/10.31219/osf.io/gj29w.
27. de Wolf, A., Phaedra, C., Perry, R. M. & Maire, M. Ultrastructural characterization of prolonged normothermic and cold cerebral ischemia in the adult rat. *Rejuvenation Res.* 23, 193–206 (2020).
28. Shibayama, H. & Kitoh, J. The postmortem changes of pyramidal neurons in the hippocampus of rats. *Psychiatry Clin. Neurosci.* 30, 73–91 (1976).
29. Bernat, J. L. A defense of the whole-brain concept of death. *Hastings Cent. Rep.* 28, 14–23 (1998).
30. Barker, R. A., Götz, M. & Parmar, M. New approaches for brain repair – from rescue to reprogramming. *Nature* 557, 329–334 (2018).

31. Epp, J. R., Silva Mera, R., Köhler, S., Josselyn, S. A. & Frankland, P. W. Neurogenesis-mediated forgetting minimizes proactive interference. *Nat. Commun.* **7**, 10838 (2016).
32. Barker, R. A., Barrett, J., Mason, S. L. & Björklund, A. Fetal dopaminergic transplantation trials and the future of neural grafting in Parkinson's disease. *Lancet Neurol.* **12**, 84–91 (2013).
33. Kawabori, M. *et al.* Cell therapy for chronic TBI: Interim analysis of the randomized controlled STEMTRA trial. *Neurology* **96**, e1202–e1214 (2021).
34. Squair, J. W. *et al.* Neuroprosthetic baroreflex controls haemodynamics after spinal cord injury. *Nature* **590**, 308–314 (2021).
35. Herron, J. A. *et al.* Cortical brain–computer interface for closed-loop deep brain stimulation. *IEEE Trans. Neural Syst. Rehabil. Eng.* **25**, 2180–2187 (2017).
36. Guggenmos, D. J. *et al.* Restoration of function after brain damage using a neural prosthesis. *Proc. Natl. Acad. Sci.* **110**, 21177–21182 (2013).
37. Berger, T. W. *et al.* A cortical neural prosthesis for restoring and enhancing memory. *J. Neural Eng.* **8**, 046017 (2011).
38. Deadwyler, S. A. *et al.* A cognitive prosthesis for memory facilitation by closed-loop functional ensemble stimulation of hippocampal neurons in primate brain. *Exp. Neurol.* **287**, 452–460 (2017).
39. Schiff, N. D. *et al.* Behavioural improvements with thalamic stimulation after severe traumatic brain injury. *Nature* **448**, 600–603 (2007).
40. Truog, R. D. Brain death – Too flawed to endure, too ingrained to abandon. *J. Law. Med. Ethics* **35**, 273–281 (2007).
41. Green, M. B. & Wikler, D. Brain death and personal identity. *Philos. Public Aff.* **9**, 105–133 (1980).
42. Agich, G. J. & Jones, R. P. Personal identity and brain death: A critical response. *Philos. Public Aff.* **15**, 267–274 (1986).
43. Merkle, R. Information-Theoretic Death. https://www.ralphmerkle.com/definitions/infodeath.html.
44. Shewmon, D. A. The brain and somatic integration: Insights into the standard biological rationale for equating brain death with death. *J. Med. Philos.* **26**, 457–478 (2001).
45. Veatch, R. M. The death of whole-brain death: The plague of the disaggregators, somaticists, and mentalists. *J. Med. Philos. Forum Bioeth. Philos. Med.* **30**, 353–378 (2005).
46. Payne, K. Physicians' attitudes about the care of patients in the persistent vegetative state: A national survey. *Ann. Intern. Med.* **125**, 104 (1996).

4. WHAT IS PERSONAL IDENTITY?

1. Bigelow, H. J. ART. I.–Dr. Harlow's case of recovery from the passage of an iron bar through the head.: REFERENCE TO PLATE. *Am. J. Med. Sci. 1827-1924* **20**, 10 (1850).
2. Harlow, J. M. Passage of an iron rod through the head. *Boston Med. Surg. J.* **39**, 389–393 (1848).
3. Harlow, J. M. Recovery from the passage of an iron bar through the head. *Publ. Mass. Med. Soc.* **2**, 329–347 (1868).
4. Innovative bill protects Whanganui River with legal personhood – New Zealand Parliament. https://www.parliament.nz/en/get-involved/features/innovative-bill-protects-whanganui-river-with-legal-personhood/ (2017).
5. Locke, J. Book 2, Chapter 27, Section 9. In *An Essay Concerning Human Understanding* (Oxford University Press, 1689).
6. Shoemaker, S. Personhood and consciousness. In *Consciousness and the Self: New Essays* (Cambridge University Press, 2011).
7. James, W. The consciousness of self. In *The Principles of Psychology* (Henry Holt and Company, 1890).
8. Gallagher, S. *Oxford Handbook on the Self*. (Oxford University Press, 2011). doi:10.1093/oxfordhb/9780199548019.003.0001.
9. Gallagher, S. Philosophical conceptions of the self: Implications for cognitive science. *Trends Cogn. Sci.* **4**, 14–21 (2000).
10. Woike, J. K., Collard, P. & Hood, B. Putting your money where your self is: Connecting dimensions of closeness and theories of personal identity. *PLOS ONE* **15**, e0228271 (2020).
11. Ari, C. & D'Agostino, D. P. Contingency checking and self-directed behaviors in giant manta rays: Do elasmobranchs have self-awareness? *J. Ethol.* **34**, 167–174 (2016).
12. Strohminger, N. & Nichols, S. The essential moral self. *Cognition* **131**, 159–171 (2014).
13. Bornstein, M. H. Human infancy . . .and the rest of the lifespan. *Annu. Rev. Psychol.* **65**, 121–158 (2014).
14. Costa, P. T. Personality across the life span. *Annu. Rev. Psychol.* **30** (2019) doi:https://doi.org/10.1146/annurev-psych-010418103244.
15. Tang, A. *et al.* Infant behavioral inhibition predicts personality and social outcomes three decades later. *Proc. Natl. Acad. Sci.* **117**, 9800–9807 (2020).
16. Bamford, S. & Danaher, J. Transfer of personality to a synthetic human ('mind uploading') and the social construction of identity. *J. Conscious. Stud.* **24**, 6–30 (2017).

17. Sender, R. & Milo, R. The distribution of cellular turnover in the human body. *Nat. Med.* 27, 45–48 (2021).
18. Melino, G. The Sirens' song. *Nature* 412, 23–23 (2001).
19. Defoiche, J. *et al.* Measurement of ribosomal RNA turnover in vivo by use of deuterium-labeled glucose. *Clin. Chem.* 55, 1824–1833 (2009).
20. Diaz, F. & Moraes, C. T. Mitochondrial biogenesis and turnover. *Cell Calcium* 44, 24–35 (2008).
21. Bulovaite, E. *et al.* A brain atlas of synapse protein lifetime across the mouse lifespan. *Neuron* 110, 4057-4073.e8 (2022).
22. Windt, J. M., Nielsen, T. & Thompson, E. Does consciousness disappear in dreamless sleep? *Trends Cogn. Sci.* 20, 871–882 (2016).
23. Altwegg-Boussac, T. *et al.* Cortical neurons and networks are dormant but fully responsive during isoelectric brain state. *Brain* 140, 2381–2398 (2017).
24. Conolly, S., Arrowsmith, J. E. & Klein, A. A. Deep hypothermic circulatory arrest. *Contin. Educ. Anaesth. Crit. Care Pain* 10, 138–142 (2010).
25. Lichterman, B. Henry Molaison. *BMJ* 338, b968 (2009).
26. Scoville, W. B. & Milner, B. Loss of recent memory after bilateral hippocampal lesions. *J. Neurol. Neurosurg. Psychiatry* 20, 11–21 (1957).
27. Bostwick, J. M., Hecksel, K. A., Stevens, S. R., Bower, J. H. & Ahlskog, J. E. Frequency of new-onset pathologic compulsive gambling or hypersexuality after drug treatment of idiopathic parkinson disease. *Mayo Clin. Proc.* 84, 310–316 (2009).
28. Dominus, S. Could conjoined twins share a mind? *The New York Times* (2011).
29. Inseparable: A Year in the Life of Tatiana and Krista Hogan, BC's Craniopagus Twins. (2017).
30. Cochrane, T. A case of shared consciousness. *Synthese* (2020) doi:10.1007/s11229-020-02753-6.
31. Andrillon, T. *et al.* Does the mind wander when the brain takes a break? Local sleep in wakefulness, attentional lapses and mind-wandering. *Front. Neurosci.* 13, 949 (2019).
32. Gazzaniga, M. S. Forty-five years of split-brain research and still going strong. *Nat. Rev. Neurosci.* 6, 653–659 (2005).
33. Schechter, E. Précis of self-consciousness and 'split' brains: The minds' I. *J. Conscious. Stud.* 29, 142–152 (2022).
34. Walker, M. J. Personal continuation: Psychological continuity and narrative theories of identity. (2010).
35. Dainton, B. & Bayne, T. Consciousness as a guide to personal persistence. *Australas. J. Philos.* 83, 549–571 (2005).

36. Shoemaker, D. & Tobia, K. Personal identity. In *The Oxford Handbook of Moral Psychology* (eds. Vargas, M. & Doris, J. M.) (Oxford University Press, 2022). doi:10.1093/oxfordhb/9780198871712.013.28.
37. Thomson, J. J. People and their bodies. In *Reading Parfit.* (ed. Dancy, J.) (Oxford: Blackwell, 1997).
38. Bourget, D. & Chalmers, D. Philosophers on Philosophy: The 2020 PhilPapers Survey. 46 (2021).
39. Nichols, S. & Bruno, M. Intuitions about personal identity: An empirical study. *Philos. Psychol.* 23, 293–312 (2010).
40. Weaver, S. & Turri, J. Personal identity and persisting as many. In *Oxford Studies in Experimental Philosophy*, vol. 2 (Oxford University Press, 2018).
41. Strohminger, N. & Nichols, S. Neurodegeneration and identity. *Psychol. Sci.* 26, 1469–1479 (2015).
42. Diamond, N. B., Armson, M. J. & Levine, B. The truth is out there: Accuracy in recall of verifiable real-world events. *Psychol. Sci.* 31 (2020).
43. Fivush, R. & Grysman, A. Accuracy and reconstruction in autobiographical memory: (Re)consolidating neuroscience and sociocultural developmental approaches. *WIREs Cogn. Sci.* 14, e1620 (2023).
44. Wagenaar, W. A. & Groeneweg, J. The memory of concentration camp survivors. *Appl. Cogn. Psychol.* 4, 77–87 (1990).
45. Baddeley, A. D. Is the study of memory unduly preoccupied with its sins? *Memory* 30, 55–59 (2022).
46. Chalmers, D. J. Uploading: A philosophical analysis. *Intell. Unbound Future Uploaded Mach. Minds* 102–118 (2014).
47. Parfit, D. *Reasons and Persons.* (Clarendon Press, Oxford, 1984).
48. Wiley, K. B. & Koene, R. A. The fallacy of favouring gradual replacement mind uploading over scan-and-copy. *J. Conscious. Stud.* 23, 212–235 (2016).
49. Wiley, K. *Nondestructive Mind Uploading and the Stream of Consciousness.* https://osf.io/sr7cf (2023) doi:10.31219/osf.io/sr7cf.
50. Goldwater, J. Uploads, faxes, and you: Can personal identity be transmitted? *Am. Philos. Q.* 58, 233–250 (2021).
51. Walker, M. Uploading and personal identity. *Intell. Unbound Future Uploaded Mach. Minds* 161–177 (2014).
52. Piccinini, G. The myth of mind uploading. In *The Mind-Technology Problem* (eds. Clowes, R. W., Gärtner, K. & Hipólito, I.) Vol. 18, 125–144 (Springer International Publishing, 2021).
53. Pigliucci, M. Mind uploading: A philosophical counter-analysis. *Intell. Unbound Future Uploaded Mach. Minds* 119–130 (2014).

5. WHAT IS CONSCIOUSNESS?

1. Abbott, A. Blind man walking. *Nature* (2008) doi:10.1038/news.2008.1328.
2. Gelder, B. *et al.* Intact navigation skills after bilateral loss of striate cortex. *Curr. Biol.* 18, R1128–R1129 (2008).
3. Pegna, A. J., Khateb, A., Lazeyras, F. & Seghier, M. L. Discriminating emotional faces without primary visual cortices involves the right amygdala. *Nat. Neurosci.* 8, 24–25 (2005).
4. Derrien, D., Garric, C., Sergent, C. & Chokron, S. The nature of blindsight: Implications for current theories of consciousness. *Neurosci. Conscious.* **2022**, niab043 (2022).
5. Weiskrantz, L. *Blindsight.* (Oxford University Press, 1990). doi:10.1093/acprof:oso/9780198521921.001.0001.
6. Seth, A. *Being You: A New Science of Consciousness.* (Dutton, 2021).
7. Nagel, T. What is it like to be a bat? *Philos. Rev.* 83, 435–450 (1974).
8. Block, N. Inverted earth. *Philos. Perspect.* 4, 53–79 (1990).
9. Thaler, L. & Goodale, M. A. Echolocation in humans: An overview. *WIREs Cogn. Sci.* 7, 382–393 (2016).
10. Chalmers, D. J. Facing up to the problem of consciousness. *J. Conscious. Stud.* 2, 200–219 (1995).
11. Levine, J. Materialism and qualia: The explanatory gap. *Pac. Philos. Q.* 64, 354–361 (1983).
12. Bourget, D. & Chalmers, D. Philosophers on Philosophy: The 2020 PhilPapers Survey. 46 (2021).
13. Klein, C., Hohwy, J. & Bayne, T. Explanation in the science of consciousness: From the neural correlates of consciousness (NCCs) to the difference makers of consciousness (DMCs). *Philos. Mind Sci.* 1, (2020).
14. Koch, C., Massimini, M., Boly, M. & Tononi, G. Neural correlates of consciousness: Progress and problems. *Nat. Rev. Neurosci.* 17, 307–321 (2016).
15. Crick, F. & Koch, C. Towards a neurobiological theory of consciousness. *Semin. Neurosci.* 2, 263–275 (1990).
16. Seth, A. K. & Bayne, T. Theories of consciousness. *Nat. Rev. Neurosci.* (2022). doi:10.1038/s41583-022-00587-4.
17. Kobes, B. W. Functionalist theories of consciousness. In *The Oxford Companion to Consciousness* (Oxford University Press, 2014).
18. Crook, R. J. Behavioral and neurophysiological evidence suggests affective pain experience in octopus. *iScience* 24, 102229 (2021).
19. Owen, A. M. Disorders of consciousness. *Ann. N. Y. Acad. Sci.* 1124, 225–238 (2008).

20. Monti, M. M. *et al.* Willful modulation of brain activity in disorders of consciousness. *N. Engl. J. Med.* 362, 579–589 (2010).
21. Owen, A. M. *et al.* Detecting awareness in the vegetative state. *Science* 313, 1402–1402 (2006).
22. Baars, B. J. Global workspace theory of consciousness: Toward a cognitive neuroscience of human experience. In *Progress in Brain Research* (ed. Laureys, S.) Vol. 150, 45–53 (Elsevier, 2005).
23. Mashour, G. A., Roelfsema, P., Changeux, J.-P. & Dehaene, S. Conscious processing and the global neuronal workspace hypothesis. *Neuron* 105, 776–798 (2020).
24. van Vugt, B. *et al.* The threshold for conscious report: Signal loss and response bias in visual and frontal cortex. *Science* 360, 537–542 (2018).
25. Deaner, R. O., Khera, A. V. & Platt, M. L. Monkeys pay per view: Adaptive valuation of social images by rhesus macaques. *Curr. Biol.* 15, 543–548 (2005).
26. Boly, M. *et al.* Consciousness in humans and non-human animals: Recent advances and future directions. *Front. Psychol.* 4 (2013).
27. Logothetis, N. K. Single units and conscious vision. *Philos. Trans. R. Soc. Lond. B. Biol. Sci.* 353, 1801–1818 (1998).
28. Portin, P. Historical development of the concept of the gene. *J. Med. Philos.* 27, 257–286 (2002).
29. Fink, S. B., Lyre, H. & Kob, L. A structural constraint on neural correlates of consciousness. *Philos. Mind Sci.* 2, (2021).
30. Lee, A. Y. Objective phenomenology. *Erkenntnis* (2022) doi:10.1007/s10670-022-00576-0.
31. Lyre, H. Neurophenomenal structuralism. A philosophical agenda for a structuralist neuroscience of consciousness. *Neurosci. Conscious.* 18 (2022).
32. Tsuchiya, N. & Saigo, H. A relational approach to consciousness: Categories of level and contents of consciousness. *Neurosci. Conscious.* 2021, niab034 (2021).
33. Zeleznikow-Johnston, A., Aizawa, Y., Yamada, M. & Tsuchiya, N. Are color experiences the same across the visual field? *J. Cogn. Neurosci.* 35, 509–542 (2023).
34. Albantakis, L. *et al.* Integrated information theory (IIT) 4.0: Formulating the properties of phenomenal existence in physical terms. Preprint at http://arxiv.org/abs/2212.14787 (2022).
35. Barbosa, L. S., Marshall, W., Streipert, S., Albantakis, L. & Tononi, G. A measure for intrinsic information. *Sci. Rep.* 10, 18803 (2020).

36. Casali, A. G. *et al.* A theoretically based index of consciousness independent of sensory processing and behavior. *Sci. Transl. Med.* 5, 198ra105-198ra105 (2013).
37. Leung, A., Cohen, D., van Swinderen, B. & Tsuchiya, N. Integrated information structure collapses with anesthetic loss of conscious arousal in drosophila melanogaster. *PLOS Comput. Biol.* 17, e1008722 (2021).
38. Aaronson, S. Why I am not an integrated information theorist (or, The unconscious expander). *Shtetl-Optimized* https://scottaaronson.blog/?p=1799 (2014).
39. Hohwy, J. *The Predictive Mind.* (Oxford University Press, 2013).
40. Metzinger, T. Minimal phenomenal experience: Meditation, tonic alertness, and the phenomenology of 'pure' consciousness. *Philosophy and the Mind Sciences.* 1(I), 7. (2020).
41. Kleiner, J. & Hoel, E. Falsification and consciousness. *Neurosci. Conscious.* **2021** (2021).
42. Francken, J. C. *et al.* An academic survey on theoretical foundations, common assumptions and the current state of consciousness science. *Neurosci. Conscious.* **2022**, niac011 (2022).
43. Chalmers, D. J. Uploading: A philosophical analysis. *Intell. Unbound Future Uploaded Mach. Minds* 102–118 (2014).
44. Godfrey-Smith, P. Mind, matter, and metabolism: *J. Philos.* 113, 481–506 (2016).
45. Ninio, J. & Stevens, K. A. Variations on the Hermann Grid: An extinction illusion. *Perception* **29**, 1209–1217 (2000).

6. WHAT ARE MEMORIES?

1. Penfield, W. Temporal lobe epilepsy. *BJS Br. J. Surg.* 41, 337–343 (1954).
2. Penfield, W. & Baldwin, M. Temporal lobe seizures and the technic of subtotal temporal lobectomy. *Ann. Surg.* 136, 625–634 (1952).
3. Penfield, W. & Perot, P. The brain's record of auditory and visual experience: A final summary and discussion. *Brain* **86**, 595–696 (1963).
4. Ségurel, L., Wyman, M. J. & Przeworski, M. Determinants of mutation rate variation in the human germline. *Annu. Rev. Genomics Hum. Genet.* 15, 47–70 (2014).
5. Polderman, T. J. C. *et al.* Meta-analysis of the heritability of human traits based on fifty years of twin studies. *Nat. Genet.* 47, 702–709 (2015).

6. Josselyn, S. A., Köhler, S. & Frankland, P. W. Finding the engram. *Nat. Rev. Neurosci.* 16, 521–534 (2015).
7. Bauman, K., Devinsky, O. & Liu, A. Temporal lobe surgery and memory: Lessons, risks, and opportunities. *Epilepsy Behav. EB* 101, 106596 (2019).
8. Teyler, T. J. & Rudy, J. W. The hippocampal indexing theory and episodic memory: Updating the index. *Hippocampus* 17, 1158–1169 (2007).
9. Liu, X. *et al.* Optogenetic stimulation of a hippocampal engram activates fear memory recall. *Nature* 484, 381–385 (2012).
10. Roy, D. S. *et al.* Brain-wide mapping reveals that engrams for a single memory are distributed across multiple brain regions. *Nat. Commun.* 13, 1799 (2022).
11. Tonegawa, S., Morrissey, M. D. & Kitamura, T. The role of engram cells in the systems' consolidation of memory. *Nat. Rev. Neurosci.* 19, 485–498 (2018).
12. Tanaka, K. Z. *et al.* Cortical representations are reinstated by the hippocampus during memory retrieval. *Neuron* 84, 347–354 (2014).
13. Kitamura, T. *et al.* Engrams and circuits crucial for systems' consolidation of a memory. *Science* 356, 73–78 (2017).
14. Yang, G., Pan, F. & Gan, W. B. Stably maintained dendritic spines are associated with lifelong memories. *Nature* 462, 920–924 (2009).
15. Girardeau, G., Benchenane, K., Wiener, S. I., Buzsáki, G. & Zugaro, M.B. Selective suppression of hippocampal ripples impairs spatial memory. *Nat. Neurosci.* 12, 1222–1223 (2009).
16. Poo, M. *et al.* What is memory? The present state of the engram. *BMC Biol.* 14, (2016).
17. Flor-García, M. *et al.* Unraveling human adult hippocampal neurogenesis. *Nat. Protoc.* 15, 668–693 (2020).
18. Sorrells, S. F. *et al.* Human hippocampal neurogenesis drops sharply in children to undetectable levels in adults. *Nature* 555, 377–381 (2018).
19. Xin, W. & Chan, J. R. Myelin plasticity: Sculpting circuits in learning and memory. *Nat. Rev. Neurosci.* 21, 682–694 (2020).
20. Lamprecht, R. & LeDoux, J. Structural plasticity and memory. *Nat. Rev. Neurosci.* 5, 45–54 (2004).
21. Berry, K. P. & Nedivi, E. Spine dynamics: Are they all the same? *Neuron* 96, 43–55 (2017).
22. Hayashi-Takagi, A. *et al.* Labelling and optical erasure of synaptic memory traces in the motor cortex. *Nature* 525, 333–338 (2015).
23. Bulovaite, E. *et al.* A brain atlas of synapse protein lifetime across the mouse lifespan. *Neuron* 110, 4057-4073.e8 (2022).
24. Suddendorf, T. & Corballis, M. C. Mental time travel across the disciplines: The future looks bright. *Behav. Brain Sci.* 30, 335–345 (2007).

25. Zeman, A., Dewar, M. & Della Sala, S. Reflections on aphantasia. *Cortex* 74, 336–337 (2016).
26. Greenberg, D. L. & Knowlton, B. J. The role of visual imagery in autobiographical memory. *Mem. Cognit.* **42**, 922–934 (2014).
27. Watkins, N. W. (A)phantasia and severely deficient autobiographical memory: Scientific and personal perspectives. *Cortex* 105, 41–52 (2018).
28. Hassabis, D., Kumaran, D., Vann, S. D. & Maguire, E. A. Patients with hippocampal amnesia cannot imagine new experiences. *Proc. Natl. Acad. Sci.* 104, 1726–1731 (2007).
29. Baddeley, A. D. Is the study of memory unduly preoccupied with its sins? *Memory* 30, 55–59 (2022).
30. Diamond, N. B., Armson, M. J. & Levine, B. The truth is out there: Accuracy in recall of verifiable real-world events. *Psychol. Sci.* 31, (2020).
31. Fivush, R. & Grysman, A. Accuracy and reconstruction in autobiographical memory: (Re)consolidating neuroscience and sociocultural developmental approaches. *WIREs Cogn. Sci.* 14, e1620 (2023).
32. Schacter, D. L. Constructive memory: Past and future. *Dialogues Clin. Neurosci.* 14, 7–18 (2012).
33. Schacter, D. L. *et al.* The future of memory: Remembering, imagining, and the brain. *Neuron* **76**, 677–694 (2012).
34. Monti, M. M. *et al.* Willful modulation of brain activity in disorders of consciousness. *N. Engl. J. Med.* **362**, 579–589 (2010).
35. Pearson, J. The human imagination: The cognitive neuroscience of visual mental imagery. *Nat. Rev. Neurosci.* **20**, 624–634 (2019).
36. Ajina, S. & Bridge, H. Blindsight and unconscious vision: What they teach us about the human visual system. *The Neuroscientist* 23, 529–541 (2017).
37. Irish, M., Addis, D. R., Hodges, J. R. & Piguet, O. Considering the role of semantic memory in episodic future thinking: Evidence from semantic dementia. *Brain* 135, 2178–2191 (2012).
38. O'Sullivan, F. & Ryan, T. If engrams are the answer, what is the question? Preprint at https://osf.io/f6amv/download/?format=pdf (2023).
39. Seung, S. *Connectome: How the Brain's Wiring Makes Us Who We Are.* (HMH, 2012).

7. HOW WE CAN SAVE SOMEONE

1. Elixson, E. M. Hypothermia: Cold-water drowning. *Crit. Care Nurs. Clin. North Am.* 3, 287–292 (1991).

2. Bauman, B. D. *et al.* Treatment of hypothermic cardiac arrest in the pediatric drowning victim, a case report, and systematic review. *Pediatr. Emerg. Care* **Publish Ahead of Print**, (2019).
3. Conolly, S., Arrowsmith, J. E. & Klein, A. A. Deep hypothermic circulatory arrest. *Contin. Educ. Anaesth. Crit. Care Pain* 10, 138–142 (2010).
4. Ziganshin, B. A. & Elefteriades, J. A. Deep hypothermic circulatory arrest. *Ann. Cardiothorac. Surg.* **2**, 303–315 (2013).
5. Seung, S. *Connectome: How the Brain's Wiring Makes Us Who We Are.* (HMH, 2012).
6. Amunts, K. *et al.* Linking brain structure, activity, and cognitive function through computation. *eNeuro* **9**, ENEURO.0316-21.2022 (2022).
7. Fricker, M., Tolkovsky, A. M., Borutaite, V., Coleman, M. & Brown, G. C. Neuronal cell death. *Physiol Rev* **98**, 68 (2018).
8. Kalimo, H., Garcia, J. H., Kamijyo, Y., Tanaka, J. & Trump, B. F. The ultrastructure of 'brain death'. *Virchows Arch. B Cell Path.* 14 (1977).
9. Petito, C. K. & Pulsinelli, W. A. Delayed neuronal recovery and neuronal death in rat hippocampus following severe cerebral ischemia: Possible relationship to abnormalities in neuronal processes. *J. Cereb. Blood Flow Metab.* **4**, 194–205 (1984).
10. de Wolf, A., Phaedra, C., Perry, R. M. & Maire, M. Ultrastructural characterization of prolonged normothermic and cold cerebral ischemia in the adult rat. *Rejuvenation Res.* **23**, 193–206 (2020).
11. Krassner, M. M. *et al.* Postmortem changes in brain cell structure: A review. (2023) doi:https://doi.org/10.31219/osf.io/gj29w.
12. Fahy, G. M. & Wowk, B. Principles of cryopreservation by vitrification. in *Cryopreservation and Freeze-Drying Protocols* (eds. Wolkers, W. F. & Oldenhof, H.) Vol. 1257 21–82 (Springer, 2015).
13. Tucker, M. & Liebermann, J. *Vitrification in Assisted Reproduction.* (CRC Press, 2015).
14. Cobo, A. & Diaz, C. Clinical application of oocyte vitrification: A systematic review and meta-analysis of randomized controlled trials. *Fertil. Steril.* **96**, 277–285 (2011).
15. de Wolf, A. & Platt, C. Cryoprotection. In *Human Cryopreservation Procedures* (Alcor, 2020).
16. Hayworth, K. Overview of 21st century medicine's cryopreservation for viability research. *The Brain Preservation Foundation* https://www.brainpreservation.org/21cm-cryopreservation-eval-page/.
17. McKenzie, A. T. *Glutaraldehyde: A review of its fixative effects on nucleic acids, proteins, lipids, and carbohydrates.* https://osf.io/8zd4e (2019) doi:10.31219/osf.io/8zd4e.

18. Winey, M., Meehl, J. B., O'Toole, E. T. & Giddings, T. H. Conventional transmission electron microscopy. *Mol. Biol. Cell* **25**, 319–323 (2014).
19. Ofer, N., Berger, D. R., Kasthuri, N., Lichtman, J. W. & Yuste, R. Ultrastructural analysis of dendritic spine necks reveals a continuum of spine morphologies. *Dev. Neurobiol.* **81**, 746–757 (2021).
20. Huebinger, J., Spindler, J., Holl, K. J. & Koos, B. Quantification of protein mobility and associated reshuffling of cytoplasm during chemical fixation. *Sci. Rep.* **8**, 17756 (2018).
21. Thorne, R. G. & Nicholson, C. *In vivo* diffusion analysis with quantum dots and dextrans predicts the width of brain extracellular space. *Proc. Natl. Acad. Sci.* **103**, 5567–5572 (2006).
22. Fulton, K. A. & Briggman, K. L. Permeabilization-free en bloc immunohistochemistry for correlative microscopy. *eLife* **10**, e63392 (2021).
23. Pallotto, M., Watkins, P. V., Fubara, B., Singer, J. H. & Briggman, K. L. Extracellular space preservation aids the connectomic analysis of neural circuits. *eLife* **4**, e08206 (2015).
24. Sjövall, P., Johansson, B. & Lausmaa, J. Localization of lipids in freeze-dried mouse brain sections by imaging TOF-SIMS. *Appl. Surf. Sci.* **252**, 6966–6974 (2006).
25. McIntyre, R. L. & Fahy, G. M. Aldehyde-stabilized cryopreservation. *Cryobiology* **71**, 448–458 (2015).
26. The Brain Preservation Foundation. Large Mammal BPF Prize Winning Announcement – The Brain Preservation Foundation. https://www.brainpreservation.org/large-mammal-announcement/ (2018).
27. *Considerations for Effective Brain Preservation* Robert McIntyre European Biostasis Foundation. (2021).
28. Meyer, C. 73001. In *Lunar Sample Compendium* (NASA, 2011).
29. Howell, E. NASA is cracking open a 50-year-old Apollo 17 moon rock sample for Artemis prep. *Space.com* https://www.space.com/nasa-opening-apollo-17-moon-rock-samples-for-artemis (2022).
30. Leibniz, G. W. De Progressione Dyadica, Pars I. In *Herrn von Leibniz' Rechnung mit Null und Einz* (Siemens Aktiengesellschaft, 1679).
31. Sandberg, A. & Bostrom, N. *Whole Brain Emulation: A Roadmap.* (Future of Humanity Institute, 2008).
32. Hayworth, K. Vitrifying the connectomic self. Preprint at https://www.brainpreservation.org/wp-content/uploads/2018/02/vitrifyingtheconnectomicself_hayworth.pdf (2018).
33. Jefferis, G., Collinson, L., Bosch, C., Costa, M. & Schlegel, P. Scaling up connectomics. https://wellcome.org/reports/scaling-connectomics (2023).

34. M'Saad, O. *et al.* All-optical visualization of specific molecules in the ultrastructural context of brain tissue. Preprint at https://www.biorxiv.org/content/10.1101/2022.04.04.486901v2.full.pdf (2022).
35. Hayworth, K. J. *et al.* Ultrastructurally smooth thick partitioning and volume stitching for large-scale connectomics. *Nat. Methods* 12, 319–322 (2015).
36. Eckstein, N. *et al.* *Neurotransmitter Classification from Electron Microscopy Images at Synaptic Sites in Drosophila Melanogaster*. http://biorxiv.org/lookup/doi/10.1101/2020.06.12.148775 (2020) doi:10.1101/2020.06.12.148775.
37. Billeh, Y. N. *et al.* Systematic integration of structural and functional data into multi-scale models of mouse primary visual cortex. Preprint at https://doi.org/10.1101/662189 (2019).
38. Fan, X. & Markram, H. A brief history of simulation neuroscience. *Front. Neuroinformatics* 13, 32 (2019).
39. Goetz, L., Roth, A. & Häusser, M. Active dendrites enable strong but sparse inputs to determine orientation selectivity. *Proc. Natl. Acad. Sci.* 118, e2017339118 (2021).
40. Menon, N. Powering an inclusive internet – Part 1 of 2. *Cisco Blogs* https://blogs.cisco.com/sp/powering-an-inclusive-internet-part-1-of-2 (2023).
41. Carlsmith, J. New report on how much computational power it takes to match the human brain. *Open Philanthropy* https://www.openphilanthropy.org/research/new-report-on-how-much-computational-power-it-takes-to-match-the-human-brain/ (2020).
42. Shapiro, L. & Spaulding, S. Embodied cognition. In *The Stanford Encyclopedia of Philosophy* (ed. Zalta, E. N.) (Stanford University, 2021).
43. Chalmers, D. J. *Reality+: Virtual Worlds and the Problems of Philosophy*. (Penguin UK, 2022).
44. Farina, D. *et al.* Toward higher-performance bionic limbs for wider clinical use. *Nat. Biomed. Eng.* (2021) doi:10.1038/s41551-021-00732-x.
45. Koch, K. *et al.* How much the eye tells the brain. *Curr. Biol.* 16, 1428–1434 (2006).
46. Findlay, G., Marshall, W., Albantakis, L. & Mayner, W. Dissociating intelligence from consciousness in artificial systems – Implications of integrated information theory. *Towards Conscious AI Systems* https://ceur-ws.org/Vol-2287/short7.pdf (2019).
47. Marković, D., Mizrahi, A., Querlioz, D. & Grollier, J. Physics for neuromorphic computing. *Nat. Rev. Phys.* 2, 499–510 (2020).
48. Pigliucci, M. Mind uploading: A philosophical counter-analysis. *Intell. Unbound Future Uploaded Mach. Minds* 119–130 (2014).

49. Godfrey-Smith, P. Mind, matter, and metabolism: *J. Philos.* 113, 481–506 (2016).
50. Kagan, B. J. *et al.* In vitro neurons learn and exhibit sentience when embodied in a simulated game-world. *Neuron* 110, 3952-3969.e8 (2022).
51. Olson, E. T. Personal identity. *Blackwell Guide Philos. Mind* 352–368 (2003).
52. Corabi, J. & Schneider, S. If you upload, will you survive? *Intell. Unbound Future Uploaded Mach. Minds* 131–145 (2014).
53. Piccinini, G. The myth of mind uploading. In *The Mind-Technology Problem* (eds. Clowes, R. W., Gärtner, K. & Hipólito, I.) Vol. 18 125–144 (Springer International Publishing, 2021).
54. Wellington, N. Whole brain emulation: Invasive vs. non-invasive methods. *Intell. Unbound Future Uploaded Mach. Minds* 178–192 (2014).
55. Feynman, R. P. There's plenty of room at the bottom. (1959).
56. Drexler, E. *Engines of Creation: The Coming Era of Nanotechnology.* (Anchor, 1987).
57. Freitas Jr, R. *Cryostasis Revival: The Recovery of Cryonics Patients through Nanomedicine.* (Alcor Life Extension Foundation, 2022).
58. Abhyankar, R. S. & Jessop, K. M. From craft to profession: The development of modern anesthesiology. *Mo. Med.* 119, 14–20 (2022).
59. Bamford, S. & Danaher, J. Transfer of personality to a synthetic human ('mind uploading') and the social construction of identity. *J. Conscious. Stud.* 24, 6–30 (2017).

8. HOW WE CAN SAVE EVERYONE

1. Philadelphia, T. C. H. of. Emily Whitehead, first pediatric patient to receive CAR T-cell therapy, celebrates cure 10 years later. https://www.chop.edu/news/emily-whitehead-first-pediatric-patient-receive-car-t-cell-therapy-celebrates-cure-10-years (2022).
2. Martin, A., Morgan, E. & Hijiya, N. Relapsed or refractory pediatric acute lymphoblastic leukemia. *Pediatr Drugs* (2012).
3. Firth, S. Jordan parents call for better vaccine access. *That's Life* (2018).
4. Pharmaceutical Benefits Scheme (PBS). Multicomponent Meningococcal Group B Vaccine, 0.5mL, injection, prefilled syringe, Bexsero® - November 2013. (2013).
5. World Bank Open Data. *World Bank Open Data* https://data.worldbank.org.

6. Ortiz-Ospina, E. Long-term perspective on government healthcare spending. *Our World in Data* https://ourworldindata.org/when-did-the-provision-of-healthcare-first-become-a-public-policy-priority (2022).
7. Gutierrez-Delgado, C. *et al.* EQ-5D-5L Health-state values for the Mexican population. *Appl. Health Econ. Health Policy.* **19**, 905–914 (2021).
8. *Recommendations Made by the PBAC – November 2022.* https://www.pbs.gov.au/pbs/industry/listing/elements/pbac-meetings/pbac-outcomes#:~:text=Recommendations%20made%20by%20the%20PBAC%20%E2%80%93%20November%202022 (2022).
9. Schwarzer, R. *et al.* Systematic overview of cost–effectiveness thresholds in ten countries across four continents. *J. Comp. Eff. Res.* **4**, 485–504 (2015).
10. *Guide to the Methods of Technology Appraisal.* https://assets.publishing.service.gov.uk/government/uploads/system/uploads/attachment_data/file/191504/NICE_guide_to_the_methods_of_technology_appraisal.pdf (2004).
11. Dakin, H. *et al.* The influence of cost-effectiveness and other factors on NICE decisions. *Health Econ.* **24**, 1256–1271 (2015).
12. Mohara, A. *et al.* Using health technology assessment for informing coverage decisions in Thailand. *J. Comp. Eff. Res.* **1**, 137–146 (2012).
13. Wang, S., Gum, D. & Merlin, T. Comparing the ICERs in medicine reimbursement submissions to NICE and PBAC – Does the presence of an explicit threshold affect the ICER proposed? *Value Health* **21**, 938–943 (2018).
14. Neumann, P. J. & Weinstein, M. C. Legislating against use of cost-effectiveness information. *N. Engl. J. Med.* **363**, 1495–1497 (2010).
15. Neumann, P. J., Cohen, J. T. & Weinstein, M. C. Updating cost-effectiveness – The curious resilience of the $50,000-per-QALY threshold. *N. Engl. J. Med.* **371**, 796–797 (2014).
16. Vanness, D. J., Lomas, J. & Ahn, H. A health opportunity cost threshold for cost-effectiveness analysis in the United States. *Ann. Intern. Med.* **174**, 25–32 (2021).
17. Shrank, W. H., Rogstad, T. L. & Parekh, N. Waste in the US health care system: Estimated costs and potential for savings. *JAMA* **322**, 1501 (2019).
18. Banzhaf, H. S. The value of statistical life: A meta-analysis of meta-analyses. *J. Benefit-Cost Anal.* **13**, 182–197 (2022).
19. Kniesner, T. J. & Viscusi, W. K. The value of a statistical life. In *Oxford Research Encyclopedia of Economics and Finance* (Oxford University Press, 2019). doi:10.1093/acrefore/9780190625979.013.138.

20. Best Practice Regulation Guidance Note: Value of Statistical Life. https://oia.pmc.gov.au/sites/default/files/2022-09/value-statistical-life-guidance-note.pdf (2022).
21. GiveWell's Cost-Effectiveness Analyses. GiveWell. https://www.givewell.org/how-we-work/our-criteria/cost-effectiveness/cost-effectiveness-models (2023).
22. Reynolds, M. Salt, sugar, water, zinc: How scientists learned to treat the 20th century's biggest killer of children. *Asterisk* https://asteriskmag.com/issues/02/salt-sugar-water-zinc-how-scientists-learned-to-treat-the-20th-century-s-biggest-killer-of-children (2023).
23. Sallnow, L. *et al.* Report of the Lancet Commission on the Value of Death: Bringing death back into life. *The Lancet* **399**, 837–884 (2022).
24. Einav, L., Finkelstein, A., Mullainathan, S. & Obermeyer, Z. Predictive modeling of U.S. health care spending in late life. *Science* **360**, 1462–1465 (2018).
25. Eisen, H. Patient education: Heart transplantation (beyond the basics). *UpToDate* https://www.uptodate.com/contents/heart-transplantation-beyond-the-basics#:~:text=Survival%20%E2%80%94%20Approximately%2085%20to%2090,of%20approximately%204%20percent%20thereafter. (2021).
26. Marasco, S. F., Summerhayes, R., Quayle, M., McGiffin, D. & Luthe, M. Cost comparison of heart transplant vs. left ventricular assist device therapy at one year. *Clin. Transplant.* 30, 598–605 (2016).
27. Ritchie, H. & Mathieu, E. How many people die and how many are born each year? *Our World in Data* https://ourworldindata.org/births-and-deaths (2023).
28. Gimigliano, S. & Barnes, D. How to Build and Operate a -80C Walk-in Freezer. http://www.stem-art.com/Library/Biobanking/Extreme%20Biobanking%20High%20Density%20Storage%20-80C.pdf
29. Alcor. Cryopreservation funding and inflation: The need for action. *Cryonics Archive* https://www.cryonicsarchive.org/library/cryopreservation-funding-and-inflation/ (2011).
30. Roser, M. & Ritchie, H. Cancer. *Our World Data* (2015).
31. *NIH Professional Judgment Budget for Alzheimer's Desease and Related Dementias for Fiscal Year 2023*. https://www.nia.nih.gov/sites/default/files/2021-07/bypass_budget_executive_summary_508.pdf.
32. Pickett, J. & Brayne, C. The scale and profile of global dementia research funding. *The Lancet* **394**, 1888–1889 (2019).
33. Jorgensen, T. J. Marie Curie and her X-ray vehicles' contribution to World War I battlefield medicine. *The Conversation* http://theconversation.com/marie-curie-and-her-x-ray-vehicles-contribution-to-world-war-i-battlefield-medicine-83941 (2017).

34. Newman, P. G. & Rozycki, G. S. The history of ultrasound. *Surg. Clin. North Am.* 78, 179–195 (1998).
35. Half a Century in CT: How Computed Tomography Has Evolved. *ISCT* https://www.isct.org/computed-tomography-blog/2017/2/10/half-a-century-in-ct-how-computed-tomography-has-evolved (2016).
36. Edelman, R. R. The history of MR imaging as seen through the pages of *Radiology*. *Radiology* 273, S181–S200 (2014).
37. Ganapati, P. Oct 25, 1955: Time to nuke dinner. *Wired* (2010).

CONCLUSION

1. Kelvin on science. The Newark Advocate 4 (1902).
2. Blair, A. Reading strategies for coping with information overload ca. 1550–1700. *J. Hist. Ideas* 64, (2003).
3. McSherry, R. Suicide and homicide, under insidious forms. *The Sanitarian* (1883).
4. Bush, J. The anti-suffrage movement. British Library https://www.bl.uk/votes-for-women/articles/the-anti-suffrage-movement (2018).
5. Where the money goes. Winners and Good Causes. The National Lottery https://www.national-lottery.co.uk/life-changing/where-the-money-goes.
6. Smith, D. M. Counting the dead: Estimating the loss of life in the Indigenous Holocaust, 1492–Present. In Native American Symposium: Representations and Realities, Southeastern Oklahoma State University (2017).
7. World population living in extreme poverty. *Our World in Data* https://ourworldindata.org/grapher/world-population-in-extreme-poverty-absolute.
8. Annual working hours per worker. *Our World in Data* https://ourworldindata.org/grapher/annual-working-hours-per-worker.
9. GDP per capita. *Our World in Data* https://ourworldindata.org/grapher/gdp-per-capita-maddison-2020.
10. Franklin, B. *Mr. Franklin, A Selection from his Personal Letters*. (Yale University Press, 1956).

APPENDICES

1. Parfit, D. *Reasons and Persons*. (Clarendon Press, 1984).
2. Blass, D. Case studies. In *Personal Identity and Fractured Selves: Perspectives from Philosophy, Ethics, and Neuroscience*. (eds. Mathews, D. J., Bok, H. & Rabins, P. V.) (JHU Press, 2009).

3. Mather, J. A. Cephalopod consciousness: Behavioural evidence. *Conscious. Cogn.* **17**, 37–48 (2008).
4. VanRullen, R. & Kanai, R. Deep learning and the global workspace theory. *Trends Neurosci.* **44**, 692–704 (2021).
5. Tsuchiya, N., Andrillon, T. & Haun, A. A reply to 'the unfolding argument': Beyond functionalism/behaviorism and towards a science of causal structure theories of consciousness. *Conscious. Cogn.* **79**, 102877 (2020).
6. Block, N. Inverted earth. *Philos. Perspect.* **4**, 53–79 (1990).
7. Akins, K. A bat without qualities? In *Consciousness: Psychological and Philosophical Essays* 345–358 (Blackwell, 1993).
8. Jackson, F. The knowledge argument, diaphanousness, representationalism. In *Phenomenal Concepts and Phenomenal Knowledge: New Essays on Consciousness and Physicalism* 52–64 (2007).
9. Lycan, W. Representational theories of consciousness. In *The Stanford Encyclopedia of Philosophy* (ed. Zalta, E. N.) (Metaphysics Research Lab, Stanford University, 2019).
10. Kawakita, G., Zeleznikow-Johnston, A., Tsuchiya, N. & Oizumi, M. Is my 'red' your 'red'?: Unsupervised alignment of qualia structures via optimal transport. (2023) doi:https://doi.org/10.31234/osf.io/h3pqm.
11. Frankish, K. Illusionism as a theory of consciousness. *J. Conscious. Stud.* **23**, 11–39 (2016).
12. Frankish, K. The meta-problem is the problem of consciousness. *J. Conscious. Stud.* **9–10**, 83–94 (2019).
13. Graziano, M. S. A. Consciousness and the attention schema: Why it has to be right. *Cogn. Neuropsychol.* 1–10 (2020) doi:10.1080/02643294.2020.1761782.
14. Kammerer, F. Can you believe it? Illusionism and the illusion meta-problem. *Philos. Psychol.* **31**, 44–67 (2018).
15. Schurger, A. & Graziano, M. Consciousness explained or described? *Neurosci. Conscious.* **2022**, niac001 (2022).
16. *David Chalmers would be an illusionist if he was a materialist.* (2023). https://www.youtube.com/watch?v=NbGKoiuKGUw.
17. Haun, A. & Tononi, G. Why does space feel the way it does? Towards a principled account of spatial experience. *Entropy* **21**, 1160 (2019).
18. Barrett, A. B. & Mediano, P. A. M. The phi measure of integrated information is not well-defined for general physical systems. *J. Conscious. Stud.* **26**, 1-2 (2019).
19. Kleiner, J. & Tull, S. The mathematical structure of integrated information theory. *Front. Appl. Math. Stat.* **6**, 602973 (2021).

20. Bayne, T. On the axiomatic foundations of the integrated information theory of consciousness. *Neurosci. Conscious.* **2018** (2018).
21. Doerig, A., Schurger, A., Hess, K. & Herzog, M. H. The unfolding argument: Why IIT and other causal structure theories cannot explain consciousness. *Conscious. Cogn.* **72**, 49–59 (2019).
22. Herzog, M. H., Schurger, A. & Doerig, A. First-person experience cannot rescue causal structure theories from the unfolding argument. *Conscious. Cogn.* **98**, 103261 (2022).
23. Knierim, J. J. & Neunuebel, J. P. Tracking the flow of hippocampal computation: Pattern separation, pattern completion, and attractor dynamics. *Neurobiol. Learn. Mem.* **129**, 38–49 (2016).
24. Rolls, E. T. Pattern separation, completion, and categorisation in the hippocampus and neocortex. *Neurobiol. Learn. Mem.* **129**, 4–28 (2016).
25. Šimić, G., Kostović, I., Winblad, B. & Bogdanović, N. Volume and number of neurons of the human hippocampal formation in normal aging and Alzheimer's disease. *J. Comp. Neurol.* **379**, 482–494 (1997).
26. Borzello, M. *et al.* Assessments of dentate gyrus function: discoveries and debates. *Nat. Rev. Neurosci.* **24**, 502–517 (2023).

Index